Surgical Pathology
of the Pituitary Gland

Volume 27 in the Series
MAJOR PROBLEMS IN PATHOLOGY

RICARDO V. LLOYD, M.D., PH.D.

Professor of Pathology
University of Michigan Medical Center
Ann Arbor, Michigan

Surgical Pathology of the Pituitary Gland

Volume 27 in the Series
MAJOR PROBLEMS IN PATHOLOGY

W. B. SAUNDERS COMPANY

Harcourt Brace Jovanovich, Inc.

PHILADELPHIA LONDON TORONTO MONTREAL SYDNEY TOKYO

W. B. SAUNDERS COMPANY
Harcourt Brace Jovanovich, Inc.

The Curtis Center
Independence Square West
Philadelphia, Pennsylvania 19106

Library of Congress Cataloging-in-Publication Data

Lloyd, Ricardo V.

Surgical pathology of the pituitary gland /
Ricardo V. Lloyd.—1st ed.

p.   cm.

ISBN 0–7216–6459–8

1. Pituitary gland—Cancer—Diagnosis.   2. Adenoma—
Histopathology.   3. Pathology, Surgical.
I. Title.   [DNLM: 1. Pituitary gland—Histopathology.
2. Pituitary Diseases—diagnosis.   3. Pituitary Gland—
pathology.   WK 550 L793s]

RC280.P5L56 1993   616.4'707—dc20

DNLM/DLC   92–7600

SURGICAL PATHOLOGY OF THE PITUITARY GLAND   ISBN 0–7216–6459–8

Printed in the United States of America.

Last digit is the print number: 9   8   7   6   5   4   3   2   1

Contributors

SYLVIA L. ASA, M.D., Ph.D.

Associate Professor of Pathology, University of Toronto, Toronto, Ontario; Pathologist, St. Michael's Hospital, Toronto, Ontario, Canada
Tissue Culture in the Diagnosis and Study of Pituitary Adenomas

MILA BLAIVAS, M.D., Ph.D.

Clinical Assistant Professor of Pathology, University of Michigan, Ann Arbor, Michigan; Staff Neuropathologist, University of Michigan Medical Center, Ann Arbor, Michigan
Neoplasms of the Sellar Region

WILLIAM F. CHANDLER, M.D.

Professor of Neurosurgery, University of Michigan Medical Center, Ann Arbor, Michigan
Surgical Treatment of Pituitary Adenomas

ALAN C. DALKIN, M.D.

Assistant Professor of Medicine (Endocrinology), University of Virginia, Charlottesville, Virginia; Attending Staff, University of Virginia Hospitals, Charlottesville, Virginia
Medical Treatment of Pituitary Adenomas

JAMIE DANANBERG, M.D.

Lecturer, Department of Medicine (Endocrinology and Metabolism), University of Michigan, Ann Arbor, Michigan; Attending Staff, University Hospital, Ann Arbor, Michigan
Medical Treatment of Pituitary Adenomas

EVA HORVATH, Ph.D.

Associate Professor of Pathology, University of Toronto, Toronto, Ontario; Research Associate, Department of Pathology, St. Michael's Hospital, Toronto, Ontario, Canada
Ultrastructural Diagnosis of Pituitary Adenomas and Hyperplasias

LONG JIN, M.D.

Research Fellow, University of Michigan Medical Center, Ann Arbor, Michigan
Metastatic Neoplasms to the Pituitary Gland

KALMAN KOVACS, M.D., Ph.D., D.Sc., FRCP(C), FCAP, FRC PATH.

Professor of Pathology, Department of Pathology, University of Toronto, Ontario; Staff Pathologist, Department of Pathology, St. Michael's Hospital, Toronto, Ontario, Canada
Light Microscopic Special Stains and Immunochemistry in the Diagnosis of Pituitary Adenomas; Ultrastructural Diagnosis of Pituitary Adenomas and Hyperplasias

RICARDO V. LLOYD, M.D., Ph.D.

Professor of Pathology, University of Michigan Medical Center, Ann Arbor, Michigan
Embryology and Anatomy of the Pituitary Gland; Cytology and Function of the Pituitary Gland; Practical

Approaches to the Diagnosis and Study of Pituitary Lesions; Frozen Sections in the Diagnosis of Pituitary Lesions; Non-Neoplastic Pituitary Lesions, Including Hyperplasia; Molecular Biological Analysis of Pituitary Disorders; Ectopic Pituitary Adenomas; Metastatic Neoplasms to the Pituitary Gland; Future Prospects in the Diagnosis and Treatment of Pituitary Adenomas

PAUL E. McKEEVER, M.D., Ph.D.

Associate Professor of Pathology, University of Michigan, Ann Arbor, Michigan; Chief of Neuro-pathology Section, University of Michigan Medical Center, Ann Arbor, Michigan
Neoplasms of the Sellar Region

PETER J. PERNICONE, M.D.

Instructor, Mayo School of Medicine, Rochester, Minnesota; Surgical Pathology, Saint Mary's Hospital and Rochester Methodist Hospital, Rochester, Minnesota
Invasive Pituitary Adenomas and Pituitary Carcinomas

BERNARD W. SCHEITHAUER, M.D.

Professor of Pathology, Mayo Graduate School of Medicine, Rochester, Minnesota
Invasive Pituitary Adenomas and Pituitary Carcinomas

ANDERS A. F. SIMA, M.D., Ph.D.

Professor of Pathology and Professor of Internal Medicine, University of Michigan, Ann Arbor, Michigan; Staff Neuropathologist, University of Michigan Medical Center and Consultant Neuro-pathologist, Veterans Administration Hospital, Ann Arbor, Michigan
Neoplasms of the Sellar Region

LUCIA STEFANEANU, Ph.D.

Assistant Professor of Pathology, Department of Pathology, University of Toronto, Ontario; Research Associate, Department of Pathology, St. Michael's Hospital, Toronto, Ontario, Canada
Light Microscopic Special Stains and Immunochemistry in Diagnosis of Pituitary Adenomas

Foreword

The general surgical pathologist is confronted with lesions of the pituitary on an infrequent basis. These lesions often present very difficult diagnostic problems.

Dr. Lloyd and his co-authors, in *Surgical Pathology of the Pituitary Gland,* have summarized a huge amount of morphological, immunohistochemical, clinical and surgical information on various lesions of the pituitary gland and its surrounding anatomic structures. The contributors to this volume include a veritable "who's who" in pituitary pathology. Virtually every topic in this area has been covered, and the work is extensively referenced and illustrated.

I predict that this monograph will rapidly become the single most important reference on surgical pathology of the pituitary gland in the near future.

VIRGINIA A. LiVOLSI, M.D.
SERIES EDITOR

Preface

The field of pituitary pathology has expanded greatly since the 1970s due to the contributions of electron microscopic and immunohistochemical analyses of pituitary adenomas. The use of hematoxylin and eosin staining without immunohistochemical and ultrastructural studies to classify pituitary adenomas does not provide the correlative information that is needed to relate the pathologic findings to the biochemical abnormalities detected by radioimmunoassays and other sophisticated tests. Molecular and cell biological approaches such as hybridization analyses, cell culture and the polymerase chain reaction are producing a great deal of new and clinically relevant information that can be used in the diagnosis, treatment and follow-up of patients with pituitary disorders.

This book combines traditional morphological approaches with more recent information derived from studies with the tools of the new biology. This integrated approach provides a foundation for making specific diagnoses of pituitary disorders but also indicates the future directions of pituitary pathology. The inclusions of chapters on the medical and surgical treatment of pituitary adenomas should provide the surgical pathologist with a balanced perspective on the approach to the patient with pituitary tumors. These chapters should also provide insight for the surgical pathologist into various aspects of the management of pituitary adenomas and other lesions that are important to the neurosurgeon and endocrinologist during the performance of frozen sections or in the diagnosis and subsequent follow-up of patients with pituitary adenomas.

The field of pituitary pathology has made significant progress because of the work of many outstanding individuals, who are too numerous to mention. However, the comprehensive and systematic studies of Eva Horvath and Kalman Kovacs over the past two decades have provided a firm foundation for the classification of human pituitary adenomas. Their contributions to this field will continue to influence other pituitary pathologists far into the future.

Contents

Abbreviations

ACE	angiotensin I–converting enzyme
ACTH	adrenocorticotropic hormone
ADH	antidiuretic hormone, or vasopressin
AIDS	acquired immunodeficiency syndrome
CALLA	common acute lymphoblastic leukemia antigen
CNS	central nervous system
CRF	corticotropin releasing factor (hormone)
CSF	cerebrospinal fluid
CT	computed tomography
EM	electron microscopy
FSH	follicle-stimulating hormone
GAP	gonadotropin releasing hormone–associated peptide
GCT	granular cell tumor
GCTB	giant cell tumor of bone
GFAP	glial fibrillary acidic protein
GH	growth hormone
GHRH	growth hormone releasing hormone
GnRH	gonadotropin releasing hormone
H & E	hematoxylin and eosin
hCG	human chorionic gonadotropin
HPS	hematoxylin phloxine-saffron
IGF I	insulin-like growth factor I
IGF II	insulin-like growth factor II
IH	immunohistochemistry
ISH	*in situ* hybridization
LH	luteinizing hormone

MRI	magnetic resonance imaging
NPC	nasopharyngeal carcinoma
NSE	neuron-specific enolase
PAS	periodic acid–Schiff
PCR	polymerase chain reaction
PLAP	placental alkaline phosphatase
POMC	proopiomelanocortin
PRL	prolactin
RER	rough endoplasmic reticulum
SNUC	sinonasal undifferentiated carcinoma
α-SU	α subunit of glycoprotein hormones (FSH, LH, TSH) and of human chorionic gonadotropin
T_3	triiodothyronine
T_4	thyroxine
TRH	thyrotropin releasing hormone
TSH	thyroid-stimulating hormone
VIP	vasoactive intestinal polypeptide

Chapter

1

EMBRYOLOGY AND ANATOMY OF THE PITUITARY GLAND

Ricardo V. Lloyd

The pituitary gland is composed of tissues of different embryological origins. The pars distalis, pars intermedia and pars tuberalis constitute the adenohypophysis (Fig. 1–1). The adenohypophysis originates from Rathke's pouch, which arises from the evagination of the stomodeal ectoderm of the primitive buccal cavity. The infundibulum, neural stalk and posterior lobe of the pituitary constitute the neural part of the pituitary and arise from the floor of the diencephalon. The pituitary can be recognized grossly by the 3rd month of gestation (1). At this time acidophilic and basophilic cells can be readily identified (Figs. 1–2 and 1–3) (1,2), and with immunohistochemical stains the various cell types can be identified in the adenohypophysis (3–5).

Detailed immunohistochemical analyses have provided insight into the chronological appearances of various cell types in the human adenohypophysis (4,5). Adrenocorticotropic hormone (ACTH)–immunoreactive cells were detected by 5 weeks of gestation by one group of investigators (4). Intense cytoplasmic positivity for ACTH and β-endorphin can be seen by 8 weeks of gestation (5). Growth hormone (GH) can also be detected by 8 weeks (Table 1–1). The α subunit of glycoprotein hormones can be detected at 9 weeks of development, and the β subunits of thyroid-stimulating hormone (TSH), follicle-stimulating hormone (FSH) and luteinizing hormone (LH) can be identified immu-

nohistochemically by 12 weeks of development. A few prolactin cells were identified by the 12th week of gestation in one study, and there was a marked increase in the number of PRL cells by term. These PRL-containing cells were different from the GH cells (6). Analysis of hormone secretion using human fetal pituitary tissues has shown GH secretion by the 5th week of gestation (6), suggesting that the immunohistochemical analyses are less sensitive in detecting hormones or, more likely, that the hormones are secreted but not stored during these early periods of gestation. Ultrastructural studies have also revealed secretory granules in ad-

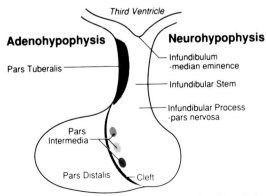

Figure 1–1. Diagram showing the relationship of the adenohypophysis and neurohypophysis. (From Lloyd RV. Endocrine Pathology. New York, Springer-Verlag, 1990.)

1

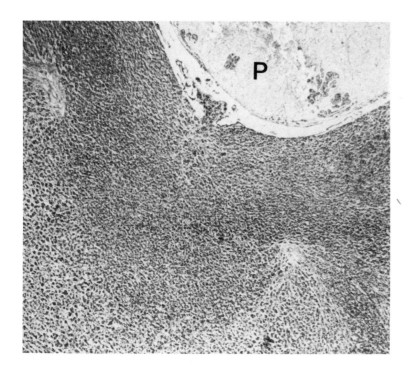

Figure 1–2. Pituitary gland tissue from a 9-week fetus. A small portion of the posterior lobe (P) and most of the anterior lobe tissue are present (×150).

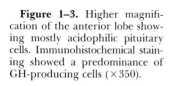

Figure 1–3. Higher magnification of the anterior lobe showing mostly acidophilic pituitary cells. Immunohistochemical staining showed a predominance of GH-producing cells (×350).

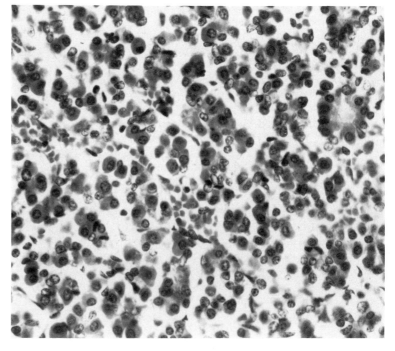

Table 1–1. Identification of Human Anterior Pituitary Hormones by Immunohistochemistry During Embryogenesis*

Hormone	Week of Gestation
ACTH	5–8
GH	8
α Subunit	9
FSH	12
LH	12
TSH	12
PRL	12

*Compiled from Osamura RY, Watanabe K. Histiogenesis of the cells of the anterior and intermediate lobes of human pituitary glands: Immunohistochemical studies. Int Rev Cytol 95:103–129, 1985; and Asa SL, et al. Human fetal adenohypophysis. Histologic and immunocytochemical analysis. Neuroendocrinology 43:308–316, 1986.

enohypophysial cells during the first trimester (7).

The posterior lobe of the pituitary has neurosecretory granules around the 5th month of gestation. These granules represent the storage sites for oxytocin and vasopressin, which are produced in the supraoptic and paraventricular nuclei of the hypothalamus.

The anterior lobe of the pituitary gland is derived from an epithelial evagination of the roof of the posterior nasopharynx. During development this tissue loses its attachment to the pharynx, migrates through the tissue that later becomes the body of the sphenoid bone, and finally comes to rest in the anlage of the sella turcica. In most individuals, small amounts of pituitary tissue can be found in the body of the sphenoid or in the pharyngeal mucosa, which is designated as the pharyngeal pituitary gland (8–11). These remnants may occasionally give rise to tumors in adults (12).

The pituitary weighs about 100 mg at birth (1) and contains all of the anterior pituitary hormones present in the adult. In the adult, the gland measures 13 mm transversely, 9 mm from anterior to posterior and 6 mm vertically. The weight of the gland in the adult ranges from 400 to 900 mg, and the anterior lobe constitutes about 80% of the pituitary. During pregnancy, there is marked PRL cell hyperplasia, and the gland may increase to over 1000 mg. The pituitary gland of multiparous women usually weighs more than the gland of nulliparous women. Abnormally developed glands, such as in anencephalic infants, contain a small pituitary gland with decreased numbers of immunoreactive ACTH cells in the anterior lobe (4). β-Endorphin is also present in the anterior pituitary gland of anencephalics, and the other anterior pituitary hormones are similar to those seen in normal neonates, indicating that the pituitary gland can differentiate functionally and process proopiomelanocortin without the influence of the hypothalamic releasing hormones from the absent central nervous system.

The pituitary gland is covered by the dura, which is a dense layer of connective tissue that covers the brain. The roof of the sella turcica is covered by the diaphragma sellae, which is a part of the dura mater. The hypophysial stalk enters to the rest of the pituitary through a small hole about 5 mm in diameter in the diaphragma sellae. When the diaphragma sellae is incomplete or absent, a condition known as the "empty sella syndrome" develops. In this condition, the diaphragma sellae is more widely opened, and there is increased cerebrospinal fluid pressure, leading to the enlargement of the sella and compression of the pituitary. The pituitary may be markedly flattened and appears like a thin layer of tissue at the bottom of the sella. This condition may be mistaken radiographically for a pituitary adenoma.

The pituitary gland has many important anatomic landmarks in its vicinity. The internal carotid artery is present in the region of the cavernous sinus lateral to the pituitary gland. The optic nerves, chiasma and optic tracts are present between the pituitary and the brain. The anterior lobe, or adenohypophysis, constitutes about 75% to 80% of the gland. It is generally darker on cut sagittal sections because of its vascularity. The posterior lobe or neurohypophysis is usually paler and is continuous with the brain by way of the infundibulum and median eminence of the tuber cinereum (13). The pars tuberalis is composed of a layer of cuboidal cells covering the stalk and adjacent areas and is richly supplied with arterial blood. The pars intermedia is composed of a thin layer of cells between the neural lobe and the pars distalis. It encloses the vestigial lumen of Rathke's pouch with central spaces filled with colloid-type material (13). The lining cells may be ciliated. The intermediate lobe is poorly developed in humans, but is well developed in other species such as rodents.

The blood supply of the adenohypophysis is from the superior hypophysial arteries via the internal carotid or posterior communicating arterial and the inferior hypophysial arteries. These are branches of the internal carotid that traverse the cavernous sinus. The stalk of adjacent parts of the anterior lobe is supplied by the branches of the superior arteries, while branches of the inferior arteries supply the posterior lobe. The pars distalis receives its blood supply via the portal system of veins. The blood from the capillaries of the pars tuberalis and adjacent stalk collects into veins that pass along the stalk and form the sinusoidal capillaries of the pars distalis (13). Branches of the superior hypophysial arteries enter the infundibulum and form a superficial plexus of vessels that gives rise to a host of capillaries and the gomitoli (14). These latter structures are composed of a central artery with a prominent muscular coat and several surrounding capillaries. Their function is unknown, but they may help to regulate blood flow, thus affecting the release of hypothalamic hormones to the adenohypophysis. Long and short portal vessels supply blood to the adenohypophysis; the long portal vessels appear to supply most of the blood.

Ultrastructural studies of the pituitary capillaries have shown that they are lined by fenestrated epithelium (1), which means that the secreted anterior pituitary hormones must pass through the basement membrane of the anterior pituitary cells, as well as that of the endothelial cells, to reach the circulation. The pars distalis has no direct nerve supply, except for a few sympathetic nerve fibers that penetrate the anterior lobe along the capillaries (15). These pericapillary nerve fibers do not regulate anterior pituitary hormone secretion but may affect blood flow to the pituitary.

The posterior pituitary lobe is composed of nerve fibers with axon terminals, pituicytes and dense core granules of stored neurosecretory proteins consisting of oxytocin, vasopressin and neurophysin. The hypothalamic tracts of the supraopticohypophyses and tubero-hypophysial fibers arise from the supraoptic and paraventricular nuclei and traverse from the hypothalamus to the stalk of the posterior pituitary lobe (1). Secretion of the posterior pituitary hormones, oxytocin and vasopressin, is greatly influenced by neural connections, since the neurohypophysis undergoes severe atrophy after stalk sectioning (16) or with injury to the axons originating in the supraoptic and paraventricular nuclei (15).

REFERENCES

1. Kovacs K, Horvath E. Tumors of the pituitary gland. In: Atlas of Tumor Pathology. Second Series. Fascicle 21. Washington, DC, Armed Forces Institute of Pathology, 1986.
2. Goodyer CG, Guyda HJ, Giroud CJP. Development of the hypothalamic-pituitary axis in the human fetus. In: Tolis G, Labrie F, Martin JB, Naftolin F (eds). Clinical Neuroendocrinology: A Pathophysiological Approach. New York, Raven, 1972, pp 199–214.
3. Baker BL, Jaffe RB. The genesis of cell types in the adenohypophysis of the human fetus as observed with immunocytochemistry. Am J Anat *143*:137–161, 1975.
4. Osamura RY, Watanabe K. Histogenesis of the cells of the anterior and intermediate lobes of human pituitary glands: Immunohistochemical studies. Int Rev Cytol *95*:103–129, 1985.
5. Asa SL, Kovacs K, Laszlo FA, Domokos I, Ezrin C. Human fetal adenohypophysis. Histologic and immunocytochemical analysis. Neuroendocrinology *43*:308–316, 1986.
6. Siler-Khodr TM, Morgenstern LL, Greenwood FC. Hormone synthesis and release from human fetal adenohypophyses in vitro. J Clin Endocrinol Metab *39*:891–905, 1974.
7. Gluckman PD, Grumbach MM, Kaplan SL. The neuroendocrine regulation and function of growth hormone and prolactin in the mammalian fetus. Endocr Rev *2*:363–395, 1981.
8. Boyd JD. Observations on the human pharyngeal hypophysis. J Endocrinol *14*:66–77, 1956.
9. Ciocca DR, Puy LA, Stati AO. Identification of seven hormone-producing cell types in the human pharyngeal hypophysis. J Clin Endocrinol Metab *60*:212–216, 1985.
10. Ciocca DR, Puy LA, Stati AO. Immunocytochemical evidence for the ability of the human pharyngeal hypophysis to respond to change in endocrine feedback. Virchows Arch (Pathol Anat) *405*:497–502, 1985.
11. Lindholm J, Korsgaard O, Rasmussen P. Ectopic pituitary function. Acta Med Scand *198*:299–302, 1975.
12. Lloyd RV, Chandler WF, Kovacs K, Ryan N. Ectopic pituitary adenomas with normal anterior pituitary gland. Am J Surg Pathol *10*:546–552, 1986.
13. Gray H. Anatomy of the Human Body. Gross CM, ed. Philadelphia, Lea and Febiger, 1966, pp 1243–1247.
14. Bergland RM, Page RB. Can the pituitary secrete directly to the brain? (Affirmative anatomical evidence). Endocrinology *102*:1325–1338, 1978.
15. Sheehan HL, Kovacs K. Neurohypophysis and hypothalamus. In: Bloodworth JMB Jr (ed). Endocrine Pathology. 2nd Ed. Baltimore, Williams and Wilkins, 1982, pp 45–99.
16. Daniel PM, Prichard MML. Studies of the hypothalamus and the pituitary gland with special reference to the effects of transection of the pituitary stalk. Acta Endocrinol (Kbh) *201*(suppl):1–216, 1975.

2

CYTOLOGY AND FUNCTION OF THE PITUITARY GLAND

RICARDO V. LLOYD

The anterior pituitary has a great variety of cell types and functions. After staining with hematoxylin and eosin (H & E), the cells of the anterior pituitary are acidophilic, basophilic and chromophobic. These histochemical stains do not reliably indicate the specific hormone that the pituitary cell or tumor is producing. Classic histochemical stains have been largely replaced by immunochemical stains in the study of normal pituitary cells and pituitary adenomas.

The synthesis and secretion of anterior pituitary hormones are regulated by hypothalamic hormones (Table 2–1; Fig. 2–1). Corticotropin releasing hormone (CRH) regulates pituitary adrenocorticotropic hormone (ACTH) secretion by interacting with membrane receptors on the ACTH-secreting cell (1). CRH is synthesized as a prohormone and is further processed enzymatically to an amidated form. Growth hormone releasing hormone (GHRH) is produced in the hypothalamus, but can be produced ectopically by many neoplasms. GHRH interacts with growth hormone (GH)–producing cells to increase GH secretion and transcription of GH messenger RNA (mRNA) (3). GHRH secretion is mediated through adenylyl cyclase–, cyclic adenosine monophosphate (cAMP)– and Ca^{2+}-dependent mechanisms (2). Glucocorticoids increase the effects of GHRH on the pituitary, while somatostatin inhibits these effects. Somatostatin inhibits GH as well as thyroid-stimulating hormone (TSH) secretion in the anterior pituitary. This peptide is present in many cells throughout the nervous system and in extraneural tissues such as the gastrointestinal tract and pancreas (4). Somatostatin receptors are present on many other tissues in addition to subsets of anterior pituitary cells (5). This peptide inhibits GH and TSH secretion, but may also decrease prolactin (PRL) and ACTH secretion. Somatostatin reduces membrane permeability to calcium and also stimulates potassium washout from cells (4).

The tripeptide thyrotropin releasing hormone (TRH) stimulates the release of TSH

Table 2–1. Hypothalamic Hormones Regulating Anterior Pituitary Secretion

Peptide/Amine	Amino Acids	Hormone Regulated
CRH	41	Stimulation of ACTH secretion
GnRH	10	Stimulation of LH/FSH secretion
GHRH	40	Stimulation of GH secretion
TRH	3	Stimulation of TSH and PRL secretion
SRIF	14	Inhibition of GH secretion
VIP	28	Stimulation of PRL secretion
Dopamine	a	Inhibition of PRL secretion

a—Amine; ACTH—adrenocorticotropic hormone; CRH—corticotropin releasing hormone; FSH—follicle-stimulating hormone; GH—growth hormone; GHRH—growth hormone releasing hormone; GnRH—gonadotropin releasing hormone; LH—luteinizing hormone; PRL—prolactin; SRIF—somatostatin; TRH—thyrotropin releasing hormone; VIP—vasoactive intestinal polypeptide.

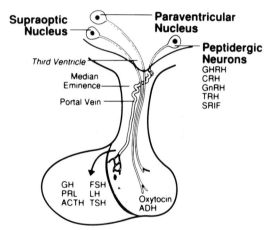

Figure 2–1. Diagram showing the peptidergic neurons with releasing hormones that regulate anterior pituitary hormone secretion and the neurons that produce oxytocin and vasopressin (antidiuretic hormone), which are stored in and released from the posterior pituitary. (From Lloyd RV. Endocrine Pathology. New York, Springer-Verlag, 1990.)

and PRL from the anterior pituitary gland. TSH is synthesized as a prohormone and is subsequently processed with amide and cyclized glutamic acid termini, which are necessary for biological activity (6,7). TRH has also been found in most regions of the brain and the spinal cord (7). TRH interacts with the membrane receptor of TSH and PRL cells, which leads to an increase in secretion of both of these hormones. Gonadotropin releasing hormone (GnRH), also known as luteinizing hormone releasing hormone (LHRH), is also synthesized as a prohormone and is subsequently cleaved and modified during processing. LHRH interacts with receptors on FSH/LH cells, which leads to increased secretion of these hormones by mobilization of intracellular calcium (8,9).

The cell types of the anterior pituitary are summarized in Tables 2–1 and 2–2 (Fig. 2–2). GH is the most common cell type and constitutes about 40% to 50% of cells (Fig. 2–3). GH cells are predominantly in the lateral wings of the anterior pituitary. The pituitary has about 5 to 10 mg of stored GH. GH has effects on skeletal and soft tissue growth associated with a positive nitrogen balance. Deficiencies in or excessive production of GH leads to striking changes in growth and body composition (Table 2–3). Some of the effects of GH are mediated through somatomedins or insulin-like growth factors (IGFs). IGF I is very low in the serum of GH-deficient individuals and is markedly elevated in acromegaly and gigantism, while IGF II is less GH dependent. In GH deficiency, serum IGF II decreases to 30% to 50% of normal, but is not elevated above normal in acromegaly or gigantism (10). Somatostatin analogues are

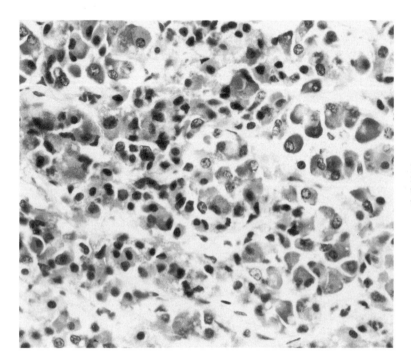

Figure 2–2. Normal anterior pituitary gland stained with hematoxylin and eosin. Various cell types with a normal acinar pattern are present (×350).

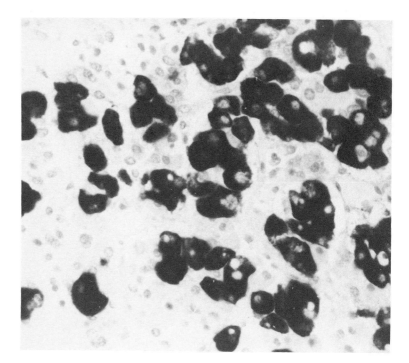

Figure 2–3. Immunostaining with a GH antiserum in a normal pituitary shows that 40% to 50% of the cells are positive for GH (×350).

effective in inhibiting GH secretion and IGF I levels in GH-producing adenomas (11).

PRL cells are the second most abundant cell type in the anterior pituitary gland and may range from 15% to 25% of total cells (Fig. 2–4). PRL cells are present throughout the pars distalis. These cells are usually acidophilic or chromophobic on H & E staining. PRL cells are numerous in late fetal life and in neonates, possibly owing to maternal estrogens. The number of PRL cells decreases after birth and remains low during child-

hood. The highest percentage of PRL cells is found during pregnancy and lactation secondary to hyperplasia (Fig. 2–5). The pituitary gland may weigh more than 1000 mg at this time. Immunochemical staining and electron microscopy of the normal pituitary reveal two types of PRL cells. One cell type stains strongly and diffusely for PRL, while the second type has a distinct juxtanuclear immunoreactive staining pattern. The first cell type has large secretory granules ranging from 500 to 700 nm in diameter on ultrastructural examination, while the cells with

Table 2–2. Cells of the Pituitary Gland

Cell Type	Molecular Size of Hormone	Approx. Cell Percentage	Secretory Granule Diameter (nm)
Growth hormone	21,800	40–50	250–600
PRL	22,500	15–25	500–700
ACTH	4500	10–20	200–350
Follicle-stimulating hormone	29,000	10*	200–300
Luteinizing hormone	29,000	10*	300–500
Thyroid-stimulating hormone	29,000	5	100–300
Folliculo-stellate cell†	None	<1	None
Antidiuretic hormone‡	1100	—	100–200
Oxytocin‡	1100	—	100–200

*Most gonadotropic cells contain both FSH and LH.
†Folliculo-stellate cells do not have secretory granules.
‡Storage in posterior pituitary.
All hormone-containing cells except antidiuretic hormone and oxytocin are in the adenohypophysis.

Table 2–3. Specific Signs/Symptoms Associated With Deficiency or Hypersecretion of Pituitary Hormones

Hormone	Deficiency	Hypersecretion
ACTH	Hypoadrenocorticism	Hyperadrenocorticism Cushing's disease
Growth hormone	Dwarfism	Gigantism/acromegaly
Prolactin	Variable—eg, failure to lactate in postpartum period	Hyperprolactinemia Amenorrhea/ galactorrhea
Thyrotropin	Hypothyroidism	Hyperthyroidism
Gonadotropin (FSH/LH)	Hypogonadism	Associated with hypogonadism
Antidiuretic hormone	Diabetes insipidus	Syndrome of inappropriate ADH secretion with hyponatremia

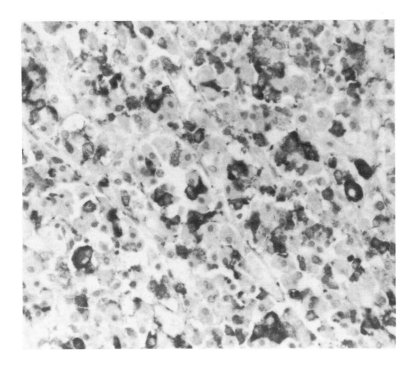

Figure 2–4. Prolactin cells in the normal pituitary constitute between 15% and 25% of the anterior pituitary cells by immunostaining (×300).

juxtanuclear staining have smaller secretory granules of 200 to 350 nm in diameter. Mixed PRL-GH or mammosomatotroph cells have been identified in the normal human pituitary by ultrastructural immunochemistry and with the reverse hemolytic plaque assay (12). This cell type is also seen in the pituitary of rodents (13).

PRL is responsible for initiating and maintaining lactation after adequate stimulation of the breast by estrogens and progesterone. These steroid hormones inhibit lactation during pregnancy in spite of the high serum levels of PRL. With the rapid decline of estrogen and progesterone levels after delivery, the unopposed action of PRL stimulates

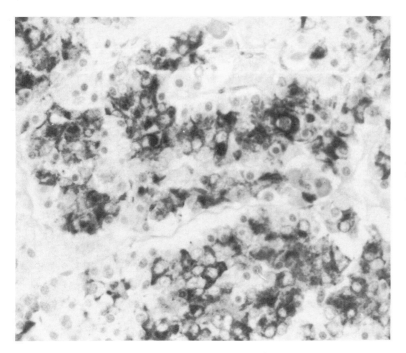

Figure 2–5. This pituitary from a 5-months-pregnant woman contains increased numbers and clusters of PRL cells, indicating PRL cell hyperplasia, which is commonly seen during pregnancy (×300).

lactation. The specific function of PRL in males is not clear, although PRL receptors are present in testes and prostate tissues, indicating that this hormone has specific effects on these target tissues. Vasoactive intestine polypeptide and TRH have a stimulatory effect on PRL secretion, while dopamine has an inhibitory effect on PRL secretion. The clinical use of dopamine agonists such as bromocriptine has been very effective in controlling PRL secretion and reducing tumor size in adenomas (14).

Corticotroph cells constitute 10% to 20% of anterior pituitary cells (Fig. 2–6). These cells are basophilic with periodic acid–Schiff (PAS)–positive cytoplasm, which is related to the glycoprotein content of proopiomelenocortin (POMC) precursors. Proopiomelanocortin is a 31K glycoprotein that is processed by proteolytic digestion into various biologically active fragments, including β-endorphin, β-lipotropin, γ-lipotropin, β-melanotropin and γ-melanotropin. The ACTH-producing cells are found mainly in the central mucoid wedge. In lower vertebrates, a separate intermediate lobe with mostly corticotrophs is present, but this is absent in humans. In older patients, corticotroph cells may infiltrate the posterior lobe, a process known as "basophil invasion" (Fig. 2–7). After immunostaining for ACTH, large perinuclear vacuoles, or "enigmatic bodies,"

that do not stain may be seen in the cytoplasm. These enigmatic bodies probably represent lysosomes. Ultrastructural studies of ACTH cells reveal moderate to large secretory granules ranging from 250 to 700 nm in diameter with abundant type I microfilaments in a perinuclear location. With glucocorticoid excess from endogenous or exogenous sources, Crooke's hyaline change becomes prominent (Fig. 2–8). These are glassy homogeneous type I keratin intermediate filaments, which accumulate in the cytoplasm and push the ACTH secretory granules to the cell periphery. ACTH acts on the adrenal cortical cells to stimulate increased steroidogenesis with increased conversion of cholesterol to pregnenolone and increases synthesis of adrenal cortical cell proteins and RNAs, leading to increased adrenal weight. ACTH has generalized effects on other tissues, including lipolysis in adipocytes and increased muscle uptake of amino acids and glucose. ACTH also stimulates increased insulin and GH secretion.

The gonadotropin hormones, follicle-stimulating hormone (FSH) and LH, are usually present in the same cell type of the adenohypophysis. These cell types make up about 10% of pars distalis cells (Figs. 2–9 and 2–10). The cells are variably PAS positive because of their glycoprotein content. A small percentage of gonadotrophs have only FSH

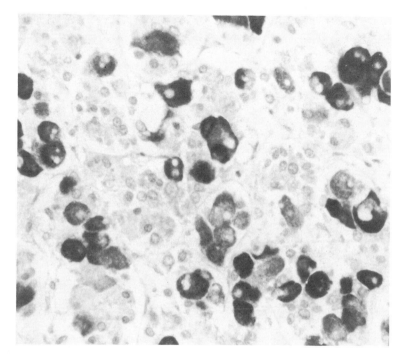

Figure 2–6. Corticotroph cells constitute about 10% to 20% of anterior pituitary cells. These cells are larger than most other anterior pituitary cells and show variable positive immunoreactivity after ACTH staining (×350).

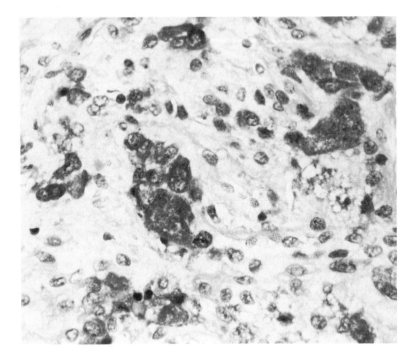

Figure 2–7. Posterior pituitary with a cluster of basophilic corticotroph cells. This phenomenon, known as "basophil invasion," increases with age and should not be mistaken for an invading neoplasm (×350).

Figure 2–8. Prominent Crooke's hyaline change *(arrows)* is present in the pituitary gland. These changes are highly specific for excess endogenous or exogenous glucocorticoids (×400).

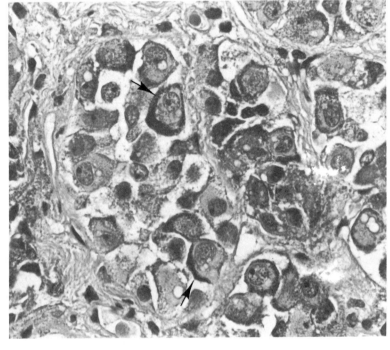

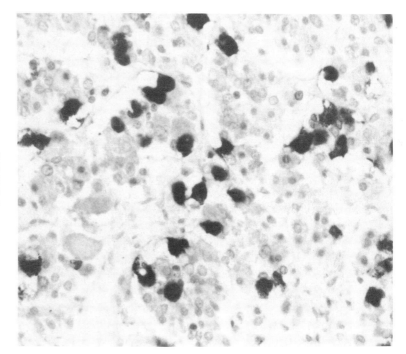

Figure 2–9. Gonadotroph cells stained for LH in the normal anterior pituitary. FSH and LH are usually present in the same cells in the normal pituitary ($\times 350$).

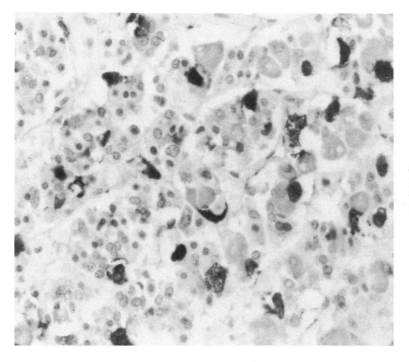

Figure 2–10. Gonadotroph cells stained for FSH in a normal pituitary. FSH/LH cells comprise about 10% of the cells in the normal pituitary ($\times 350$).

or LH (15). FSH and LH cells are present in the mucoid area, and a small percentage of these cells may be found in the pars distalis, which is covered by arachnoid membranes. These are two granule populations in the gonadotrope cells. These measure 200 to 300 nm and 300 to 500 nm in diameter. After removal of the gonads, distinct cells with widely dilated rough endoplasmic reticulum (ER) and decreased numbers of secretory granules in which the nucleus is pushed to the periphery by the expanded rough ER, which are known as "castration" cells or "signet ring" cells, become prominent. FSH and LH have a variety of biological functions, primarily in reproduction. FSH stimulates spermatogenesis by its actions on the Sertoli cells. FSH also increases the LH receptors on the Leydig cells and thus potentiates the actions of LH (10). In females, FSH stimulates granulosa cells with increased estrogen synthesis and development of follicles. LH acts on the Leydig cells in males and has a stimulatory effect on testosterone production, while in females, LH has an important role in the rupture of the follicle at ovulation and in the luteinization of the corpus luteum. A mid-cycle peak in FSH secretion is also present, but is less than the LH peak (16).

The glycoprotein hormone TSH constitutes about 5% of anterior pituitary cells (Fig. 2–11). These PAS-positive cells are often angular. On ultrastructural examination, they have secretory granules ranging in size from 100 to 300 nm in diameter, and the granules are usually adjacent to the cell membrane (Fig. 2–12). Thyroidectomy cells consist of enlarged thyrotropic cells with prominent Golgi complexes, markedly dilated rough ER and decreased numbers of secretory granules. These cells are present with chronic hypothyroidism but can be induced in experimental animals after treatment with propylthiouracil or related drugs. TSH has many effects on various physiological functions via its actions on the thyroid gland. Direct effects on the thyroid include increased weight and vascularity of the gland, increased height of the follicular epithelium and decreased stored colloid. Acute effects of TSH include activation of thyroid metabolism, with increases in glucose metabolism, nucleotide formation and phospholipid turnover (17). Chronic effects include increased protein kinase, increased RNA and protein synthesis (17). The effects of TSH on the thyroid cell are initiated by interaction with specific cell membrane receptors and activation of the adenylyl cyclase system, which is a common primary mode of action for many anterior pituitary hormones.

The folliculo-stellate cells of the anterior

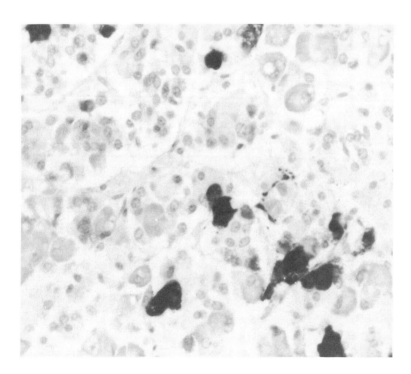

Figure 2–11. TSH cells constitute about 5% of normal pituitary cells. After immunostaining for TSH, many of the positive TSH cells have an angular shape (×350).

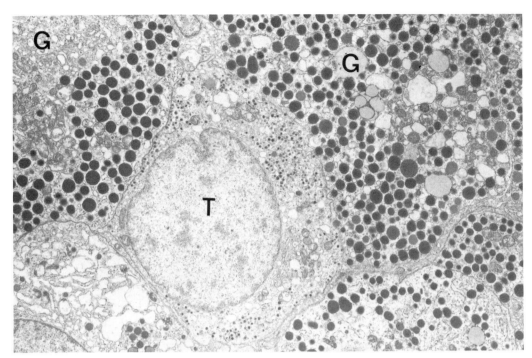

Figure 2–12. Ultrastructural features of normal pituitary gland cells. A thyrotroph cell (T) with small secretory granules 100 to 300 nm in diameter is present. Several GH cells (G) with secretogranules ranging from 500 to 700 nm in diameter are also seen (×5000).

pituitary have a distinct morphological appearance with irregular processes that extend between the hormone-producing cells (Figs. 2–13 and 2–14). Ultrastructural examination reveals few organelles and no secretory granules in these cells. Cell junctions are often seen between folliculo-stellate and secretory cells in the anterior pituitary. These cells have been reported to have many functions, including phagocytic functions, sustentacular or supporting and paracrine functions (18,19). Some workers consider these cells to be degenerating secretory cells (20). Studies of folliculo-stellate cells in other species have indicated that these cells regulate pituitary hormone release by paracrine mechanisms (21). Other studies have shown that the cultured bovine folliculo-stellate cells are capable of producing basic fibroblast growth factor (22), as well as a growth factor for vascular endothelial cells (23).

The hormones of the posterior pituitary include vasopressin (also known as antidiuretic hormone, or ADH) and oxytocin, which are transported from the supraoptic and paraventricular nuclei to the neurohypophysis for storage. These hormones are present in the dilated axon terminals within

secretory granules that range from 100 to 200 nm in diameter. These octapeptides all have sulfhydryl bonds between the cysteine residues and are in a ring conformation. These hormones are bound to neurophysins, which are sulfur-rich proteins of about 10 kd. Most of the secreted ADH and oxytocin are present in the unbound form. The principal cell in the posterior pituitary is the pituicyte, which is the glial cell of the posterior lobe. It has supportive and phagocytic functions. The posterior lobe is highly vascularized, and the capillaries are lined by fenestrated endothelium. The high degree of vascularity from the direct arterial blood supply may account for the higher incidence of metastatic tumors to the posterior lobe compared to the anterior lobe.

ADH secretion is regulated by osmotic and volume-mediated nonosmotic stimuli. Osmotic stimuli produce linear increases in vasopressin release with normal blood volume, while a 10% or greater depletion of blood volume leads to an exponential increase in ADH secretion (24). Many chemical agents, such as morphine, nicotine, barbiturates and cyclophosphamide, enhance ADH release, while others, like phenytoin, alcohol

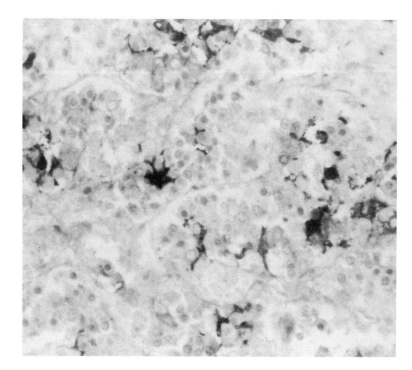

Figure 2–13. Staining of this pituitary gland for S-100 acidic protein reveals folliculo-stellate cells. These cells have irregular processes that extend between the hormone-producing cells. Folliculo-stellate cells are increased in number in the pituitary gland during pregnancy (×350).

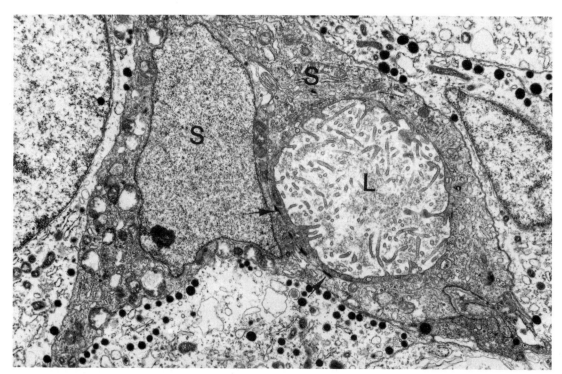

Figure 2–14. Ultrastructural features of two folliculo-stellate (S) cells. These cells do not have secretory granules. Desmosomes (*arrows*) are present, and there is a central lumen (L) with microvilli (×8600).

and narcotic antagonists, suppress ADH release (24). Oxytocin release is stimulated by mechanical distention of the reproductive tract and suckling of the nipples. This hormone stimulates uterine contraction during delivery and increases intramammary pressure during suckling. Release of oxytocin is also stimulated by plasma hypertonicity (24).

MISCELLANEOUS PEPTIDES PRODUCED BY THE ANTERIOR PITUITARY

A variety of peptide hormones, in addition to the classic hormones, have been detected in the anterior pituitary by immunohistochemistry, radioimmunoassay and other analytical methods (25–44) (Table 2–4). While the functions of many of these substances are not known, some of these that are widely distributed in the pituitary probably have specific functions in various cell types. Substances such as neuron-specific enolase, chromogranins and synaptophysin can be used in diagnostic pathology as broad-spectrum markers for neuroendocrine cells, including those of the anterior pituitary gland. The chromogranins show a variable distribution in the anterior pituitary, since prolactinomas express chromogranin B but not chromogranin A, while gonadotroph cells express both chromogranins A and B (27). Likewise, neural cell adhesion molecules (NCAMs) are expressed by many anterior pituitary cells, but prolactinomas have fewer NCAMs than some other adenomas (28).

Normal and neoplastic ACTH cells have been associated with various other peptides, including cholecystokinin (34) and galanin (36). The presence of these peptides in ACTH cells suggests that they may have a role in ACTH secretion. The presence of TRH and TRH-binding sites in human pituitary null cell adenomas (41) suggests that this and other hypothalamic peptides may have autocrine and paracrine effects on pituitary adenomas. The TSH cell has also been associated with specific peptides, including methionine-enkephalin and substance P (33,37), and there may be a physiological role for these substances in regulating thyroid function, such as positive autocrine feedback influences to increase TRH-stimulated TSH release.

The localization of many peptides in the anterior pituitary has been very controversial. The specificity of the detection system utilized, including the antibodies used for immunochemical detection, has been questioned, and there has been a great deal of species variation for the localization of specific peptides in the gland or within certain cell types. The physiological significance of many of the reported observations is unknown, and the report that specific peptides are present in neoplasms but not in the normal pituitary cells suggests that this may be ectopic rather than eutopic peptide/hormone expression. Analysis of growth factors, oncogenes and other peptides expressed in the anterior pituitary is a rapidly changing area, and new findings will contribute to further understanding of the regulatory functions of these substances in the normal pituitary and in pituitary neoplasms.

Table 2–4. Some Peptides/Hormones Detected in the Anterior Pituitary

Peptide/Hormone	Specific Cell Type	Reference
Chromogranins	Many cell types	25,26
Neural cell adhesion molecule	Many cell types	27,28
Neuron-specific enolase	Many cell types	29
Synaptophysin	Many cell types	30
Protein 7B2	Many cell types	31
Substance P	TSH	32
Cholecystokinin	ACTH	33
Renin	PRL	34,35
Galanin	ACTH	36
Methionine-enkephalin	TSH	37
Insulin-like peptide	—	38
Chorionic gonadotropin	—	39
Alpha-transforming growth factor	Prolactin*	40
Thyrotropin releasing hormone	Null cell adenoma	41
Fibroblast growth factor	Many adenoma cells	43
	Folliculo-stellate cells†	22,43
Vascular endothelial growth factor	Folliculo-stellate cells†	23
Calcitonin	—	42
Lipocortin-1	Folliculo-stellate cells† Some ACTH cells	44
mAB lu-5	ACTH	45

*Bovine pituitary tissue.
†Cultured bovine cells.

REFERENCES

1. Vale W, Rivier C, Brown MR, Spiess J, Koob G, Swanson L, Bilezikjian L, Bloom F, Rivier J. Chemical and biological characterization of corticotropin releasing factor. Recent Prog Horm Res *39*:245–270, 1983.

2. Shibasaki T, Shizume K, Masudu A, Nakahara M, Hizuka N, Miyakawa M. Plasma growth hormone response to growth hormone-releasing factor in acromegalic patients. J Clin Endocrinol Metab 58:215–217, 1984.

3. Barinaga M, Yamonoto G, Rivier C, Vale W, Evans R, Rosenfeld MG. Transcriptional regulation of growth hormone gene expression by growth hormone-releasing factor. Nature 306:84–85, 1983.

4. Reichlin S. Neuroendocrinology. In: Wilson JD, Foster DW (eds). Williams' Textbook of Endocrinology. 7th Ed. Philadelphia, WB Saunders, 1985, pp 492–567.

5. Reubi JC, Maurer R, Von Werder K, Torhorst J, Klijn JGM, Lamberts SWJ. Somatostatin receptors in human endocrine tumors. Cancer Res 47:551–558, 1987.

6. Sandow J, Konig W. Chemistry of the hypothalamic hormones. In: Jeffcoate SL, Hutchinson JSM (eds). The Endocrine Hypothalamus. London, Academic Press, 1978, pp 149–211.

7. Jackson IM. Thyrotropin-releasing hormone. N Engl J Med 306:145–155, 1982.

8. Clayton RN, Catt KJ. Gonadotropin-releasing hormone receptors: Characterization, physiological regulation, and relationship to reproductive function. Endocr Rev 2:186–209, 1981.

9. Conn PM, Marian JM, McMillian M, Stern J, Rogers D, Hamby M, Penna A, Grant E. Gonadotropin-releasing hormone action in the pituitary: A three step mechanism. Endocr Rev 2:174–185, 1981.

10. Daughaday WH. The anterior pituitary. In: Wilson JD, Foster DW (eds). Williams' Textbook of Endocrinology. Philadelphia, WB Saunders, 1985, pp 568–613.

11. Barkan AL, Lloyd RV, Chandler WF, Hatfield MK, Gebarski SS, Kelch RP, Beitins IZ. Preoperative treatment of acromegaly with long-acting somatostatin analog SMS 201-995: Shrinkage of invasive pituitary macroadenomas and improved surgical remission rate. J Clin Endocrinol Metab 67:1040–1048, 1988.

12. Lloyd RV, Anagnostou D, Cano M, Barkan AL, Chandler WF. Analysis of mammosomatotropic cells in normal and neoplastic human pituitary tissues by the reverse hemolytic plaque assay and immunocytochemistry. J Clin Endocrinol Metab 66:1103–1110, 1988.

13. Nikitovitch-Winer MB, Atkin J, Maley BE. Colocalization of prolactin and growth hormone within specific adenohypophyseal cells in male, female and lactating female rats. Endocrinology 121:625–630, 1987.

14. Tindall GT, Kovacs K, Horvath E, Thorner MO. Human prolactin-producing adenomas and bromocriptine: A histological, immunocytochemical, ultrastructural and morphometric study. J Clin Endocrinol Metab 55:1178–1183, 1982.

15. Pelletier G, Robert F, Hardy J. Identification of human anterior pituitary cells by immunoelectron microscopy. J Clin Endocrinol Metab 46:534–542, 1978.

16. Ross GJ, Gargille CM, Lipsett MB, Rayford PL, Marshall JR, Strott CA, Rodbard O. Pituitary and gonadal hormones in women during spontaneous and induced ovulatory cycles. Recent Prog Horm Res 26:1–62, 1970.

17. Carazen P, Amra S. Mechanisms of thyroid regulation. In: DeGroot LJ (ed). Endocrinology. Vol 1.

2nd Ed. Philadelphia, WB Saunders, 1989, pp 530–540.

18. Morris CS, Hitchcock E. Immunocytochemistry of folliculo-stellate cells of normal and neoplastic human pituitary gland. J Clin Pathol 38:481–488, 1985.

19. Stokreef JC, Reifel CS, Shin SH. A possible phagocytic role for folliculo-stellate cells of anterior pituitary following estrogen withdrawal from primed male rats. Cell Tissue Res 243:255–261, 1986.

20. Bergland RM, Torack RM. An ultrastructural study of follicular cells in the human anterior pituitary. Am J Pathol 57:273–297, 1969.

21. Baes M, Allaerts W, Denef C. Evidence for functional communication between folliculo-stellate cells and hormone-secreting cells in perfused anterior pituitary cell aggregates. Endocrinology 120:685–691, 1987.

22. Ferrara N, Schweigerer L, Neufeld G, Mitchell R, Gospodarowicz D. Pituitary follicular cells produce basic fibroblast growth factor. Proc Natl Acad Sci USA 84:5773–5777, 1987.

23. Ferrara N, Henzel WJ. Pituitary follicular cells secrete a novel heparin-binding growth factor specific for vascular endothelial cells. Biochem Biophys Res Commun 161:851–858, 1989.

24. Culpepper RM, Hebert SC, Andreali TE. The posterior pituitary and water metabolism. In: Wilson JD, Foster DW (eds). Williams' Textbook of Endocrinology. Philadelphia, WB Saunders, 1985, pp 614–652.

25. Lloyd RV, Wilson BS, Kovacs K, Ryan N. Immunohistochemical localization of chromogranin in human hypophyses and pituitary adenomas. Arch Pathol Lab Med 109:515–517, 1985.

26. Lloyd RV, Cano M, Rosa P, Hille A, Huttner WB. Distribution of chromogranin A and secretogranin I (chromogranin B) in neuroendocrine cells and tumors. Am J Pathol 130:296–304, 1988.

27. Aletsee-Ufrecht MC, Langley K, Gratzl O, Gratzl M. Differential expression of the neural cell adhesion molecule N-CAM 140 in human pituitary tumors. FEBS Lett 272:45–49, 1990.

28. Jin L, Hemperly JJ, Lloyd RV. Expression of neural cell adhesion molecule (N-CAM) in normal and neoplastic human neuroendocrine tissues. Am J Pathol 138:961–969, 1991.

29. Asa SL, Ryan N, Kovacs K, Singer W, Marangos PJ. Immunohistochemical localization of neuron-specific enolase in the human hypophysis and pituitary adenomas. Arch Pathol Lab Med 108:40–43, 1984.

30. Stefaneanu L, Ryan N, Kovacs K. Immunocytochemical localization of synaptophysin in human hypophyses and pituitary adenomas. Arch Pathol Lab Med 112:801–804, 1988.

31. Seidah NG, Hsi KL, De Serres G, Rochemont J, Hamelin J, Antakly T, Cantin M, Chretien M. Isolation and NH$_2$-terminal sequence of a highly conserved human and porcine pituitary protein belonging to a new superfamily. Immunocytochemical localization in pars distalis and pars nervosa of the pituitary and in the supraoptic nucleus of the hypothalamus. Arch Biochem Biophys 225:525–534, 1983.

32. Roth KA, Krause JE. Substance-P is present in a subset of thyrotrophs in the human pituitary. J Clin Endrinol Metab 71:1089–1095, 1990.

33. Rehfeld JF, Lindholm J, Andersen BN, Bardram L,

Cantor P, Fenger M, Ludecke DK. Pituitary tumors containing cholecystokinin. N Engl J Med *316*:1244–1247, 1987.

34. Mizuno K, Ojima M, Hashimoto S, Watari H, Tani M, Satoh M, Fukuchi S. Multiple forms of immunoreactive renin in human pituitary tissue. Life Sci *37*:2297–2304, 1985.

35. Saint-Andre J-P, Rohmer V, Alhenic-Gelas F, Menard J, Bigorgne J-C, Corvol P. Presence of renin, antiotensinogen and converting enzyme in human pituitary lactotroph cells and prolactin adenomas. J Clin Endocrinol Metab *63*:231–237, 1986.

36. Vrontakis ME, Sono T, Kovacs K, Friesen HG. Presence of galanin-like immunoreactivity in nontumorous corticotrophs and corticotroph adenomas of the human pituitary. J Clin Endocrinol Metab *70*:747–751, 1990.

37. Roth KA, Lorenz RG, McKeel DW, Leykam J, Barchas JD, Tyler AN. Methionine-enkephalin and thyrotropin-stimulating hormone are intimately related in the human anterior pituitary. J Clin Endocrinol Metab *66*:804–810, 1988.

38. Budd GC, Pansky B, Budd NJ. Insulin or insulin-like peptides in the human pituitary. Ann Clin Lab Sci *17*:111–115, 1987.

39. Odell WD, Griffin J, Hildegarde M, Snyder PJ. Secretion of chorionic gonadotropin by cultured human pituitary cells. J Clin Endocrinol Metab *71*:1318–1321, 1990.

40. Kobrin MS, Asa SL, Samsoondar J, Kudlow JE. α-Transforming growth factor in the bovine anterior pituitary gland: Secretion by dispersed cells and immunohistochemical localization. Endocrinology *121*:1412–1416, 1987.

41. Le Dafniet M, Grouselle D, Li JY, Kujas M, Bression D, Barret A, Tixier-Vidal A, Peillon F. Evidence of thyrotropin-releasing hormone (TRH) and TRH-binding sites in human nonsecreting pituitary adenomas. J Clin Endocrinol Metab *65*:1014–1019, 1987.

42. Deftos LJ. Pituitary cells secrete calcitonin in the reverse hemolytic plaque assay. Biochem Biophys Res Commun *146*:1350–1356, 1987.

43. Silverlight JJ, Prysor-Jones RA, Jenkins JS. Basic fibroblast growth factor in human pituitary tumours. Clin Endocrinol *32*:669–676, 1990.

44. Johnson MD, Gray ME, Pepinsky RB, Stahlman MT. Lipocortin-1 immunoreactivity in the human pituitary gland. J Histochem Cytochem *38*:1841–1845, 1990.

45. Kovacs K, Ryan N, Stefaneanu L. Identification of corticotrophs in the human pituitary with mAB lu-5, a novel immunocytochemical marker. Pathol Res Pract *182*:775–779, 1987.

3

PRACTICAL APPROACHES TO THE DIAGNOSIS AND STUDY OF PITUITARY LESIONS

Ricardo V. Lloyd

The diagnosis of pituitary lesions requires close clinicopathologic and radiologic correlations in addition to sophisticated morphological studies. The presurgical evaluation of the patient should be complete, with assessment of hormonal abnormalities in the serum by appropriate radioimmunoassays and other immunological studies. Radiologic studies, including computed tomography (CT) scans, magnetic resonance imaging (MRI) and additional analyses as required, can be of great assistance to the surgeon in planning the surgical approach, in grading adenomas and in detecting unusual cases such as adenomas in ectopic locations and assessment of empty sella or partial empty sella syndrome.

Most pituitary surgical procedures are performed transsphenoidally. The value of frozen sections at the time of surgery varies among different institutions and countries and is discussed in more detail in Chapter 4. Frozen sections may be used to confirm the presence of an adenoma, but are used less often by the experienced neurosurgeon. Frozen sections have been used to evaluate possible margins of resection of adenomas. Some experienced pathologists maintain that the establishment of surgical margins by histopathologic techniques is often unrealistic (1). However, in some unusual circumstances this approach may be necessary (2). Freezing only a portion of the adenoma or performing touch preparations can help to avoid some of the problems with freezing artifacts for subsequent routine light microscopic, immunohistochemical and ultrastructural analyses. Frozen sections or touch preparations are very useful when there is some doubt on gross examination that the tissue represents a pituitary adenoma.

As with examination of most tissue specimens, delay in fixation and drying of artifacts makes subsequent interpretations very difficult. The tissue should be transported to the surgical suite after excision as rapidly as possible on a pad moistened with saline solution. The tissues should not be immersed in saline during transportation because of the numerous artifacts that develop with such treatment.

Depending on the size of the specimen and interest of the pathologists and others involved in the evaluation of pituitary abnormalities, the minimal amount of tissue for processing should involve fixing some of the tissue in neutral buffered formalin (Fig. 3–1). Some investigators prefer to fix some of the tissue in paraformaldehyde, Bouin's or Zamboni's fixative as well, but neutral buffered formalin is probably the best all-around fixative for most light microscopic studies. For electron microscopic studies, tissues should be fixed in buffered glutaraldehyde using at least two 1- to 2-mm pieces of tissue

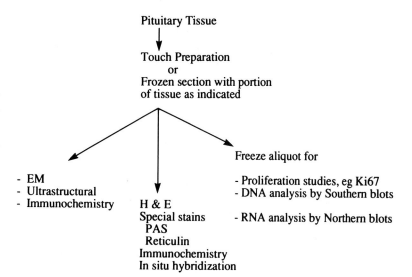

Figure 3–1. Flow chart summarizing one possible approach for examining and processing pituitary tissues obtained immediately after biopsy or excision of a neoplasm. The number of studies that can be done is determined by the size of the adenoma.

from two different locations if possible. Depending on the size of the specimen and interest of the pathologist, other tissue aliquots can be used for cell culture studies, and frozen for biochemical, molecular biological and other studies.

The most important routine stain for diagnosis of pituitary adenomas is the hematoxylin and eosin (H & E) preparation. Periodic acid–Schiff (PAS) staining can be helpful, since it is positive in adrenocorticotropic hormone (ACTH)–producing adenomas and in some glycoprotein-producing tumors. Reticulin stains can be helpful with small neoplasms in which it is difficult to distinguish between a hyperplastic nodule and a small adenoma. Some authors have used the term "tumorlette" to characterize lesions that are between hyperplasia and a true adenoma (1,3). In the tumorlette, reticulin staining reveals that the acinar pattern is preserved, although expanded, and the cells are almost monomorphous.

Immunohistochemical stains for pituitary hormones performed routinely on pituitary adenomas include stains for prolactin (PRL), growth hormone (GH), luteinizing hormone (LH), follicle-stimulating hormone (FSH), thyroid-stimulating hormone (TSH) and ACTH. To diagnose null cell adenomas or other clinically nonfunctioning adenomas that may express only glycoprotein hormones focally (4), staining with broad-spectrum neuroendocrine markers such as chromogranin A, neuron-specific enolase or synaptophysin should be performed. In addition, staining for the α subunit of gonadotropin and β-

endorphin is often done by some laboratories. The use of frozen sections for immunochemistry is more sensitive than paraffin sections, but the morphological details of the specimens are often suboptimal. Tissues that have been used for frozen sections and then thawed and processed in paraffin after formalin fixation often provide suboptimal immunostaining results that may be difficult to interpret; these should be avoided.

The use of routine ultrastructural studies is essential in the diagnosis of some adenomas, such as oncocytomas, and is useful in the diagnosis of null cell adenomas and various subtypes of silent corticotropic adenomas. Tissues fixed in glutaraldehyde and post-fixed in osmium tetroxide can be used for these purposes. When performing ultrastructural immunochemistry, post-fixation in osmium tetroxide should be avoided. Certain hormones such as PRL, GH and ACTH are well preserved in glutaraldehyde-fixed tissues, and post-embedding immunostaining is often successful for adenomas producing these hormones. However, the glycoprotein hormones FSH, LH and TSH are poorly preserved and are best demonstrated by pre-embedding immunostaining (5).

Lectin binding to pituitary cells at the light microscope level can be studied with frozen sections or formalin-fixed, paraffin-embedded tissue sections. For ultrastructural analysis of lectin binding to secretory granules, glutaraldehyde-fixed tissues without post-fixation with osmium tetroxide are usually used (6).

DNA-ploidy analysis of pituitary adenomas

has been reported by various investigators (7–10). Most studies have revealed a low incidence of aneuploidy in pituitary adenomas, and aneuploid tumors have usually been associated with PRL- and GH-producing tumors. The clinical significance of these studies is unclear at this time, and prospective studies are needed to further evaluate the clinical utility of this technique. While most flow cytometric studies have used fresh tissues, formalin-fixed tissues have also been utilized. Comparison of the DNA content in fresh and fixed specimens has shown a higher frequency of aneuploidy and a lower estimate of S-phase fractions when fresh tumors are analyzed (8,9).

Cell culture studies have contributed to our understanding of the regulation of pituitary adenomas *in vitro,* and some of these observations can be extrapolated to *in vivo* events. Fresh tissues are needed for these studies. Tissues can be placed in tissue culture media and maintained at room temperature or at 4°C for a few hours with a high degree of viability of the tumor cells retained. Ideally the tissues should be processed for cell or organ culture as rapidly as possible.

Molecular biological analysis is usually carried out with fresh tissue. Techniques such as restriction fragment length polymorphism (RFLP) and Southern and Northern analysis yield the best results with fresh tissues. *In situ* hybridization (ISH) analysis is best done with frozen tissue sections. However, the use of paraffin-embedded sections provides greater morphological detail in spite of the loss of some RNA or DNA during tissue processing.

Although pituitary tumors are generally benign, invasive growth may be present in a significant portion of these neoplasms (11). Analysis of the proliferative rate of adenomas may provide some useful information about the biological behavior of these tumors. Use of bromodeoxyuridine and the monoclonal antibody Ki-67 (12,13) can provide useful information about proliferation. Frozen tissues are required for Ki-67 studies, while bromodeoxyuridine studies require *in vitro* administration or analysis of the tumor cells in culture before performing immunostaining (14). Studies with Ki-67 have shown that invasive pituitary adenomas had almost twice as many Ki-67–positive cells as the non-invasive adenomas (12). The use of another proliferation marker, cyclin, or proliferating cell nuclear antigen (PCNA), enables the investigator to analyze proliferation using paraffin-embedded tissue sections (15).

The development of a tumor bank of frozen pituitary tissues can be very useful for analysis of a large series of cases in which paraffin-embedded sections do not prove adequate, such as with some immunochemical staining procedures with an antibody such as Ki-67. Tissues can be rapidly frozen in liquid nitrogen and kept at −70°C for many years. Tissues should be carefully wrapped to prevent desiccation. Although optimal cutting temperature (OCT) compound has been used to embed some of these tissues to decrease desiccation, the OCT may interfere with some subsequent analyses and should not be used for the entire sample.

REFERENCES

1. Scheithauer BW. The pituitary and sellar region. In: Sternberg SS (ed). Diagnostic Surgical Pathology. New York, Raven, 1989, pp 371–393.
2. Lang H-D, Saeger W, Ludecke DK, Muller D. Rapid frozen section diagnosis of pituitary tumors. Endocr Pathol *1*:116–122, 1990.
3. Scheithauer BW, Kovacs K, Randall RV, Ryan N. Pituitary glands in hypothyroidism: Histologic and immunocytologic study. Arch Pathol Lab Med *109*:499–504, 1985.
4. Black PM, Hsu DW, Klibanski A, Kliman B, Jameson JL, Ridgway EC, Hedley-Whyte ET, Zervas NT. Hormone production in clinically nonfunctioning pituitary adenomas. J Neurosurg *66*:244–250, 1987.
5. Horvath E, Lloyd RV, Kovacs K. Propylthiouracil-induced hypothyroidism results in reversible transdifferentiation of somatotrophs into thyroidectomy cells. A morphologic study of the rat pituitary including immunoelectron microscopy. Lab Invest *63*:511–520, 1990.
6. Hori T, Nishiyama F, Anno Y, Adachi S, Numata H, Hokama Y, Muraoka K, Hiranol H. Difference of lectin binding sites of secretory granules between normal pituitary and adenoma cells. Acta Neuropathol (Berl) *66*:177–183, 1985.
7. Anniko M, Tribukait B, Wersall J. DNA ploidy and cell phase in human pituitary tumors. Cancer *53*:1708–1713, 1984.
8. Frierson HF. Flow cytometric analysis of ploidy in solid neoplasms: Comparison of fresh with formalin-fixed paraffin-embedded specimens. Hum Pathol *19*:290–294, 1988.
9. Camplejohn RS, Macartney JC. Comparison of DNA flow cytometry from fresh and paraffin-embedded samples of non-Hodgkin's lymphoma. J Clin Pathol *38*:1096–1099, 1985.
10. Fitzgibbons PL, Appley AJ, Turner RR, Bishop PC, Parker JW, Breeze RE, Weiss MH, Apuzzo MLJ. Flow cytometric analysis of pituitary tumors. Correlation of nuclear antigen p105 and DNA content with clinical behavior. Cancer *62*:1556–1560, 1988.
11. Landolt AM. Biology of pituitary microadenomas. In: Faglia G, Giovanelli MA, MacLeod RM (eds).

Pituitary Microadenomas. London, Academic Press, 1980, pp 107–122.

12. Landolt AM, Shibata T, Kleihues P. Growth rate of human pituitary adenomas. J Neurosurg *67:*803–806, 1987.

13. Knosp E, Kitz K, Perneczky A. Proliferation activity in pituitary adenomas: Measurement by monoclonal antibody Ki-67. Neurosurgery *25:*927–930, 1989.

14. Nishizaki T, Orita T, Saiki M, Furutani Y, Aoki H. Cell kinetics studies of human brain tumors by *in vitro* labeling using anti Br dU monoclonal antibody. J Neurosurg *69:*371–374, 1988.

15. McNicol AM, Sheperd M, Lane OP. Cell proliferation in pituitary adenomas; correlation with hormonal immunoreactivity. Abstract 14. J Endocrinol Invest *14*(suppl 1):55, 1991.

4

FROZEN SECTIONS IN THE DIAGNOSIS OF PITUITARY LESIONS

Ricardo V. Lloyd

Intraoperative frozen section examination of pituitary tissues can be helpful to the surgeon. The two major topics that are addressed with the frozen section approach include (1) whether an adenoma is present and (2) examination of the margin of the neoplasm. Frozen section analysis can also be helpful in distinguishing between a pituitary adenoma and other primary lesions in the region of the sella turcica, such as craniopharyngiomas, germinomas and metastatic tumors to the pituitary (Figs. 4–1 and 4–2). The difficulties of examining adenoma margins by frozen section have been discussed by various authors (1,2). It is usually more difficult to define the margins of an adenoma than to make the diagnosis of an adenoma on frozen section. The borders of an adenoma are usually poorly defined, and in most cases, a fibrous capsule does not separate the adenoma from the non-tumorous pituitary tissues.

Features that are helpful in establishing the diagnosis of adenoma include cellular monomorphism and uniform staining of tumor cells. Although most adenomas are composed of one cell type, rare tumors may consist of two or three cell types. Cytological smears or touch preparations can be helpful in making the diagnosis of adenoma at the time of frozen section (3–6). The advantages of cytological preparations include (1) they are more rapid than cutting frozen sections, (2) the artifacts associated with freezing portions of the tissue are avoided and (3) the cellular details are more distinct. Disadvantages of the cytological touch preparation include (1) loss of architectural detail, (2) difficulty in assessing the presence of invasion and (3) difficulty in evaluating the margins of the neoplasm. The presence of pleomorphism, nuclear atypia and mitotic figures are helpful features to diagnose adenomas on cytological touch preparations.

Various stains have been used to evaluate pituitary frozen sections. These include the orange G–PAS and orange G–hematoxylin stains, which aid in identifying secretory granules in the cytoplasm (6). Adelman and Post (6) used 16-μm- rather than 8-μm-thick sections, which increased the reliability of the technique. Adjustment of staining time to distinguish between adenoma and normal pituitary was also recommended (5). Reticulin stains have also been used to distinguish between adenoma and non-tumorous pituitary tissue with frozen section; however, technical difficulties with this technique make it less desirable as a rapid frozen section technique (6,7).

McKeever *et al.* (8) reported on the use of stromal and nuclear markers for rapid identification of pituitary adenomas on frozen sections. The fluoresceinated lectin, *Ricinus communis* agglutinin 120 (RCA 120), was used to localize vascular stroma by its ability to bind galactose. Propidium iodide, which binds nucleic acids, was used to stain the cell

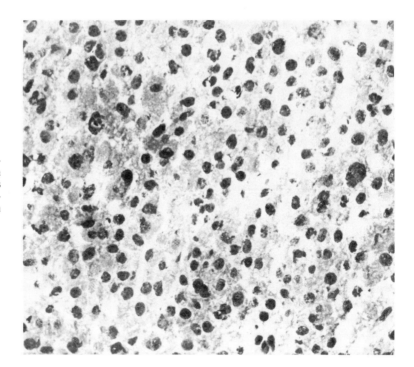

Figure 4–1. Frozen section examination of a pituitary adenoma from a patient with Cushing's disease. There is a moderate degree of nuclear pleomorphism (×350).

nuclei. Analysis of stromal configuration, nuclear morphology and cell-to-stroma ratios was used to distinguish adenoma from nontumorous adenohypophysis in a study of 35 lesions biopsied by a transsphenoidal approach. The necessity of having a fluorescence microscope available for this analysis has limited the widespread application of this approach. More recent techniques for the rapid diagnosis of adenomas have included intraoperative hormone measurement to localize microadenomas, such as in Cushing's disease (9).

In general the accuracy rates of pituitary

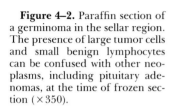

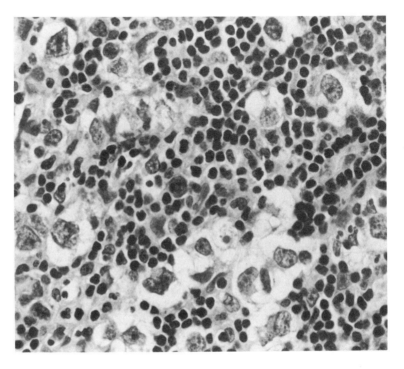

Figure 4–2. Paraffin section of a germinoma in the sellar region. The presence of large tumor cells and small benign lymphocytes can be confused with other neoplasms, including pituitary adenomas, at the time of frozen section (×350).

frozen section, which range from 80% to 90%, have been much lower than those of many other tissues in surgical pathology; these latter rates are usually greater than 90% in most laboratories. In an analysis of rapid frozen section diagnosis of pituitary tumors by Lang *et al.*, an overall accuracy of 83.1% was reported (10). Major problems that contributed to this relatively low accuracy rate included (1) abundant connective tissue or reaction of tissues to cell necrosis, leading to fibrosis and architectural distortion; (2) presence of granulation tissue as in intrasellar craniopharyngiomas; (3) freezing and other artifacts and (4) sections that were too thick or too small, with insulating cell clusters. Of 163 transsphenoidal surgical operations at the University of Michigan between 1985 and 1989, 64, or 39.3%, of these cases were analyzed by frozen section. The percentage of frozen sections done on specimens varied from year to year. In 1985, 50% of the specimens were examined by frozen sections, while in 1988 and 1989, 31.4% and 41% of cases, respectively, were examined by intraoperative frozen sections. The eight false-negative cases resulted in part from inadequate sampling at the time of frozen section and failure to recognize hyperplasia on frozen section biopsy. The two false-positive diagnoses of adenomas consisted of a small sample of a craniopharyngioma and one of a germinoma (Table 4–1; Fig. 4–2). In this retrospective analysis, the small size of the biopsy specimens and the technical quality of the hematoxylin and eosin (H & E) staining were the principal reasons for incorrect diagnosis at the time of frozen section.

Table 4–1. Transsphenoidal Surgical Biopsies Analyzed by Intraoperative Frozen Sections at The University of Michigan Hospitals Between 1985 and 1989

Number of Cases	Interpretation of Biopsy at Frozen Section*	Final Diagnosis With Immunohistochemistry
42	Adenoma	Adenoma
2	Deferred diagnosis	Adenoma
1	Adenohypophysis	Hyperplasia
7	Normal pituitary	Adenoma
3	Neurohypophysis	Neurohypophysis
2	Inflammation	Abscess
1	Craniopharyngioma	Adenoma
1	Adenoma	Germinoma
5	Normal pituitary	Normal pituitary

*All results based on H & E staining at the time of frozen section.

To ensure the best results for intraoperative frozen section diagnosis, some recommendations would include the following:

1. Perform touch preparation for good cytological details and to preserve most tissues for other analyses.
2. When performing frozen section, be sure that the sample is adequate and representative of the lesion. Be sure that the technical aspects of cutting and staining are well controlled.
3. Clinicopathologic and radiologic correlations are essential, especially in difficult cases.
4. Inform the surgeon about the limitations of determining tumor margins on frozen sections.
5. Do not attempt to make a definitive diagnosis if there are technical problems with the preparation, inadequate samples for analysis or ambiguous staining results.

The accuracy of these procedures improves with the experience of the pathologists and the surgeons. Because of the above limitations, intraoperative frozen sections of pituitary lesions should be done only when they are absolutely necessary.

REFERENCES

1. Kovacs K, Horvath E. Tumors of the pituitary gland. In: Atlas of Tumor Pathology. Second Series. Fascicle 21. Washington, DC, Armed Forces Institute of Pathology, 1986, pp 51–56.
2. Scheithauer BW. The pituitary and sellar region. In: Sternberg SS (ed). Diagnostic Surgical Pathology. New York, Raven, 1989, pp 371–393.
3. Adams H, Graham DI, Doyle D. Brain Biopsy. The Smear Technic for Neurosurgical Biopsies. Philadelphia, JB Lippincott, 1981.
4. Marshall LF, Adams H, Doyle D, Graham DI. The histological accuracy of the smear technique for neurosurgical biopsies. J Neurosurg 39:82–88, 1973.
5. Martinez A-J, Moossy J. Cytological diagnosis of pituitary adenomas. J Neuropathol Exp Neurol 42:307–311, 1983.
6. Adelman LS, Post KD. Intra-operative frozen section technique for pituitary adenomas. Am J Surg Pathol 3:173–175, 1979.
7. Velasco ME, Sindely SO, Roessmann U. Reticulum stain for frozen-section diagnosis of pituitary adenomas. J Neurosurg 46:548–550, 1977.
8. McKeever PE, Laverson S, Oldfield EH, Smith BH, Gadille D, Chandler WF. Stromal and nuclear markers for rapid identification of pituitary adenomas at biopsy. Arch Pathol Lab Med 109:509–514, 1985.
9. Ludecke DK. Intraoperative measurement of adrenocorticotropic hormone in peripituitary blood in Cushing's disease. Neurosurgery 24:201–205, 1989.
10. Lang H-D, Saeger W, Ludecke DK, Muller D. Rapid frozen section diagnosis of pituitary tumors. Endocr Pathol 1:116–122, 1990.

5

NON-NEOPLASTIC PITUITARY LESIONS, INCLUDING HYPERPLASIA

RICARDO V. LLOYD

CONGENITAL DISORDERS

Pituitary Agenesis or Aplasia

Congenital absence of the anterior pituitary gland is a very rare condition, with only a few reported cases in the literature (1–3). This condition is usually associated with hypoplasia of the thyroid, gonads and adrenal glands. Most neonates with pituitary aplasia survive only for a few hours (1–5). Rare cases of pituitary agenesis have been reported in older children, but these cases may represent hypoplasia (4). In some cases, normal posterior pituitary gland tissue may be present (2), indicating that the posterior pituitary can develop independently of the anterior pituitary gland. It is often difficult to separate failure of tissue development from atrophy during late fetal life. During normal pituitary development, the primitive pharynx forms Rathke's pouch and joins the infundibular process from the floor of the diencephalon. The important process for normal pituitary development appears to be the fusion of Rathke's pouch with the infundibular process (6).

Pituitary Hypoplasia

Hypoplastic pituitary glands not associated with anencephaly have been reported in a few cases (7,8). Hypoplastic pituitaries are usually associated with hypoplastic adrenal gland tissues as well. Anencephaly is an uncommon congenital malformation of the brain in humans. This condition, which is more common in female infants, is associated with hypoplasia or absence of the calvaria. The infants may have a disorganized brain stem in the posterior fossa and some glial nodules. The sella turcica is frequently flat and is filled with spongy vascular tissue. The pituitary is hypoplastic and has decreased numbers of immunoreactive adrenocorticotropic hormone (ACTH) cells, while the other anterior pituitary gland cells are usually normal in number (9–12). Ultrastructural studies of the ACTH cells show degenerative changes. The infants usually die hours to days after birth. They have hypoplastic adrenal glands with small fetal adrenal cortical zones, while the thyroid and gonads are usually within normal limits.

Intrasellar Cysts

Various types of cysts can occur in the pituitary gland. Rathke's cleft cysts are probably the most common. These cysts arise from remnants of Rathke's pouch (13) and are present between the anterior and posterior lobes (Figs. 5–1 to 5–3). Small cysts are present in 20% to 50% of pituitaries (13–15). They are slow-growing lesions that may range up to 1 cm in diameter. The cysts are

25

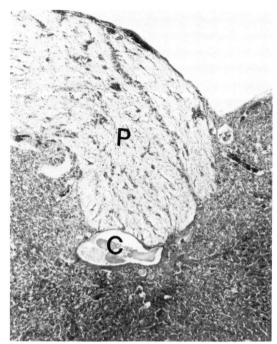

Figure 5–1. Rathke's cleft cyst (C) located between the anterior and posterior (P) lobes of the pituitary (× 150).

lined by columnar or cuboidal ciliated epithelium and may have goblet cells. Mucoid colloid material is often present in the lumen. Although they are usually asymptomatic, cysts that are 1 cm or larger may cause

symptoms and mimic pituitary adenomas. Compression of the pituitary stalk and secondary hyperprolactinemia may also develop. In Cornelia de Lange's syndrome, cysts of Rathke's pouch may lead to compression of the adenohypophysis and result in atrophy of the pituitary (15).

Persistence of the craniopharyngeal canal with lack of contact between Rathke's pouch and the infundibulum is usually not associated with any specific endocrinologic syndromes. However, the pituitary can be displaced and may protrude into the craniopharyngeal canal (16).

CIRCULATORY DISORDERS

Adenohypophysial Infarction and Necrosis

Pituitary infarction can be seen with various conditions associated with vascular occlusion or simply hypoperfusion, leading to ischemia and cell death. Small pituitary infarcts may be seen in up to 8% of cases at the time of autopsy. The adenohypophysis is very resistant to cell loss. Loss of fewer than 50% of the anterior lobe cells is usually asymptomatic and can be detected only by histological examination. With infarction and loss of 60% to 75% of anterior pituitary tissue, moderate

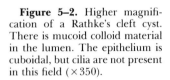

Figure 5–2. Higher magnification of a Rathke's cleft cyst. There is mucoid colloid material in the lumen. The epithelium is cuboidal, but cilia are not present in this field (× 350).

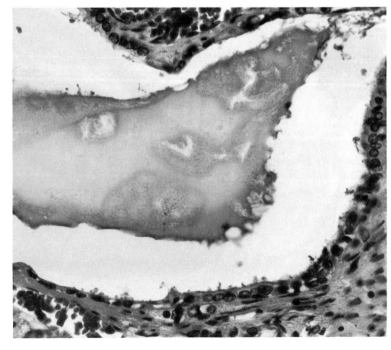

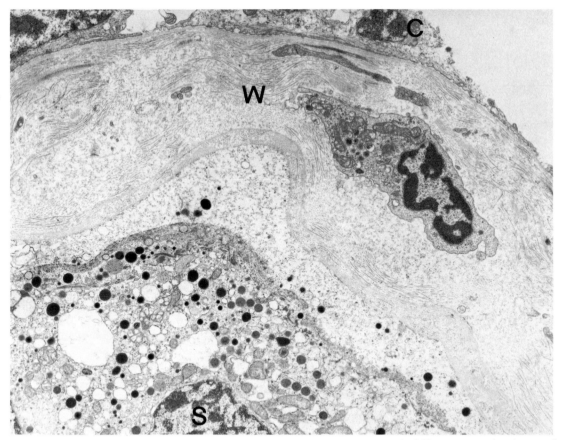

Figure 5–3. Ultrastructure of a Rathke's cleft cyst. The cyst wall (W) is composed of fibrous connective tissue and is lined by cuboidal cells (C). The underlying compressed adenohypophysis with a secretory cell (S) is also seen (×7000).

symptoms of hypopituitarism develop, while severe hypophysial insufficiency becomes apparent when a loss of more than 90% of hormone-producing cells occurs (15). Adenohypophysial infarction may occur with traumatic head injury, diabetes mellitus, acute cerebrovascular lesions, elevated intracranial pressure, epidemic hemorrhagic fever and sustained use of assisted ventilation with hypoperfusion of the central nervous system (20–25). Infarction of the anterior lobe can also occur with transection or other severe damage of the hypophysial stalk resulting in decreased perfusion of the anterior lobe.

Sheehan's syndrome is a special form of pituitary necrosis occurring in the postpartum period with massive adenohypophysial infarction resulting in permanent anterior pituitary hormone insufficiency (26). Vasospasm may be the initiating trigger of ischemia leading to infarction (26). Necrosis may be focal to very extensive, involving more

than 90% of the adenohypophysis. The posterior pituitary with its rich arterial blood supply, which is independent of the portal vasculature, is usually not severely affected (27), although necrotic foci may be present in the posterior pituitary and hypophysial stalk (27). During the process of healing, fibrosis with scar formation is present in the anterior pituitary, and the gland becomes atrophic with extensive loss of hormone-producing cells (28).

Hemorrhage in the pituitary may occur with traumatic head injury, with massive cerebrovascular accidents, with severe disseminated intravascular coagulation and in patients with marked thrombocytopenia. In some cases, adenomas have been associated with extensive hemorrhagic infarction; this is referred to as pituitary "apoplexy." Although pituitary apoplexy has been associated in many cases with growth hormone (GH)–producing adenomas (29), with dramatic improvement of the patient's symptoms after infarction of the adenoma, it is commonly associated with many large adenomas, including the frequently occurring null cell and oncocytic adenomas.

INFLAMMATORY LESIONS OF THE PITUITARY

Acute inflammation of the pituitary is uncommon. Patients who have septicemia may develop purulent hypophysitis, with development of an abscess leading to secondary loss of adenohypophysial cells. Pituitary cysts may be a predisposing factor for abscess development (30). Purulent inflammation in the anatomic structures adjacent to the pituitary, such as the sphenoid bone; osteomyelitis; sphenoid sinusitis; bacterial meningitis and purulent otitis media could lead to acute suppurative inflammation in the pituitary (15,30–32).

The pituitary gland may be involved by a variety of granulomatous processes, including sarcoidosis, fungal infections and tuberculosis (33,34). The histological appearance of the pituitary with multinucleated giant cells is similar to the changes seen in the lung and other tissues (Fig. 5–4). Culture, microbiological and/or immunohistochemical and other special stains can be used to characterize the infectious agent before initiating treatment. Syphilis (35) as well as tuberculosis involving the pituitary can lead to extensive destruction of the adenohypophysis and to hypopituitarism in some cases. Sarcoidosis involving the anterior and/or posterior pituitary is a diagnosis of exclusion. Sarcoidosis may also involve the hypothalamus, leading to pituitary insufficiency with destruction of the neurons producing various pituitary regulatory peptides. Sarcoidosis has been associated with amenorrhea, galactorrhea and hyperprolactinemia (15).

Giant cell granuloma is a rare idiopathic inflammatory disorder of the pituitary gland. It may be associated with similar findings in the adrenal cortex, gonads or thyroid. The adenohypophysis is usually the only organ involved with the non-caseating granulomas. Unlike sarcoidosis, this disorder is limited to the adenohypophysis and does not involve the neurohypophysis and hypothalamus (33,36). Necrosis is absent, and special stains for organisms are negative.

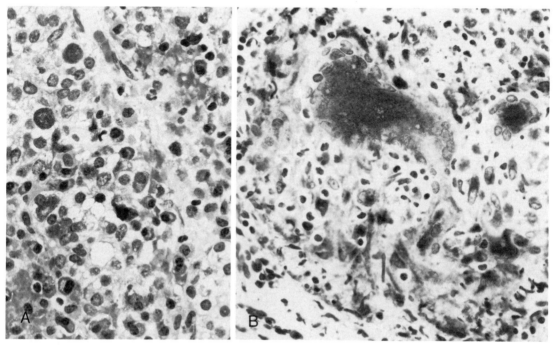

Figure 5–4. *A,* Mixed inflammatory infiltrate of lymphocytes and plasma cells is present in this pituitary biopsy specimen (×350). B, Adjacent areas showed a few multinucleated giant cells. Special stains and culture for organisms were negative. The multinucleated giant cells stained positively with monoclonal antibody KP1 (CD68) (×350).

Lymphocytic hypophysitis is an inflammatory disorder of the pituitary that has been recognized with increased frequency since the 1980s (37–42). The lesion, which affects mostly young women, often causes enlargement of the pituitary gland and may mimic a tumor. Most patients are pregnant or in the postpartum period at the onset. Antipituitary antibodies have been identified in some cases, supporting an autoimmune etiology. In some patients this condition may be associated with inflammatory disorders of the thyroid, adrenals and other endocrine tissues. Although most of the earlier cases were diagnosed at autopsy, many cases are now diagnosed by pituitary biopsy (37). Histological features include cellular infiltrates consisting mostly of lymphocytes with some plasma cells. Lymphoid follicles and germinal center formation may be present. Immunofluorescence studies have failed to show immune complex deposition (37).

In a survey of 18 cases by Meichner *et al.* (42), all patients were women from 22 to 74 years old. Thirty-seven percent had pre-existing endocrine disorders, and 22% of cases were associated with autoimmune-related conditions. All patients presented within 1 year post partum or during pregnancy except for a 59- and a 74-year-old woman who were diagnosed at autopsy. Treatment with immunosuppressive drugs directed at T-cell function to prevent endocrine failure after diagnosis has been proposed (42).

Pituitary autoantibodies have been detected by a variety of methods in such conditions as hypopituitarism, specific hormone deficiencies and empty sella syndrome and in adenomas (43,44). In a study of patients with the primary empty sella syndrome, antibodies against specific pituitary cell lines were present in 44% to 75% of patients, while only 10% to 14% of patients with various types of pituitary adenomas had antibodies. In this study, a small group of patients with systemic lupus erythematosus and autoimmune adrenal failure did not have anti-pituitary antibodies, although three of six patients with idiopathic diabetes insipidus had antibodies reacting with the pituitary cell lines used in the assay.

MISCELLANEOUS CONDITIONS

The morphology of the pituitary has been examined in patients with anorexia nervosa who died of complications of this disease (45). When the pituitaries of these patients were compared to those from patients who died of organic disease associated with inanition, there was relative hypogranulation of the ACTH and of the GH cells. Minimal hyperplasia of GH and/or gonadotroph cells was noted in some patients. However, there were no specific abnormalities present in the pituitaries of patients with anorexia nervosa, indicating that a primary pituitary abnormality was not present (45).

Studies of the pituitary gland of patients with the acquired immunodeficiency syndrome (AIDS) revealed acute necrotic foci in a few cases (4 of 49), while 12% of cases had infectious involvement (46). However, no significant changes in the anterior pituitary cells were found when compared to age-matched controls (46). Common infections involving the pituitary gland in AIDS patients included cytomegalovirus and *Pneumocystis carinii* infection and a possible case of *Toxoplasma gondii* infection. In all cases there was systemic involvement with these infectious agents.

A variety of substances deposited in the pituitary gland have been reported. Some of these have been associated with systemic disease or with pituitary neoplasms. Amyloid deposition has been reported in the pituitary with systemic disease and with pituitary adenomas (47–49). Prolactinomas have been the most common type of neoplasms associated with amyloid deposits. Some investigators have described two types of amyloid deposits in pituitary adenomas, but the significance of these subtypes is unknown. Patients who have hemosiderosis or hemochromatosis may have increased iron accumulation in the pituitary gland. Analysis of the individual cells with iron deposits reveals that gonadotrophs have the highest levels of iron deposition (15,50). Varying degrees of adenohypophysial fibrosis may develop with iron deposition and may be associated with pituitary insufficiency.

Calcification and calcium deposits may be present in the pituitary glands. Some adenoma subtypes, especially prolactinomas, are frequently associated with calcification including psammoma bodies (51). Macrophages or xanthomatous cells may accumulate in the pituitary gland in specific diseases such as histiocytosis X, leading to destruction of some pituitary cells and pituitary insufficiency (52). When the xanthoma cells are present in the neurohypophysis and hypothalamus, patients can develop diabetes insipidus.

The empty sellae syndrome results from a reduction in the volume of the contents of the sellae. This condition may be primary or secondary. The primary lesion is characterized by an incomplete or absent diaphragma sellae, which leads to increased cerebrospinal fluid pressure and compression of the sphenoid bone. There is subsequent enlargement of the hypophysial fossa with flattening and remodeling of the hypophysis. The sellae may be enlarged, and the pituitary becomes very compressed and flattened, appearing as a thin layer of tissue at the bottom of the hypophysial fossa. Immunohistochemical studies have shown that all adenohypophysial cells are present (53,54). Autopsy studies have found that about 50% of adults have a defect in the diaphragma sellae of 5 mm or more. In large autopsy series, about 5% of individuals have a primary empty sella (55). In the secondary empty sella syndrome, the pituitary gland is absent or very small; this occurs in conditions such as surgical hypophysectomy, infarction and necrosis of the pituitary with atrophy and fibrosis.

PITUITARY HYPERPLASIA

Hyperplasia of the adenohypophysis is an uncommon disorder. The diagnosis is often difficult to make on small biopsy specimens. Hyperplasia may be primary, idiopathic or secondary to neoplasms producing hypothalamic releasing hormone, hypothalamic hamartomas producing releasing hormones or end-organ failure (56–69).

Hyperplasia may be dispersed, nodular or diffuse (see also Chapter 7). The nodular form of hyperplasia is easiest to recognize histologically (Figs. 5–5 and 5–6). Special stains, including reticulin and immunohistochemical stains, are helpful in making the diagnosis. Reticulin stains often show expansion of the acini with retention of the acinar unit. Immunohistochemical stains reveal enlarged cells of a specific lineage admixed with other cell types. Difficulties in establishing the diagnosis of hyperplasia arise because of the variable distribution of different cell types in the anterior pituitary. For example, corticotroph cells are more numerous in the mucoid wedge, so small biopsies from this area may lead to an erroneous diagnosis of ACTH cell hyperplasia.

Although prolactin (PRL) cell hyperplasia can be readily induced by estrogens in some experimental animals such as rodents, there is no evidence that this can occur in the human pituitary gland. Interestingly, the human pituitary can increase in weight by more than 100% during pregnancy with hyperplasia of PRL cells, indicating that this gland is capable of proliferating in response to spe-

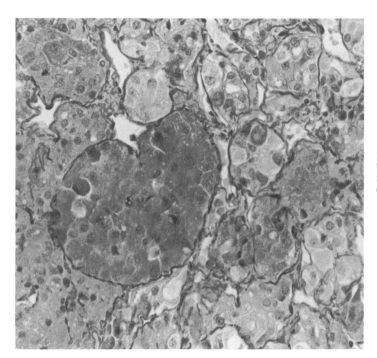

Figure 5–5. Corticotroph cell hyperplasia. The reticulin stain accentuates the hyperplastic nodule in this pituitary from a patient with Cushing's disease (×350).

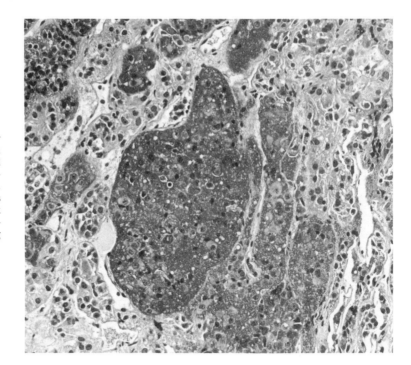

Figure 5–6. Staining for ACTH in the same patient as in Figure 5–5 with corticotroph-cell hyperplasia. Nodules of ACTH-positive cells are prominent. Some cells within the nodules were negative for ACTH but positive for GH and other hormones after immunostaining (×300).

cific stimuli (67). Hyperplasia of PRL cells is rare in humans (6), although increased numbers of PRL cells have been noted in the pituitary adjacent to PRL cell adenomas (68).

ACTH cell hyperplasia may be diffuse or nodular. In nodular hyperplasia, there is an increase in the size of acini and in the size of ACTH cells and distortion of the reticulin pattern (69). Diffuse hyperplasia is characterized by an increase in the number of ACTH cells, especially in the mucoid wedge, without significant distortion of the acinar pattern (70). The ACTH cells are increased in size and show Crooke's hyaline changes. Patients with Addison's disease can develop diffuse or nodular hyperplasia of ACTH-producing cells (69), and patients with chronic hypothyroidism can develop hyperplasia of thyroid-stimulating hormone (TSH)- and PRL-producing cells (66).

GH cell hyperplasia is commonly associated with ectopic growth hormone releasing hormone (GHRH) production (58,60–63). Histological features of GH cell hyperplasia include a distorted reticulin pattern with enlargement of the pituitary acini and increased numbers of immunoreactive GH cells. Bihormonal cells with GH and PRL may be present (70). Ultrastructural studies often show heavily granulated cells with large secretory granules; well-developed, rough endoplasmic reticulum and large Golgi complexes (70).

Hyperplasia of TSH cells may be nodular or diffuse. Nodular hyperplasia is characterized by expanded acini with enlarged TSH cells, which have weak immunoreactivity by immunostaining, suggesting minimal storage of TSH hormone. Diffuse hyperplasia is characterized by increased numbers of TSH cells with strong immunoreactivity for TSH and minimal attention of the acinar architecture. TSH microadenomas may be associated with both nodular and diffuse hyperplasia in patients with chronic hypothyroidism (72).

Hyperplasia of gonadotroph cells is very uncommon and has not been documented in surgically resected pituitaries. Chronic primary hypogonadism may lead to hyperplasia. Gonadotroph hyperplasia may be present in pituitary glands with PRL-producing adenomas (70).

Because of the difficulties involved in diagnosing pituitary hyperplasia, a great deal of caution must be used in making this diagnosis on small surgical biopsy specimens. When the entire pituitary is available for examination in autopsy cases, the diagnosis of hyperplasia can be made with more confidence after immunohistochemical staining and quantitation of the various cell types.

REFERENCES

1. Blizzard RM, Alberts M. Hypopituitarism, hypoadrenalism and hypogonadism in the newborn infant. J Pediatr *48:*782–792, 1956.
2. Brewer D. Congenital absence of the pituitary gland and its consequences. J Pathol Bacteriol *73:*59–67, 1957.
3. Reid JD. Congenital absence of the pituitary gland. J Pediatr *56:*658–664, 1960.
4. Steiner MM, Boggs JD. Absence of pituitary gland, hypothyroidism, hypoadrenalism and hypogonadism in a 17-year-old dwarf. J Clin Endocrinol Metab *25:*1591–1598, 1965.
5. Moncrieff MW, Hill DS, Archer J, Arthur LJ. Congenital absence of pituitary gland and adrenal hypoplasia. Arch Dis Child *47:*136–137, 1972.
6. Gilbert MS. Some factors influencing the early development of mammalian hypophysis. Anat Rec *62:*337–360, 1935.
7. Mosier HD. Hypoplasia of the pituitary and adrenal cortex. J Pediatr *48:*633–639, 1956.
8. Ehrlich RM. Ectopic and hypoplastic pituitary with adrenal hypoplasia; case report. J Pediatr *51:*377–384, 1957.
9. Osamura RY, Watanabe K. Histogenesis of the cells of the anterior and intermediate lobes of human pituitary glands: Immunohistochemical studies. Int Rev Cytol *95:*103–129, 1985.
10. Osamura RY. Functional prenatal development of anencephalic and normal anterior pituitary glands. I. Human and experimental animals studied by peroxidase-labeled antibody method. Acta Pathol Jpn *27:*495–509, 1977.
11. Hatakeyama S. Electron microscopic study of the anencephalic adenohypophysis with reference to the adrenocorticotrophs and their correlation with the functional differentiation of the hypothalamus during the foetal life. Endocrinol Jpn *16:*187–203, 1969.
12. Salazar H, MacAulay MA, Charles D, Pardo M. The human hypophysis in anencephaly. I. Ultrastructure of the pars distalis. Arch Pathol *87:*201–211, 1969.
13. Steinberg GK, Koenig GH, Golden JB. Symptomatic Rathke's cleft cysts: A report of two cases. J Neurosurg *56:*290–295, 1982.
14. Weber EL, Vogel FS, Odom GL. Cysts of the sella turcica. J Neurosurg *33:*48–53, 1970.
15. Horvath E, Kovacs K. Pathology of the pituitary gland. In: Ezrin C, Horvath E, Kaufman B, Kovacs K, Weiss MH (eds). Pituitary Diseases. Boca Raton, FL, CRC Press, 1980, p 1–83.
16. Warner NE. Pituitary gland. In: Anderson WAD, Kissane JM (eds). Pathology. Vol 2. 7th Ed. St Louis, CV Mosby, 1977, p 1601.
17. Plaut A. Pituitary necrosis in routine necropsies. Am J Pathol *28:*883–900, 1952.
18. Kovacs K. Necrosis of anterior pituitary in humans. Neuroendocrinology *4:*170–199, 1969.
19. Kovacs K. Adenohypophysial necrosis in routine autopsies. Endokrinologie *60:*309–316, 1972.
20. Sheehan HL, Davis JC. Pituitary necrosis. Br Med Bull *24:*59–70, 1968.
21. Wolman L. Pituitary necrosis in raised intracranial pressure. J Pathol Bacteriol *72:*575–586, 1956.
22. McCormick WF, Halmi NS. The hypophysis in patients with coma depasse ("respirator brain"). Am J Clin Pathol *54:*374–383, 1970.
23. Daniel PN, Spicer EJ, Treip CS. Pituitary necrosis in patients maintained on mechanical respirators. J Pathol *111:*135–138, 1973.
24. Kovacs K, Bilbao JM. Adenohypophysial necrosis in respirator-maintained patients. Pathol Microbiol *41:*275–282, 1974.
25. Towbin A. The respirator brain death syndrome. Hum Pathol *4:*583–594, 1973.
26. Sheehan HL, Stanfield JP. The pathogenesis of post-partum necrosis of the anterior lobe of the pituitary gland. Acta Endocrinol (Copenh) *37:*479–510, 1961.
27. Sheehan HL, Whitehead R. The neurohypophysis in post-partum hypopituitarism. J Pathol Bacteriol *85:*145–169, 1963.
28. Sheehan HL. The repair of post-partum necrosis of the anterior lobe of the pituitary gland. Acta Endocrinol (Copenh) *48:*40–60, 1965.
29. Rovit RL, Fein JM. Pituitary apoplexy: A review and reappraisal. J Neurosurg *37:*280–288, 1972.
30. Obenchain TG, Becker DP. Abscess formation in a Rathke's cleft cyst. Case report. J Neurosurg *36:*359–362, 1972.
31. Lindholm J, Rasmussen P, Korsgaard O. Intrasellar or pituitary abscess. J Neurosurg *38:*616–619, 1973.
32. Domingue JN, Wilson CB. Pituitary abscesses. Report of seven cases and review of the literature. J Neurosurg *46:*601–608, 1977.
33. Rickards AG, Harvey PW. "Giant cell granuloma" and the other pituitary granulomata. Q J Med *47:*425–440, 1954.
34. Vesely DL, Maldonodo A, Levey GS. Partial hypopituitarism and possible hypothalamic involvement in sarcoidosis: Report of a case and review of the literature. Am J Med *62:*425–431, 1977.
35. Oelbaum MH. Hypopituitarism in male subjects due to syphilis. Q J Med *45:*249–266, 1952.
36. Doniach I. Histopathology of the pituitary. Clin Endocrinol Metab *14:*765–789, 1985.
37. Asa SL, Bilbao JM, Kovacs K, Josse RG, Kreines K. Lymphocytic hypophysitis of pregnancy resulting in hypopituitarism: A distinct clinicopathologic entity. Ann Intern Med *95:*166–171, 1981.
38. Jensen MD, Handwerger BS, Scheithauer BW, Carpenter PC, Mirakian R, Banks PM. Lymphocytic hypophysitis with isolated corticotropin deficiency. Ann Intern Med *105:*200–203, 1986.
39. Portocarrero CJ, Robinson AG, Taylor AL, Klein I. Lymphoid hypophysitis: An unusual cause of hyperprolactinemia and enlarged sella turcica. JAMA *246:*1811–1812, 1981.
40. Sobrinho-Simoes M, Brandao A, Paiva ME, Vilela B, Fernandes E, Carneiro-Chaves F. Lymphoid hypophysitis in a patient with lymphoid thyroiditis, lymphoid adrenalitis and idiopathic retroperitoneal fibrosis. Arch Pathol Lab Med *109:*230–233, 1985.
41. Mayfield RK, Levine JH, Gordon L, Powers J, Galbraith RM, Rawe SE. Lymphoid adenohypophysitis presenting as a pituitary tumor. Am J Med *69:*619–623, 1980.
42. Meichner RH, Riggio S, Manz HJ, Earll JM. Lymphocytic adenohypophysitis causing pituitary mass. Neurology *37:*158–161, 1987.
43. Pouplard A. Pituitary autoimmunity. Horm Res *16:*289–297, 1982.
44. Komatsu M, Kondo T, Yamauchi K, Yokokawa N, Ichikawa K, Ishihara M, Aizawa T, Yamada T, Imai Y, Tanaka K, Taniguchi K, Watanabe T, Takahashi Y. Antipituitary antibodies in patients with primary empty sella syndrome. J Clin Endocrinol Metab *67:*633–638, 1988.

45. Scheithauer BW, Kovacs KT, Jariwala LK, Randall RV, Ryan N. Anorexia nervosa: An immunohistochemical study of the pituitary gland. Mayo Clin Proc *63*:23–28, 1988.

46. Sano T, Kovacs K, Scheithauer BW, Rosenblum MK, Petito CK, Greco CM. Pituitary pathology in acquired immunodeficiency syndrome. Arch Pathol Lab Med *113*:1066–1070, 1989.

47. Bilbao JM, Horvath E, Hudson AR, Kovacs K. Pituitary adenoma producing amyloid-like substance. Arch Pathol *99*:411–415, 1975.

48. Bilbao J, Kovacs K, Horvath E, Higgins HP, Horsey WJ. Pituitary melanocorticotrophinoma with amyloid deposition. Can J Neurol Sci *2*:199–202, 1975.

49. Landolt AM, Kleihues P, Heitz PU. Amyloid deposits in pituitary adenomas. Differentiation of two types. Arch Pathol Lab Med *111*:453–458, 1987.

50. Bergeron C, Kovacs K. Pituitary siderosis. A histologic, immunocytologic and ultrastructural study. Am J Pathol *93*:295–309, 1978.

51. Zahra M, Sengupta RP. An unusual case of chromophobe adenoma with conspicuous calcifications. Acta Neurochir *38*:279–283, 1977.

52. Ezrin C, Chaikoff R, Hoffman H. Panhypopituitarism caused by Hand-Schuller-Christian disease. Can Med Assoc J *89*:1290–1293, 1963.

53. Bergeron C, Kovacs K, Bilbao JM. Primary "empty sella." A histologic and immunocytologic study. Arch Intern Med *139*:248–249, 1979.

54. Domingue JN, Wing SD, Wilson CB. Coexisting pituitary adenomas and partially empty sellas. J Neurosurg *48*:23–28, 1978.

55. Bergland RM, Ray BS, Torack RM. Anatomical variations in the pituitary gland and adjacent structures in 225 human autopsy cases. J Neurosurg *28*:93–99, 1968.

56. Asa SL, Penz G, Kovacs K, Ezrin C. Prolactin cells in the human pituitary. A quantitative immunocytochemical analysis. Arch Pathol Lab Med *106*:360–363, 1982.

57. Asa SL, Kovacs K, Tindall GT, Barrow DL, Horvath E, Vecsei P. Cushing's disease associated with an intrasellar gangliocytoma producing corticotrophin-releasing factor. Ann Intern Med *101*:789–793, 1984.

58. Asa SL, Scheithauer BW, Bilbao JM, Horvath E, Ryan N, Kovacs K. A case for hypothalamic acromegaly: A clinicopathological study of six patients with hypothalamic gangliocytomas producing growth hormone-releasing factor. J Clin Endocrinol Metab *58*:796–803, 1984.

59. Judge DM, Kulin HE, Page R, Santen R, Trapukdi S. Hypothalamic hamartoma: A source of luteinizing hormone-releasing factor in precocious puberty. N Engl J Med *296*:7–10, 1977.

60. Scheithauer BW, Kovacs K, Randall RV, Horvath E, Okazaki H, Laws ER Jr. Hypothalamic neuronal hamartoma and adenohypophyseal neuronal chor-

61. Garcia-Luna PP, Leal-Cerro A, Montero C, Scheithauer BW, Campanario A, Dieguez C, Astorga R, Kovacs K. A rare cause of acromegaly: Ectopic production of growth hormone-releasing factor by a bronchial carcinoid tumor. Surg Neurol *27*:563–568, 1987.

62. Scheithauer BW, Carpenter PC, Bloch B, Brazeau P. Ectopic secretion of a growth hormone-releasing factor: Report of a case of acromegaly with bronchial carcinoid tumor. Am J Med *76*:605–616, 1984.

63. Thorner MO, Perryman RL, Cronin MJ, Rogol AD, Draznin M, Johanson A, Vale W, Horvath E, Kovacs K. Somatotroph hyperplasia: Successful treatment of acromegaly by removal of the pancreatic islet tumor secreting a growth hormone-releasing factor. J Clin Invest *70*:965–977, 1982.

64. Lloyd RV, Chandler WF, McKeever PE, Schteingart DE. The spectrum of ACTH-producing pituitary lesions. Am J Surg Pathol *10*(9):618–626, 1986.

65. Thorner MO, Perryman RL, Cronin MJ, Rogol AD, Draznin M, Johanson A, Vale W, Horvath E, Kovacs K. Somatotroph hyperplasia. Successful treatment of acromegaly by removal of a pancreatic islet tumor secreting a growth hormone-releasing factor. J Clin Invest *70*:965–977, 1982.

66. Pioro EP, Scheithauer BW, Laws ER Jr, Randall RV, Kovacs K, Horvath E. Combined thyrotroph and lactotroph cell hyperplasia simulating prolactin-secreting pituitary adenoma in long-standing primary hypothyroidism. Surg Neurol *29*:218–226, 1988.

67. Kovacs K, Ilse G, Ryan N, McComb DJ, Horvath E, Chen HJ, Walfish PG. Pituitary prolactin cell hyperplasia. Horm Res *12*:87–95, 1980.

68. Saeger W, Ludecke DK. Pituitary hyperplasia. Definition, light and electron microscopic structures and significance in surgical specimens. Virchows Arch Pathol Anat *399*:277–287, 1983.

69. McKeever PE, Koppelman MC, Metcalf D, Quindlen E, Kornblith PL, Strott CA, Howard R, Smith BH. Refractory Cushing's disease caused by multinodular ACTH-cell hyperplasia. J Neuropathol Exper Neurol *41*:490–499, 1982.

70. Scheithauer BW, Kovacs K, Randall RV. The pituitary gland in untreated Addison's disease. A histologic and immunocytologic study of 18 adenohypophyses. Arch Pathol Lab Med *107*:484–487, 1983.

71. Horvath E, Kovacs K. The adenohypophysis. In: Kovacs K, Asa SL (eds). Functional Endocrine Pathology. Boston, Blackwell Scientific Publications, 1991, pp 245–281.

72. Scheithauer BW, Kovacs K, Randall RV, Ryan N. Pituitary gland in hypothyroidism. Histologic and immunocytologic study. Arch Pathol Lab Med *109*:499–504, 1985.

6

LIGHT MICROSCOPIC SPECIAL STAINS AND IMMUNOCHEMISTRY IN THE DIAGNOSIS OF PITUITARY ADENOMAS

Lucia Stefaneanu
Kalman Kovacs

The pituitary gland, a main conductor of the endocrine orchestra, has a rather complicated structure and possesses many important functions that affect practically the entire body. Diseases of the pituitary are diverse, and some of them exert a major impact on the patient's health. In this chapter, only adenomas of the pituitary will be dealt with; other diseases, such as ischemic or inflammatory conditions or additional tumors, are beyond the scope of this review.

Pituitary adenomas are benign, epithelial neoplasms originating in and consisting of adenohypophysial cells. They are common, representing approximately 10% of all intracranial neoplasms. At unselected adult autopsies, pituitary adenomas are found in approximately 6% to 22% of cases, depending on how many sections have been examined. Pituitary adenomas may cause endocrine and local symptoms and may lead to elevation of pituitary hormone levels and target gland hormone levels in the blood. Local symptoms include visual disturbances, cranial nerve palsies, headache, nausea and other complications of increased intracranial pressure. Pituitary adenomas either grow expansively or invade adjacent structures. In the former

case, the tumors are usually small, well demarcated and restricted to the pituitary or the sella turcica. Invasive adenomas usually have a more rapid growth rate, spreading into neighboring tissues such as the sphenoid sinus, the optic nerve, the cavernous sinus or, in some cases, the brain. Endocrine symptoms include acromegaly or gigantism resulting from growth hormone excess, the amenorrhea-galactorrhea syndrome, infertility, decreased libido and impotence secondary to prolactin (PRL) hypersecretion, Cushing's disease due to increased adrenocorticotropic hormone (ACTH) release and, rarely, hyperthyroidism as a result of thyroid-stimulating hormone (TSH) overproduction. Excessive secretion of follicle-stimulating hormone (FSH) and/or luteinizing hormone (LH) usually is unassociated with significant clinical symptoms. Oversecretion of the α subunit of the glycoprotein hormones causes no endocrine abnormalities. It should be mentioned here that pituitary adenomas, by destroying the hormone-secreting cells of the nontumorous adenohypophysis or by interfering with the synthesis, discharge and adenohypophysial transport of the hypothalamic regulating hormones, can lead to various degrees of hypopituitarism from mild hypofunction of one hormone to severe panhypopituitarism. Hyperprolactinemia may also occur due to the decreased delivery of dopamine to pituitary PRL cells.

Numerous attempts have been made to classify pituitary adenomas and separate them into distinct clinical or pathologic entities. Pathologically, a previously widely used classification divided pituitary adenomas on the basis of tinctorial characteristics of the cell cytoplasm. This classification, which was applied for a long period of time, divided pituitary adenomas into acidophilic (or eosinophilic), basophilic or chromophobic tumors. Acidophilic adenomas, often accompanied by acromegaly or gigantism, were assumed to secrete growth hormone (GH); basophilic adenomas were claimed to produce ACTH and cause Cushing's disease; chromophobic adenomas were thought to have no hormonal function and were regarded as endocrinologically inactive tumors.

As many cases accumulated and clinicopathologic comparisons were made, it became apparent that this classification had outlived its usefulness. Pathologists and endocrinologists realized that classifications based on the staining affinity of the cell cytoplasm did not permit correlations between structural features and endocrine activity. It became clear that acidophilic adenomas, in some cases, produced no GH but did produce PRL, or they were unaccompanied by endocrine hyperfunction. Some basophilic adenomas failed to cause ACTH excess and were unassociated with Cushing's disease. The study of many cases clearly indicated that chromophobic adenomas contained secretory granules and possessed all the necessary cytoplasmic constituents needed for hormone secretion. Indeed, it became evident that many chromophobic adenomas produced various hormones in excess and resulted in the development of clinical symptoms and biochemical abnormalities secondary to hormone oversecretion.

Unprecedented progress has been achieved with the introduction of several novel morphological and biochemical techniques. From the pathologist's point of view, the most important methods are transmission electron microscopy and immunocytochemistry. Ultrastructural investigation of pituitary adenomas enables the visualization of subcellular features of the cells and helps obtain a deeper insight into the secretory process. Immunocytochemistry has achieved specific, sensitive, reliable and reproducible localization of hormones and other cellular products in the cell cytoplasm. Based primarily on transmission electron microscopy and immunocytochemistry, a new pituitary adenoma classification has been developed that separates pituitary adenoma types on the basis of fine structural features, hormone content, cellular composition, differentiation and origin (1). This new classification has been adopted by many laboratories. The various tumor types and their frequency are shown in Table 6–1.

In this chapter, we will review the application of histological stains and immunocytochemical methods used in the diagnosis and classification of pituitary adenomas. It is our view that detailed immunocytochemical investigation should be carried out in every case of surgically removed pituitary adenoma. Immunocytochemical examination of autopsy-obtained pituitary adenomas also provides very valuable information. It is well known that pituitary adenomas obtained at autopsy are suitable for immunocytochemical investigation.

In past decades, a very large number of antibodies have been produced. Specific antibodies, raised against all known pituitary hormones, are commercially available. The testing of the surgically removed adenomas for GH, PRL, ACTH, TSH, FSH, LH and α subunit is mandatory. Numerous other antibodies have been raised; some are essential,

Table 6–1. Frequency of Adenoma Types in Unselected Surgical Material of 1043 Biopsies

Cell Type	%
GH cell adenoma	
Densely granulated	6.7
Sparsely granulated	7.3
PRL cell adenoma	
Densely granulated	0.6
Sparsely granulated	26.7
Mixed GH cell–PRL cell adenoma	4.8
Acidophil stem cell adenoma	2.2
Mammosomatotroph adenoma	1.5
Corticotroph cell adenoma	8.0
Silent ("corticotroph") adenoma	5.9
TSH cell adenoma	1.0
Gonadotroph cell adenoma	6.4
Null cell adenoma	
Non-oncocytic	16.3
Oncocytic	9.0
Plurihormonal adenoma	3.7

whereas many others are not useful in pituitary-related studies. In previous reviews, the immunocytochemical approach to pituitary tumors was discussed according to the various tumor types and the immunocytochemical profile of various adenoma types has been described. In this chapter we will follow a different approach. We will deal with individual antibodies and their value to the surgical pathology of pituitary adenomas. This approach has the advantage that pathologists can decide which antibodies they wish to use in pituitary studies.

HISTOLOGICAL STAINS

Pituitary adenomas exhibit different growth patterns, including diffuse, papillary and sinusoidal types, that are unrelated to their hormone production and biological behavior (1–4). Silver stains for the demonstration of reticulin fibers are often useful in distinguishing among normal adenohypophysis, hyperplasia and adenoma. In many cases, the reticulin fibers form a pseudocapsule at the border of the adenoma due to the compression of surrounding tissue. In adenomas, the regular fiber network that delineates acinar structures in the normal gland is missing or is disrupted and irregular (Fig. 6–1), whereas

in hyperplasia the acinar structures are maintained but enlarged, and the reticulin fiber network is slightly distorted (Fig. 6–2).

Conventional histological stainings differentiate acidophilic, basophilic and chromophobic adenomas, but such tinctorial affinities do not provide information about cellular derivation and hormone content. The hematoxylin and eosin (H & E), hematoxylin-phloxine (HP) or hematoxylin-phloxine-saffron (HPS) and periodic acid–Schiff (PAS) methods are useful for routine histological examination of pituitary lesions. They should be used in every case to ensure histological diagnosis. The capricious trichrome stains have been abandoned, since they have no value in pituitary adenoma diagnosis. It should be stressed that tinctorial properties of pituitary tumors, depending on fixation, processing and staining variant used, can give misleading results.

Acidophilic adenomas, previously associated exclusively with GH overproduction and acromegaly or gigantism, can produce GH or PRL or may lack hormones (1,5,6). Acidophilic adenomas producing GH and composed of densely granulated GH cells are intensely stained with acidic dyes, such as eosin, phloxine or orange G. Strongly eosinophilic adenomas, composed of densely granulated PRL cells, are rare; they often

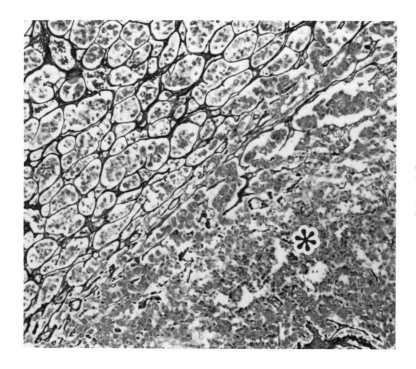

Figure 6–1. Pituitary adenoma (*asterisk*) shows disruption of reticulin fiber network that surrounds acinar structures in the normal gland. Gordon-Sweet technique (× 100).

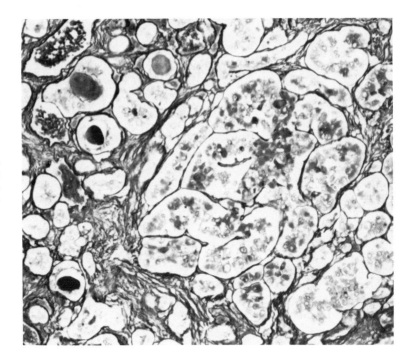

Figure 6–2. Reticulin stain demonstrates enlarged acini in a hyperplastic area of the pituitary. Gordon-Sweet technique (×100).

stain positively with Herlant's erythrosin or Brooke's carmoisin method. Mixed GH cell–PRL cell adenomas may be acidophilic or partly acidophilic depending on the granularity of the composing cells. Mammosomatotroph adenomas exhibit strong or moderate acidophilia with HE or HPS, but are negative with Brooke's carmoisin method. Acidic dyes also stain some adenomas composed of oncocytes, because mitochondria take up the dyes. Pituitary tumors contain smaller oncocytes when compared with those arising in the thyroid, parathyroid or salivary glands and are characterized by abundance of enlarged mitochondria. Oncocytic transformation can occur in some cells of other pituitary adenoma types and can prevail in acidophil stem cell tumors.

Pituitary adenomas that derive from corticotrophs and glycoprotein- (TSH-, FSH-, LH-) producing cells stain with PAS and lead hematoxylin. The most reliable way to diagnose corticotroph adenomas at the light microscopic level is the PAS method (1). The strong PAS affinity of corticotrophs is due to the carbohydrate moiety present in the pro-opiomelanocortin (POMC) molecule—the precursor of ACTH and other POMC-related peptides (7). Rarely, corticotroph adenomas contain cells with a few secretory granules, and consequently, a few or no PAS- or lead hematoxylin–positive granules. Among silent corticotroph adenomas, the subtype 1 variant cannot be distinguished from the functioning variant based on histological stainings or other morphological criteria. The silent subtype 2 adenoma shows moderate or slight PAS and lead hematoxylin staining. The silent subtype 3 adenoma, considered an independent entity with unknown cell type derivation, may contain very fine PAS-positive granules.

Adenomas originating in thyrotrophs are chromophobic by H & E and may contain a varying number of PAS- or aldehyde thionin–positive granules. Gonadotroph adenomas may contain very fine PAS-positive granules, often visible only with an oil immersion objective.

Chromophobic adenomas represent both functioning and endocrine-inactive tumors originating in any adenohypophysial cell type, or they may consist of undifferentiated cells or oncocytes. Chromophobic GH cell adenomas contain a varying number of slightly acidophilic cells and frequently a globular body, the so-called "fibrous body" in the concavity of nuclei. They are recognized as unstained images with H & E or HPS and have diagnostic significance. Chromophobic PRL cell adenomas may contain fine acidophilic granules by H & E and HPS. The rare secretory granules in some tumors may stain bright red with Herlant's erythrosin or

Brooke's carmoisin method. Chromophobic adenomas composed of other cell types, such as acidophilic stem cells, oncocytes or unclassified cell types, are encountered as well.

Calcifications are fairly common in PRL-producing adenomas and occur occasionally in other types of pituitary adenomas.

Endocrine amyloid deposits are reported to be present in 5% of PRL cell adenomas (1) and in 74% to 79% of GH cell and PRL cell adenomas (8,9). Amyloid can be stained with Congo red and is birefringent under Polaroid light.

IMMUNOCYTOCHEMISTRY

Hormonal Markers

Immunocytochemical methods specifically demonstrate the hormonal content of pituitary cells and their adenomas. As soon as immunocytochemistry for all adenohypophysial hormones was applied to a large number of pituitary adenomas, it became evident that the majority of adenomas produce one or more hormones. The percentage of completely immunonegative tumors is relatively low. Clinically, adenomas immunoreactive for one or more hormones can be endocrine active due to hormone overproduction or "silent" when, despite their hormone content, the blood hormone levels remain within the normal range.

Based on immunocytochemistry results, the cellular derivation of pituitary adenomas cannot be reliably established. The correct morphological diagnosis of pituitary adenomas relies on histological, immunocytochemical and ultrastructural correlations. At the ultrastructural level, monomorphous and plurimorphous (mixed) adenomas are evident. By correlating immunocytochemical and electron microscopy results, it was found that a monomorphous adenoma can produce one or more hormones. Plurimorphous adenomas are composed of two or more cell types, each having the capability to produce one or more hormones. Thus, for example, an adenoma immunoreactive for GH and PRL can be a mixed tumor composed of GH cells and PRL cells or GH cells and mammosomatotrophs—bihormonal cells producing both GH and PRL; it can represent a monomorphous adenoma composed of bihormonal acidophil stem cells or mammoso-

matotrophs. Clinically, in all cases, endocrine symptoms can be encountered due to overproduction of one or both hormones.

GH-immunoreactive Adenomas. Before the immunocytochemistry era, it was assumed that acidophilic tumors were accompanied by acromegaly or gigantism due to GH overproduction and were composed of GH cells (somatotrophs). Besides acidophilic adenomas causing acromegaly, chromophobic tumors capable of GH secretion were added as a result of correlative immunocytochemical, ultrastructural and clinical studies. Moreover, electron microscopy proved that GH-producing adenomas are a heterogeneous group and include monomorphous and plurimorphous tumors (1,6).

About one third of acromegalic patients have an acidophilic adenoma with a diffuse, trabecular or sinusoidal pattern. The GH immunoreactivity is strong all over the cytoplasm of adenoma cells owing to the abundance of secretory granules (Fig. 6–3). Ultrastructurally, the acidophilic adenoma corresponds to a densely granulated GH cell adenoma (1,6). Most such adenomas contain a variable percentage of cells immunoreactive for PRL as well; these represent mammosomatotrophs. They can release enough PRL to cause mild hyperprolactinemia (10–12). Many densely granulated GH cell adenomas (57%) express α subunit (α-SU) immunoreactivity of glycoprotein hormones, and a few of them express TSH as well. Usually, TSH production does not result in hyperthyroidism (13).

With approximately the same frequency, acromegaly is caused by chromophobic adenomas, exhibiting a rather scanty immunopositivity for GH in the cytoplasm of adenoma cells (Fig. 6–4); the immunoreactivity pattern differs from that in acidophilic tumors, being localized predominantly in the Golgi area or around the negative image of the fibrous body. Occasionally, scattered cells immunoreactive for PRL are noted. By electron microscopy, they correspond to sparsely granulated GH cell adenomas (1,6). Rarely, this type of adenoma is "silent"—i.e., unaccompanied by acromegaly—and the blood GH level is normal (14).

Rarely, acromegaly can be caused by a strongly or a moderately acidophilic adenoma that shows intense GH immunoreactivity and usually a less intense or even negative PRL immunopositivity. These tumors resem-

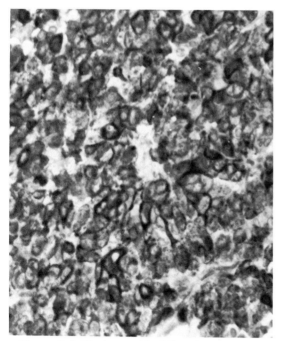

Figure 6–3. Pituitary acidophilic adenoma exhibits strong immunoreactivity for GH in most cells. Ultrastructurally, this tumor was composed of densely granulated GH cells (×250).

ble acidophilic, densely granulated GH cell adenomas, and only by electron microscopy can they be diagnosed as densely granulated mammosomatotroph adenomas (1,15).

Infrequently, acromegaly can be produced by a chromophobic or acidophilic adenoma that is immunoreactive for both GH and PRL. Usually, PRL immunopositivity prevails over that of GH. The serum GH level is slightly elevated or normal. Ultrastructurally, the acidophil stem cell adenoma is diagnosed (1,16). At the light microscopic level, it is difficult to distinguish it from PRL cell adenoma.

Approximately one third of adenomas with GH overproduction are bimorphous tumors composed of two cell populations that are immunoreactive for GH and PRL, respectively. The pattern of immunoreactivity corresponds to the proportion and distribution of the two cell types that can be acidophilic or chromophobic by conventional stainings and sparsely or densely granulated GH cells and sparsely granulated PRL cells by electron microscopy (1,17). Some cells can be bihormonal mammosomatotrophs. At the light microscopic level, bihormonal mammosomato-

trophs are demonstrated on serial mirror sections consecutively immunostained for GH and PRL; their presence is shown more reliably by electron microscopy using the immunogold technique.

Acromegaly can develop in patients with thyrotroph adenomas that coproduce GH in addition to TSH (18). GH-immunoreactive cells can occur in association with other hormones in monomorphous or mixed plurihormonal adenomas.

PRL-immunoreactive Adenomas. The majority of PRL-producing pituitary adenomas are chromophobic, monomorphous adenomas. Sometimes a few acidophilic granules or a slight basophilia—probably due to extensive rough endoplasmic reticulum rich in RNA content—is evident. In small adenomas found incidentally at autopsy, the papillary pattern predominates, whereas in surgical biopsy specimens, the diffuse disposition is frequently seen (1,13,19). By immunocytochemistry, most adenoma cells show a typical globular PRL positivity in the Golgi area (Fig. 6–5). Rarely, α-SU immunoreactivity is seen as well (20). Ultrastructurally, this type of PRL adenoma is composed of sparsely granulated PRL cells.

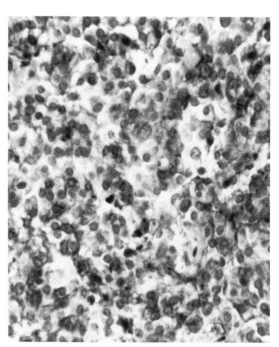

Figure 6–4. Pituitary adenoma belonging to a sparsely granulated GH cell type shows a moderate to weak immunoreactivity for GH (×250).

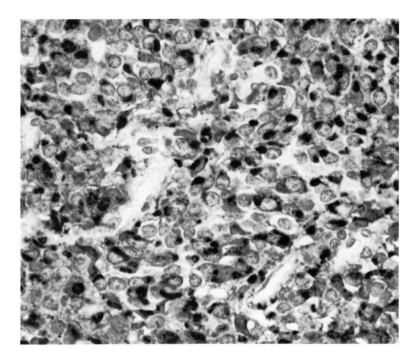

Figure 6–5. Sparsely granulated PRL cell adenoma immunostained for PRL contains characteristic globular immunoreactivity in the Golgi area (×400).

Strongly acidophilic adenomas with a diffuse PRL immunoreactivity over all the cytoplasm and corresponding to densely granulated PRL cell adenomas are rare (1,13,19).

In many patients, dopamine agonist therapy results in reduction of serum PRL to normal levels and in tumor shrinkage (21,22). By light microscopy, the responsive adenoma cells become extremely closely apposed owing to the strong decrease in their cytoplasm. The nuclei are heterochromatic. Extensive perivascular and interstitial fibrosis is often present (23–25). Immunocytochemistry indicates a low level or lack of PRL in these markedly suppressed cells (Fig. 6–6). In some adenomas the response is not as intense, or populations of markedly suppressed cells alternate with groups of large cells with euchromatic nuclei and characteristic PRL immunopositivity in the Golgi area. Such a pattern can also be seen in adenomas from patients in whom bromocriptine therapy was interrupted at least 2 months before surgery, indicating the persistence of inhibited cells (26).

About 10% of surgically removed pituitary adenomas produce both PRL and GH. The two hormones can be localized in the same cell in monomorphous adenomas such as mammosomatotroph and acidophil stem cell adenomas, or in two distinct cells in mixed PRL cell–GH cell adenomas. The mammo-

somatotroph adenomas are associated with mild hyperprolactinemia, whereas acidophil stem cell adenomas produce predominantly PRL. Since most of these tumors produce GH as well and are also accompanied by acromegaly, their immunocytochemistry has been described under GH-immunoreactive adenomas.

PRL-immunoreactive cells are found in association with other hormones in some plurihormonal adenomas and are rarely associated with elevated PRL blood levels. Such adenomas are discussed separately.

ACTH-immunoreactive Adenomas. Most of the pituitary adenomas secreting ACTH and associated with Cushing's disease are small, basophilic tumors with a sinusoidal disposition (1,4,27,28). The cytoplasm of adenoma cells shows a diffuse or peripheral immunoreactivity for ACTH, β-lipotropin and β-endorphin derived from the same precursor molecule, proopiomelanocortin (POMC). In some adenomas, ACTH immunoreactivity is almost negative, while β-endorphin is intensely positive (Fig. 6–7). Ultrastructurally, they are composed of densely granulated corticotrophs. A few adenomas exhibit massive Crooke's hyalinization (29,30). The adenoma cells possess a ring of basophilia and ACTH immunoreactivity at the periphery of the cytoplasm where the secretory granules are pushed by the

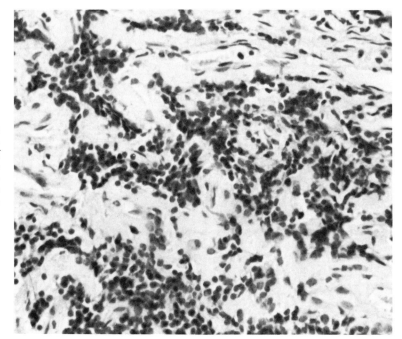

Figure 6–6. PRL cell adenoma from a patient treated with bromocriptine up to the time of surgery is composed of PRL-immunonegative cells with heterochromatic nuclei surrounded by marked interstitial and perivascular fibrosis (×250).

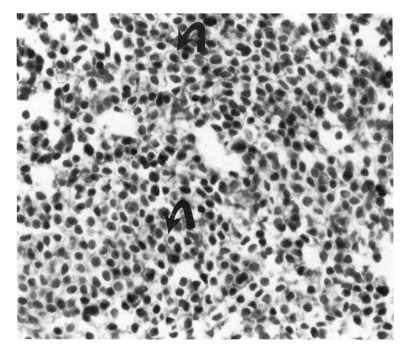

Figure 6–7. Functioning corticotroph adenoma immunostained for β-endorphin displays immunoreactivity at the periphery of the cytoplasm *(arrows)* (×400).

abundant microfilaments. Such tumors, composed of Crooke's cells, appear to maintain the capacity to secrete ACTH, since adenoma removal leads to cure of Cushing's disease. The nontumorous adenohypophysis contains Crooke's cells that are suppressed corticotrophs due to glucocorticoid excess (Fig. 6–8).

Rarely, ACTH-producing adenomas are chromophobic and may be accompanied by insidious Cushing's disease. The adenomas have a diffuse pattern and a weak ACTH immunoreactivity. Ultrastructurally, they correspond to sparsely granulated corticotroph adenomas (1). The reported incidence of multiple immunoreactivities in functioning corticotroph adenomas is variable. The co-production of PRL, α-SU or β subunit (β-SU) of glycoprotein hormones can occur. In our experience, such cases are rare, and the second hormone is restricted to certain groups of cells (20,21–33).

Some adenomas containing ACTH-immunoreactive cells are unassociated with elevated blood ACTH levels and endocrine symptoms (1,13,34,35). They are divided into three types and called "silent corticotroph

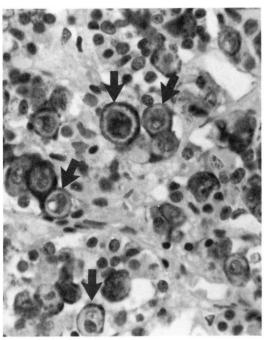

Figure 6–8. The nontumorous adenohypophysis removed with a functioning corticotroph adenoma contains many Crooke's cells *(arows)*; ACTH immunoreactivity corresponds to the secretory granules pushed to the periphery of cells by hyaline material, which is ACTH immunonegative (×400).

adenoma." They are monomorphous adenomas with well-defined ultrastructural features.

Silent subtype 1 adenomas, as already mentioned, resemble functioning corticotroph adenomas composed of well-differentiated, densely granulated corticotrophs. However, silent subtype 1 adenomas are large, often with infarcted areas, and the recurrence rate is relatively high (14%). Crooke's hyalinization may involve a varying percentage of adenoma cells. By the pattern of ACTH and other POMC-derived peptides and the ultrastructural features, these adenomas cannot be distinguished from functioning variant ones. The nontumorous adenohypophysis contains no Crooke's cells owing to the lack of glucocorticoid excess in such patients.

Silent subtype 2 adenomas have a diffuse or sinusoidal pattern, and ACTH, β-endorphin and β-lipotropin immunoreactivities are present in varying degrees. No Crooke's change is noticed in this group of adenomas. The diagnosis of silent subtype 2 is based on ultrastructural features.

Silent subtype 3 adenomas show a diffuse or trabecular arrangement. By immunocytochemistry, the ACTH immunopositivity can be diffuse, patchy or absent. Scattered cells positive for any adenohypophysial hormone, especially for GH, PRL and α-SU, may be seen. Some adenomas are completely immunonegative. By immunocytochemistry, the silent subtype 3 adenomas can mimic a plurihormonal or a null cell adenoma. Despite this inconsistent immunocytochemical profile, by electron microscopy they are monomorphous adenomas, showing some resemblance to glycoprotein-producing tumors (36). The morphological diagnosis of silent subtype 3 adenoma is possible only at the ultrastructural level.

Some patients bearing silent subtype 2 or 3 adenomas have mild to moderate hyperprolactinemia, oligomenorrhea and/or amenorrhea and galactorrhea and are misdiagnosed as having prolactinomas. Most probably the nontumorous stimulated PRL cells are the source of excessive PRL. In silent subtype 3 adenomas it is possible that adenoma cells immunoreactive for PRL can contribute to PRL production as well (37).

TSH-immunoreactive Adenomas. TSH-producing pituitary adenomas are associated with long-standing primary hypothyroidism, secondary hyperthyroidism or euthyroidism (38–42). Patients with hyperthyroidism secondary to TSH-secreting pituitary adenomas are rare. Frequently such patients are treated for primary thyroid overactivity, and their tumors are large and invasive at the time of surgery. The blood TSH level can be either elevated and nonsuppressible or in the normal range but with increased biological activity (43,44). Free α-SU is elevated in the blood as well. By histology, TSH-secreting adenomas present a diffuse or sinusoidal pattern with pseudorosettes of elongated cells around capillaries. Immunocytochemistry demonstrates β-TSH and α-SU in the cytoplasm of adenoma cells in varying amounts. Rarely, TSH immunoreactivity is intense and even over the entire tumor. More frequently, TSH and α-SU are present in groups of cells or isolated cells (Fig. 6–9) (1,13,42,45,46). Scattered immunoreactivity for GH is common (17). When many cells produce GH, patients develop acromegaly. Sometimes TSH immunoreactivity is faint or absent. There is no correlation between immunocytochemical results and blood TSH and α-SU levels. Ultrastructurally, some adenomas are composed of TSH cells resembling nontumorous cells, whereas other TSH cells are similar to those of null cell adenomas. In the latter situation, the diagnosis of TSH cell adenoma is based

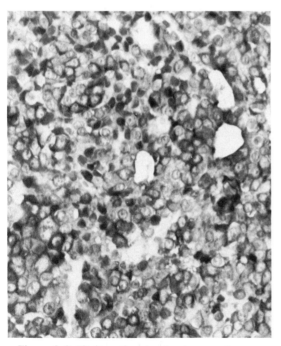

Figure 6–9. Pituitary thyrotroph adenoma shows variable intensity of TSH immunostaining in adenoma cells (×250).

on clinical and biochemical data showing elevated blood TSH levels (1,13).

TSH immunoreactivity is also found in different amounts in some densely granulated GH cell adenomas, null cell adenomas, oncocytomas and some plurimorphous plurihormonal adenomas.

FSH/LH-immunoreactive Adenomas. Variable degrees of immunoreactivity for FSH, LH and α-SU are present in gonadotroph adenomas, null cell adenomas and oncocytomas (1,13). By light microscopy, these three types of adenomas can have a sinusoidal pattern, with elongated cells forming pseudorosettes resembling thyrotroph adenomas. They can display a diffuse disposition as well. Adenomas composed of gonadotrophs contain FSH and/or LH and α-SU in most cells (Fig. 6–10) or, more frequently, in groups of cells. Elevation of blood FSH, and rarely LH, levels is frequent in men and may develop as a consequence of long-standing hypogonadism. Many cases have no history of gonadal hypofunction. In women, gonadotroph adenomas are "silent," or, if they secrete some FSH into the blood, this is difficult to demonstrate, especially at menopause (47–50). Elevation of α-SU levels in the blood is a more reliable marker for gonadotroph adenomas (51). Some gonadotroph adenomas show no immunopositivity for FSH and/or LH, and sometimes pronase predigestion can provide positive staining. Ultrastructurally, "male" and "female" types of gonadotroph adenomas are described (52). Electron microscopy is helpful in women but is inconsistent in men, since some gonadotroph adenomas may resemble null cell adenomas. In such cases, the diagnosis of gonadotroph tumors relies on clinical and biochemical data (13).

Alpha-SU-immunoreactive Adenomas. α-SU of glycoprotein hormones is found in association with their β-SU and other hormones, especially GH but rarely PRL and ACTH in different types of adenohypophysial adenomas.

Adenomas exclusively immunoreactive for α-SU are relatively rare and clinically endocrine inactive. The role of free α-SU is unknown at present. The adenomas containing only α-SU are very small obtained at autopsy or large in surgical material corresponding to null cell adenomas or oncocytomas by electron microscopy (53).

Adenomas With Multiple Hormonal Immunoreactivities (Plurihormonal Adeno-

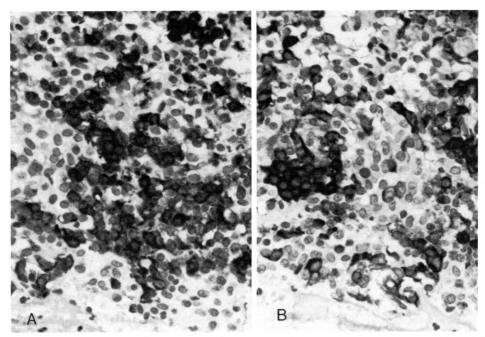

Figure 6–10. Gonadotroph adenoma exhibits LH immunoreactivity *(A)* and α-SU immunoreactivity *(B)* in many groups of cells (×250).

mas). Pituitary adenomas producing two or more hormones are called "plurihormonal adenomas." Systematic immunocytochemical investigations revealed that plurihormonal adenomas are frequently encountered. By correlating ultrastructural features with hormonal immunoreactivities, it became evident that multiple immunoreactivities are seen in (1) well-defined adenoma entities composed of a single cell type, (2) mixed adenomas in which two or more cell types are seen and (3) adenomas composed of a single cell type with no resemblance to any adenohypophysial cell.

In the first group, multiple immunoreactivities occur frequently in densely granulated GH cell adenomas and occasionally in sparsely granulated GH cell adenomas, mammosomatotroph adenomas, acidophil stem cell adenomas, corticotroph adenomas, thyrotroph adenomas, gonadotroph adenomas and silent subtype 3 adenomas. The mechanism responsible for the multiple hormonality of such adenomas is speculative at present. It is possible that this phenomenon is just a reflection of a process occurring in human nontumorous adenohypophysial cells. New data have demonstrated the presence of mammosomatotroph, bihormonal cells coproducing GH and PRL. The percentage of GH cells coexpressing α-SU is not well established. By the immunogold method PRL immunoreactivity was found at the ultrastructural level in some corticotrophs and gonadotrophs (56). In the rat rendered hypothyroid, the transdifferentiation of GH cells into TSH cells has been demonstrated (57). These emerging data will change the present classification of adenohypophysial cells in well-established cell types, and in the near future, proof of interconvertibility of other cell types is expected.

In the second group, the most representative mixed adenomas are GH cell–PRL cell adenomas. Adenomas composed of two or three cell types, such as GH cells, PRL cells, mammosomatotrophs, TSH cells or glycoprotein cells, are described and can be immunoreactive for GH, TSH, PRL, β-FSH, β-LH and α-SU in any combination (58–62). When one cell type predominates, oversecretion of its hormone is manifest in endocrine symptoms, including acromegaly, hyperprolactinemia or, rarely, hyperthyroidism. More commonly, plurimorphous plurihormonal adenomas are not associated with elevation of plasma hormone levels. It is believed that this group of mixed adenomas originates in a multipotential stem cell, the common progenitor cell of the embryonal human pituitary. Another possibility is the pluriclonal origin of such adenomas in different functionally committed cell types.

The origin of monomorphous plurihormonal adenomas that cannot be classified in any tumor type is unknown (63).

Nonimmunoreactive Adenomas. Most of the pituitary adenomas displaying no immunoreactivity for any adenohypophysial hormones are represented by null cell adenomas, oncocytomas and transitional forms between these two types (64–66). They represent up to 25% of surgically removed pituitary adenomas and are unassociated with clinical and biochemical evidence of hormone excess. When more sensitive immunocytochemical methods are applied, it becomes evident that scanty or focal immunopositivity for glycoprotein hormones (FSH, LH, TSH and α-SU) is not a rare finding (Figs. 6–11 and 6–12). Less commonly, other pituitary hormones, such as GH and/or PRL, are present. By histological pattern and immunoreactivity, as already mentioned, it is difficult to distinguish gonadotroph adenomas or glycoprotein-producing adenomas from null cell adenomas and oncocytomas. Ultrastructural and biochemical data contribute to the correct diagnosis of nonimmunoreactive adenomas. The results of reverse hemolytic plaque assay and tissue culture studies support the hypothesis that some null cell adenomas orig-

inate in or differentiate to gonadotrophs (67–70). The potential for multidirectional differentiation of null cell adenomas is indicated by a case in which scattered immunoreactivity for GH, PRL, TSH, FSH and α-SU correlated with the presence of mammosomatotrophs and thyrotroph-like cells at the ultrastructural level (71). These findings suggest that some null cell adenomas may originate in uncommitted precursor cells capable of differentiating into different cell types. It may be that null cell adenomas are a heterogeneous group with varying histogenesis.

Non-adenohypophysial Hormonal Markers

The presence of a large number of peptides, other than adenohypophysial hormones, has been investigated in the pituitary gland and its adenomas. These peptides include epithelial markers, neuroendocrine markers with a broad distribution, enzymes, releasing factors, mediators, receptors and other peptides. These immunocytochemical markers are distributed in many organs and tissues, including the pituitary, and most of them have no major diagnostic importance in pituitary adenomas.

Cytokeratins. Cytokeratins are constituents

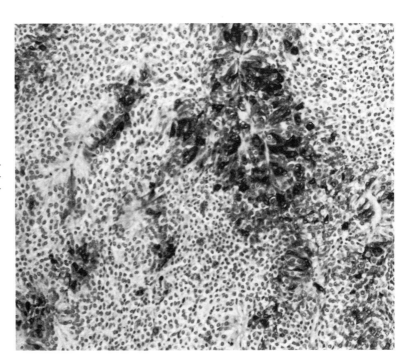

Figure 6–11. Null cell adenoma presents focal immunoreactivity for α-SU of glycoprotein hormones (×100).

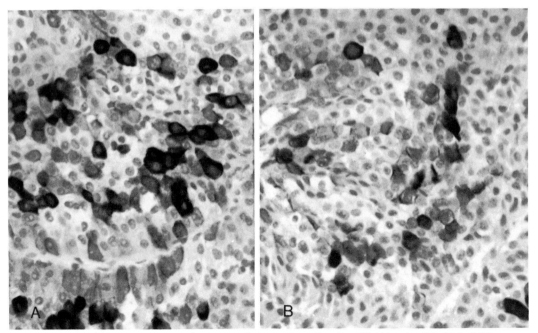

Figure 6–12. Oncocytoma contains some cells immunopositive for LH *(A)* and α-SU *(B)* (×250).

of intermediate filaments and are represented by 19 different polypeptides, with the molecular weight ranging from 40,000 to 70,000 daltons. Low- and intermediate-molecular-weight subunit cytokeratins are present in GH cells, PRL cells, ACTH cells and ACTH cells with Crooke's hyaline change. In corticotroph adenomas, the intermediate-molecular-weight subunit is consistently present, whereas the low-molecular-weight subunit is present only occasionally (72–74). In GH cell adenomas, cytokeratin immunopositivities are located in fibrous bodies, and possibly they can be related to some cytokeratin polypeptides associated with nuclear DNA as well (72,75). In PRL cell adenomas, cytokeratin immunopositivity is present in 10-nm microfilaments distributed throughout the cytoplasm.

mAB lu-5. mAB lu-5, a panepithelial monoclonal antibody raised against a lung cancer cell line, shows distinct immunoreactivity in pituitary corticotrophs and corticotroph adenomas (76). The mAB lu-5 antiserum also immunostains Crooke's hyaline material in nontumorous and adenoma cells. The mAB lu-5 antibody is very useful in identifying corticotroph adenomas in which ACTH immunoreactivity is not satisfactory (Fig. 6–13). The pattern of mAB lu-5 immunostaining is similar to that of cytokeratins

but is stronger and more distinct with less background.

The fibrous bodies of sparsely granulated GH cell adenomas are immunoreactive for this antibody as well (Fig. 6–14) (76). It should be noted that this panepithelial marker is present in many epithelial tumors of other organs.

Neuron-specific Enolase (NSE). NSE, a glycolytic enzyme enolase found in high amounts in the nervous system and neuroendocrine cells (77), has limited value in the diagnosis of neuroendocrine tumors owing to the lack of specificity, since it is present in some non-neuroendocrine tumors (78). In the pituitary, NSE is demonstrated by immunocytochemistry in all adenohypophysial cells and most pituitary adenomas and has no value in identifying any tumor type (79).

Synaptophysin. This intrinsic membrane protein of neuronal synaptic vesicles is also found in many endocrine cells and is recommended as a broad-range immunocytochemical marker for neuroendocrine tumors (80). In the pituitary, all types of adenohypophysial cells and the majority of tested adenomas are immunoreactive for synaptophysin (81). Therefore, synaptophysin, as NSE, cannot be used as an immunocytochemical marker for the diagnosis of different adenoma types.

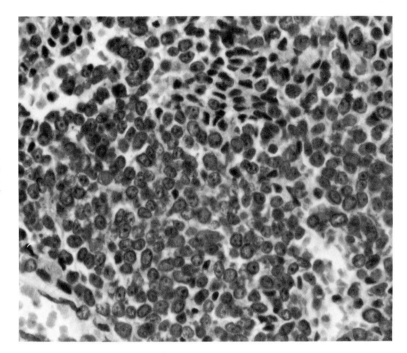

Figure 6–13. Corticotroph adenoma associated with Cushing's disease is intensely immunopositive for panepithelial marker mAB lu-5 (×400).

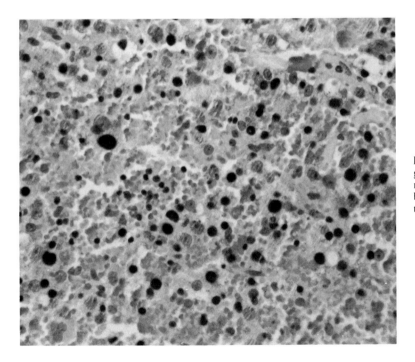

Figure 6–14. Sparsely granulated GH cell adenoma contains globular immunopositivity for mAB lu-5, corresponding to fibrous bodies at the ultrastructural level (×250).

Chromogranins. Chromogranins, which are acidic proteins associated with the secretory granules of neuroendocrine cells, are divided into three families: A, 68–75 kd; B (secretogranin I), 105 kd; and C (secretogranin II), 86 kd (82). Their role is still speculative. Chromogranin A is recommended as an excellent marker of neuroendocrine tumors (83). In the normal pituitary, it is localized in glycoprotein-producing cells. In pituitary adenomas, chromogranin A is present in tumors producing TSH, FSH/LH or FSH/LH/TSH and null cell adenomas. GH cells, PRL cells and ACTH cells and their adenomas are consistently negative for chromogranin A. Chromogranin B is detected in PRL cell, gonadotroph and null cell adenomas (84). An increased plasma level of chromogranin A in patients with nonfunctioning pituitary adenomas has been found, suggesting its use as a marker for such tumors (85).

S-100 Protein. S-100 protein was considered a marker for glial cells and Schwann cells (86) before being demonstrated in other cell types (87). In the pituitary, S-100 protein is present in folliculo-stellate cells (88). In our experience, S-100 immunoreactive cells are present in all types of pituitary adenomas, with a greater frequency in gonadotroph adenomas. The number of folliculo-stellate cells differs from case to case and they can even be absent. In some adenomas, both folliculo-stellate cells and groups of adenoma cells are immunostained for S-100 protein (89a).

Galanin. Galanin, a 29–amino acid peptide isolated from porcine intestine (89), was demonstrated by immunocytochemistry in the nervous system, adrenal medulla and other organs. In the rat pituitary, estrogen administration induces galanin synthesis in PRL cells and, to a lesser extent, in GH cells (90,91). In the human pituitary, galanin-like immunoreactivity was found in corticotrophs, Crooke's cells and basophils spreading into the posterior lobe. Some corticotroph adenomas are also immunoreactive for galanin. No other types of pituitary adenomas reacted with anti-galanin (92). The function of galanin in the pituitary is obscure.

Neurophysins. The carrier proteins of oxytocin and vasopressin identified in the hypothalamic nuclei have been found in human corticotrophs and corticotroph adenomas associated with Cushing's disease. Some GH cell adenomas contain scattered neurophysin immunoreactive cells as well (93). Their role is unknown.

Proteins of the Renin-Angiotensin System. Renin, angiotensinogen and angiotensin I converting enzymes have been localized in the human pituitary in PRL cells, PRL cell adenomas and mixed PRL cell–GH cell adenomas. Since angiotensin II promotes PRL release, it is possible that the renin-angiotensin system plays an autocrine role in the pituitary (94).

Other Antigens. Other peptides distributed in the nervous system and endocrine tissues, such as vasoactive intestinal peptide and gastrin (95,96), were demonstrated by immunocytochemistry in pituitary cells and some of their adenomas. It is possible that they have a paracrine and/or autocrine role.

REFERENCES

1. Kovacs K, Horvath E. Tumors of the pituitary gland. In: Atlas of Tumor Pathology. Fascicle 21. 2nd Series. Washington, DC, Armed Forces Institute of Pathology, 1986, pp 1–269.
2. Mukai K. Pituitary adenomas. Immunocytochemical study of 150 tumors with clinicopathologic correlations. Cancer 52:648–653, 1983.
3. Saeger W. Pathology of the pituitary gland. In: Belchetz PE (ed). Management of Pituitary Disease. London, Chapman and Hall, 1982, pp 253–289.
4. McNicol AM. Pituitary adenomas. Histopathology 11:995–1011, 1987.
5. Kovacs K, Horvath E, Ryan N. Immunocytology of the human pituitary. In: DeLellis RA (ed). Diagnostic Immunocytochemistry. New York, Mason, 1981, pp 17–35.
6. Kovacs K, Horvath E. Pathology of growth hormone-producing tumors of the human pituitary. Semin Diagn Pathol 3:18–33, 1986.
7. Herbert E, Roberts J, Phillips M, Allen R, Hinman M, Budarf M, Policastro P, Rosa P. Biosynthesis, processing and release of corticotropin, β-endorphin, and melanocyte-stimulating hormone in pituitary cell culture systems. In: Martini L, Ganong WF (eds). Frontiers in Neuroendocrinology. Vol 6. New York, Raven, 1980, pp 67–101.
8. Landolt AM, Heitz PU. Differentiation of two types of amyloid occurring in pituitary adenomas. Pathol Res Pract 183:552–554, 1988.
9. Voight C, Saeger W, Gerigk C, Ludecke DK. Amyloid in pituitary adenomas. Pathol Res Pract 183:555–557, 1988.
10. Bassetti M, Arosio M, Spada A, Buna M, Bazzoni N, Faglia G, Giannatasio G. Growth hormone and prolactin secretion in acromegaly: Correlation between hormonal dynamics and immunocytochemical findings. J Clin Endocrinol Metab 67:1195–1204, 1988.
11. Robert F, Pelletier G, Serri O, Hardy J. Mixed growth hormone and prolactin-secreting human pi-

tuitary adenomas. A pathologic, immunocytochemical, ultrastructural and immunoelectron microscopic study. Hum Pathol *19:*1327, 1988.

12. Giannattasio G, Bassetti M. Human pituitary adenomas. Recent advances in morphological studies. Review article. J Endocrinol Invest *13:*435–453, 1990.

13. Horvath E, Kovacs K. The adenohypophysis. In: Kovacs K, Asa SL (eds). Functional Endocrine Pathology. Vol 1. Boston, Blackwell Scientific, 1990, pp 245–281.

14. Kovacs K, Lloyd R, Horvath E, Asa SL, Stefaneanu L, Killinger DW, Smyth S. Silent somatotroph adenomas of the human pituitary. A morphologic study of three cases including immunocytochemistry, electron microscopy, in vitro examination, and in situ hybridization. Am J Pathol *134:*345–353, 1989.

15. Horvath E, Kovacs K, Killinger DW, Smyth HS, Weiss MH, Ezrin C. Mammosomatotroph cell adenoma of the human pituitary: A morphologic entity. Virchows Arch (A) *398:*277–289, 1983.

16. Horvath E, Kovacs K, Singer W, Ezrin C, Kerenyi NA. Acidophil stem cell adenoma of the human pituitary. Arch Pathol Lab Med *101:*594–599, 1977.

17. Corenblum B, Sirek AMT, Horvath E, Kovacs K, Ezrin C. Human mixed somatotrophic and lactotrophic pituitary adenomas. J Clin Endocrinol Metab *42:*857–863, 1976.

18. Kovacs K, Horvath E, Ezrin C, Weiss MH. Adenoma of the human pituitary producing growth hormone and thyrotropin. A histologic, immunocytologic and fine-structural study. Virchows Arch (A) *395:*59–68, 1982.

19. Horvath E, Kovacs K. Pathology of prolactin cell adenomas of the human pituitary. Semin Diagn Pathol *3:*417, 1986.

20. Heitz PU, Landolt AM, Zenklusen H-R, Kasper M, Reubi JC, Oberholzer M, Roth J. Immunocytochemistry of pituitary tumors. J Histochem Cytochem *35:*1005–1011, 1987.

21. Thorner MO, Schran HF, Evans WS, Rogol AD, Morris JL, MacLeod RM. A broad spectrum of prolactin suppression by bromocriptine in hyperprolactinemic women: A study of serum prolactin and bromocriptine levels after acute and chronic administration of bromocriptine. J Clin Endocrinol Metab *50:*1026–1033, 1980.

22. Thorner MO, Perryman RL, Rogol AD, Conway BP, MacLeod RM, Login IS, Morris JL. Rapid changes of prolactinoma volume after withdrawal and reinstitution of bromocriptine. J Clin Endocrinol Metab *53:*480–483, 1981.

23. Tindall GT, Kovacs K, Horvath E, Thorner MO. Human prolactin-producing adenomas and bromocriptine: A histologic, immunocytological, ultrastructural and morphometric study. J Clin Endocrinol Metab *55:*1178–1183, 1982.

24. Bassetti M, Spada A, Pezzo G, Giannattasio G. Bromocriptine treatment reduces the cell size in human macroprolactinomas: A morphometric study. J Clin Endocrinol Metab *58:*268–273, 1984.

25. Landolt AM, Osterwalder V. Perivascular fibrosis in prolactinoma: Is it increased by bromocriptine. J Clin Endocrinol Metab *58:*1179–1183, 1984.

26. Kovacs K, Stefaneanu L, Horvath E, Lloyd RV, Lancranjan I, Buchfelder M, Fahlbusch R. Effect of dopamine agonist medication on prolactin producing pituitary adenomas. A morphologic study including immunocytochemistry, electron microscopy

and in situ hybridization. Virchows Arch (A) *418:*439–446, 1991.

27. Horvath E, Kovacs K. Pathology of the hypothalamus and pituitary gland. In: Mendelsohn G (ed). Diagnosis and Pathology of Endocrine Diseases. Philadelphia, JB Lippincott, 1988, pp 377–412.

28. Scheithauer BW. The pituitary and sellar region. In: Sternberg SS (ed). Diagnostic Surgical Pathology. New York, Raven, 1989, pp 371–393.

29. Felix IA, Horvath E, Kovacs K. Massive Crooke's hyalinization in corticotroph cell adenomas of the human pituitary. A histological, immunocytological, and electron microscopic study of three cases. Acta Neurochir (Wien) *58:*235–243, 1982.

30. Horvath E, Kovacs K, Josse R. Pituitary corticotroph cell adenoma with marked abundance of microfilaments. Ultrastruct Pathol *5:*249–255, 1983.

31. Bigos ST, Robert F, Pelletier G, Hardy J. Cure of Cushing's disease by transsphenoidal removal of a microadenoma from a pituitary gland despite a radiologically normal sella turcica. J Clin Endocrinol Metab *45:*1251–1258, 1977.

32. Sano T, Kovacs K, Asa SL, Smyth HS. Immunoreactive luteinizing hormone in functioning corticotroph adenomas of the pituitary. Immunohistochemical and tissue culture studies of two cases. Virchows Arch (A) *417:*361–367, 1990.

33. Berg KK, Scheithauer BW, Felix I, Kovacs K, Horvath E, Klee GC, Laws ER Jr. Pituitary adenomas producing ACTH and alpha subunit: A clinicopathologic, immunohistochemical, ultrastructural and immunoelectron microscopical study of nine cases. Neurosurgery *26:*337–403, 1989.

34. Horvath E, Kovacs K, Killinger DW, Smyth HS, Platts ME, Singer W. Silent corticotropic adenomas of the human pituitary gland: A histologic, immunocytologic and ultrastructural study. Am J Pathol *98:*617–638, 1980.

35. Hassoun J, Charpin C, Jaquet P, Lissitzky JC, Grisoli F, Toga M. Corticotropin immunoreactivity in silent chromophobe adenomas: A light and electron microscopic study. Arch Pathol Lab Med *106:*25–30, 1982.

36. Horvath E, Kovacs K, Smyth HS, Killinger DW, Scheithauer BW, Randall R, Laws ER Jr, Singer W. A novel type of pituitary adenoma: Morphological features and clinical correlations. J Clin Endocrinol Metab *66:*1111–1118, 1988.

37. Lloyd RV, Fields K, Jin L, Horvath E, Kovacs K. Analysis of endocrine active and clinically silent corticotroph adenomas by in situ hybridization. Am J Pathol *137:*479–488, 1990.

38. Samaan NA, Osborne BM, Mackay B, Leavens ME, Duello T, Halmi NS. Endocrine and morphologic studies of pituitary adenomas secondary to primary hypothyroidism. J Clin Endocrinol Metab *45:*903–911, 1977.

39. Katz MS, Gregerman RI, Horvath E, Kovacs K, Ezrin E. Thyrotroph cell adenoma of the human pituitary gland associated with primary hypothyroidism: Clinical and morphological features. Acta Endocrinol (Copenh) *95:*41–48, 1980.

40. Afrasiabi A, Valenta L, Gwinup GA. A TSH-secreting pituitary tumor causing hyperthyroidism: Presentation of a case and review of the literature. Acta Endocrinol (Copenh) *92:*448–454, 1979.

41. Grisoli F, Leclerq T, Winteler JP, Jaquet P, Guibout M, Diaz-Vasquez P, Hassoun J, Nayak R. Thyroid-

stimulating hormone pituitary adenomas and hyperthyroidism. Surg Neurol 25:361–368, 1986.

42. Girod C, Trouillas J, Claustrat B. The human thyrotropic adenoma: Pathologic diagnosis in five cases and critical review of the literature. Semin Diagn Pathol 3:58–68, 1986.

43. Beck-Peccoz P, Piscitelli G, Amr S, Ballabio M, Bassetti M, Giannattasio G, Spada A, Nissim M, Weintraub BD, Faglia G. Endocrine, biochemical, and morphological studies of a pituitary adenoma secreting growth hormone, thyrotropin (TSH), and α-subunit: Evidence for secretion of TSH with increased bioactivity. J Clin Endocrinol Metab 62:704–711, 1986.

44. Gesundheit N, Petrick PA, Nissim M, Dahlberg PA, Doppman JL, Emerson CH, Braverman LE, Oldfield EH, Weintraub BD. Thyrotropin-secreting pituitary adenomas: Clinical and biochemical heterogeneity. Case reports and follow-up of nine patients. Ann Intern Med 111:827–835, 1989.

45. Saeger W, Ludecke DK. Pituitary adenomas with hyperfunction of TSH. Frequency, histological classification, immunocytochemistry and ultrastructure. Virchows Arch (A) 394:255–267, 1982.

46. Samuels MH, Wood WM, Gordon DF, Kleinschmidt-DeMasters BK, Lillehei K, Ridgway EC. Clinical and molecular studies of a thyrotropin-secreting pituitary adenoma. J Clin Endocrinol Metab 68:1211–1215, 1982.

47. Kovacs K, Horvath E, Van Loon GR, Rewcastle NB, Ezrin C, Rosenbloom AA. Pituitary adenomas associated with elevated blood follicle-stimulating hormone levels. A histologic, immunocytologic and electron microscopic study of two cases. Fertil Steril 29:622–628, 1978.

48. Trouillas J, Girod C, Sassolas G, Claustrat B, Lheritier M, Dubois MP, Goutelle A. Human pituitary gonadotropic adenomas: Histologic, immuocytochemical, ultrastructural and hormonal studies in eight cases. J Pathol 135:315–336, 1981.

49. Snyder PJ. Gonadotroph cell adenomas of the pituitary. Endocrinol Rev 6:552–563, 1985.

50. Nicolis G, Shimshi M, Allen C, Halmi NS, Kourides IA. Gonadotropin-producing pituitary adenoma in a man with long-standing primary hypogonadism. J Clin Endocrinol Metab 66:237–241, 1988.

51. Demura R, Jibiki K, Kubo O, Odagiri E, Demura H, Kitamura K, Shizume K. The significance of α-subunit as a tumor marker for gonadotropin-producing pituitary adenomas. J Clin Endocrinol Metab 63:564–569, 1986.

52. Horvath E, Kovacs K. Gonadotroph adenomas of the human pituitary: Sex-related fine structural dichotomy. A histologic, immunocytochemical and electron microscopic study of 30 cases. Am J Pathol 117:429–440, 1984.

53. Landolt AM, Heitz PU. Alpha-subunit-producing pituitary adenomas. Immunocytochemical and ultrastructural studies. Virchows Arch (A) 409:417–431, 1986.

54. Horvath E, Kovacs K. Fine structural cytology of the adenohypophysis in rat and man. J Electron Microsc Technol 8:401–432, 1988.

55. Lloyd RV. Analysis of mammosomatotropic cells in normal and neoplastic human pituitaries. Pathol Res Pract 183:577–579, 1988.

56. Newman GR, Jasani B, Williams ED. Multiple hormone storage by cells of the human pituitary. J Histochem Cytochem 37:1183–1192, 1989.

57. Horvath E, Lloyd RV, Kovacs K. Propylthiouracyl-induced hypothyroidism results in reversible transdifferentiation of somatotrophs into thyroidectomy cells. A morphologic study of the rat pituitary including immunoelectron microscopy. Lab Invest 63:511–520, 1990.

58. Duello TM, Halmi NS. Pituitary adenoma producing thyrotropin and prolactin. An immunocytochemical and electron microscopic study. Virchows Arch (A) 376:255–265, 1977.

59. Heitz PU. Multihormonal pituitary adenomas. Horm Res 10:1–13, 1979.

60. Carlson HE, Linfoot JA, Braunstein GD, Kovacs K, Young RT. Hyperthyroidism and acromegaly due to a thyrotropin- and growth hormone-secreting pituitary tumor. Lack of hormonal response to bromocriptine. Am J Med 74:915–923, 1983.

61. Horvath E, Kovacs K. Pituitary adenomas producing growth hormone, prolactin, and one or more glycoprotein hormones: A histologic, immunohistochemical, and ultrastructural study of four surgically removed tumors. Ultrastruct Pathol 5:171–183, 1983.

62. Scheithauer BW, Horvath E, Kovacs K, Laws ER, Randall RV, Ryan N. Plurihormonal pituitary adenomas. Semin Diagn Pathol 3:69–82, 1986.

63. McComb DJ, Bayley TA, Horvath E, Kovacs K, Kourides IA. Monomorphous plurihormonal adenoma of the human pituitary. A histologic, immunocytologic and ultrastructural study. Cancer 53:1538–1544, 1984.

64. Kovacs K, Horvath E, Ryan N, Ezrin C. Null cell adenoma of the human pituitary. Virchows Arch (A) 387:165–174, 1980.

65. Kovacs K, Horvath E. Pituitary "chromophobe" adenoma composed of oncocytes. A light and electron microscopic study. Arch Pathol 95:235–239, 1973.

66. Landolt AM, Oswald UW. Histology and ultrastructure of an oncocytic adenoma of the human pituitary. Cancer 31:1099–1105, 1973.

67. Yamada S, Asa SL, Kovacs K, Muller P, Smyth HS. Analysis of hormone secretion by clinically nonfunctioning human pituitary adenomas using the reverse hemolytic plaque assay. J Clin Endocrinol Metab 66:73–80, 1989.

68. Surmont DWA, Winslow CLJ, Loizon M, White MC, Adams FF, Mashiter K. Gonadotropin and alpha subunit secretion by human "functionless" pituitary adenomas in cell cultures: Long term effects of luteinizing hormone releasing hormone and thyrotropin releasing hormone. Clin Endocrinol 19:325–336, 1983.

69. Asa SL, Gerrie BM, Singer W, Horvath E, Kovacs K, Smyth HS. Gonadotropin secretion in vitro by human pituitary null cell adenomas and oncocytomas. J Clin Endocrinol Metab 62:1011–1019, 1986.

70. Yamada S, Asa SL, Kovacs K. Oncocytomas and null cell adenomas of the human pituitary: Morphometric and in vitro functional comparison. Virchows Arch (A) 413:333–339, 1988.

71. Kontogeorgos G, Horvath E, Kovacs K, Killinger DW, Smyth HS. Null cell adenoma of the pituitary with features of plurihormonality and plurimorphous differentiation. Arch Pathol Lab Med 115:61–64, 1991.

72. Ironside IW, Royds JA, Jefferson AA, Timperley WR. Immunolocalization of cytokeratins in the normal and neoplastic human pituitary gland. J Neurol Neurosurg Psychiatry 50:57–65, 1987.

73. Hofler H, Denk H, Walter GF. Immunohistochemical demonstration of cytokeratins in endocrine cells of the human pituitary gland and in pituitary adenomas. Virchows Arch (A) *404:*359–368, 1984.

74. Neumann PE, Horoupian DS, Goldman JE, Hess MA. Cytoplasmic filaments of Crooke's hyaline change belong to the cytokeratin class. Am J Pathol *116:* 142–222, 1984.

75. Ward WS, Schmidt WN, Schmidt CA, Hnilica LS. Association of cytokeratin p39 with DNA in intact Novikoff hepatoma cells. Proc Natl Acad Sci USA *81:*419–423, 1984.

76. Kovacs K, Ryan N, Stefaneanu L. Identification of corticotrophs in the human pituitary with mAB lu-5, a novel immunocytochemical marker. Pathol Res Pract *182:*775–779, 1987.

77. Schmechel D, Marangos PJ, Brightman M. Neuron-specific enolase is a molecular marker for peripheral and central neuroendocrine cells. Nature *276:*834–836, 1978.

78. Pahlman S, Esscher T, Nitsson K. Expression of α-subunit of enolase, neuron-specific enolase, in human non-neuroendocrine tumors and derived cell lines. Lab Invest *54:*554–560, 1986.

79. Asa SL, Ryan N, Kovacs K, Singer W, Marangos PJ. Immunohistochemical localization of neuron-specific enolase in the human hypophysis and pituitary adenomas. Arch Pathol Lab Med *108:*40–43, 1984.

80. Gould VE, Wiedenmann B, Lee I, Schwechheimer K, Dockhorn-Dworniczak B, Radosevich JA, Moll R, Franke WW. Synaptophysin expression in neuroendocrine neoplasms as determined by immunocytochemistry. Am J Pathol 126:243–257, 1987.

81. Stefaneanu L, Ryan N, Kovacs K. Immunocytochemical localization of synaptophysin in human hypophyses and pituitary adenomas. Arch Pathol Lab Med *112:*801–804, 1988.

82. Rindi G, Buffa R, Sessa F, Tortora O, Solcia E. Chromogranin A, B and C immunoreactivities of mammalian endocrine cells. Distribution, distinction from costored hormones/prohormones and relationship with the argyrophil component of secretory granules. Histochemistry *85:*19–28, 1986.

83. Lloyd RV, Cano M, Rosa P, Hille A, Huttner WB. Distribution of chromogranin A and secretogranin I (chromogranin B) in neuroendocrine cells and tumors. Am J Pathol *130:*296–304, 1988.

84. Lloyd RV, Wilson BS, Kovacs K, Ryan N. Immunohistochemical localization of chromogranin in human hypophyses and pituitary adenomas. Arch Pathol Lab Med *109:*515–547, 1985.

85. Deftos LJ, O'Connor DT, Wilson CB, Fitzgerald PA. Human pituitary tumors secrete chromogranin A. J Clin Endocrinol Metab *68:*869–872, 1989.

86. Moore BW. A soluble protein characteristic of nervous system. Biochem Biophys Res Commun *19:*739–744, 1965.

87. Cocchia D, Michetti F, Donato R. Immunochemical and immunocytochemical localization of S-100 antigen in normal human skin. Nature *294:*85–87, 1981.

88. Lauriola L, Cocchia D, Sentinelli S, Maggiario N, Maira G, Michetti F. Immunohistochemical detection of folliculo-stellate cells in human pituitary adenomas. Virchows Arch (B) *47:*189–197, 1984.

89. Tatemoto K, Rokaeus A, Jornvall H, McDonald TJ, Mutt V. Galanin, a novel biological active peptide from porcine intestine. FEBS Lett *164:*124–128, 1983.

89a. Marin F, Kovacs K, Stefaneanu L, Horvath E, Cheng Z. S-100 protein immunopositivity in human nontumorous hypophyses and pituitary adenomas. Endocr Pathol (in press).

90. Vrontakis M, Peden L, Duckworth ML, Friesen HG. Isolation and characterization of a complementary DNA (galanin) clone from estrogen induced pituitary tumor messenger RNA. J Biol Chem *262:*1655–1658, 1987.

91. Kaplan LM, Gabriel SM, Koenig JI, Sunday ME, Spindel ER, Martin JB, Chin WW. Galanin is an estrogen-inducible, secretory product of the rat anterior pituitary. Proc Natl Acad Sci USA *85:*7408–7412, 1988.

92. Vrontakis ME, Sano T, Kovacs K, Friesen HG. Presence of galanin-like immunoreactivity in nontumorous corticotrophs and corticotroph adenomas of the human pituitary. J Clin Endocrinol Metab *70:*747–751, 1990.

93. Kimura N, Andoh N, Sasano N, Sasaki A, Mouri T. Presence of neurophysins in the human pituitary corticotrophs, Cushing's adenomas, and growth hormone-producing adenomas detected by immunohistochemical study. Am J Pathol 125:269–275, 1986.

94. Saint-Andre J-P, Rohmer V, Alhenc-Gelas F, Menard J, Bigorgne J-C, Corvol P. Presence of renin, angiotensinogen, and converting enzyme in human pituitary lactotroph cells and prolactin adenomas. J Clin Endocrinol Metab *63:*231–237, 1986.

95. Hsu DW, Riskind PN, Hedley-Whyte TE. Vasoactive intestinal peptide in the human pituitary gland and adenomas. Am J Pathol *135:*329–338, 1989.

96. Holm R, Nesland JM, Attramadal A, Halse J, Johannessen JV. Null cell adenomas of the pituitary gland, an immunohistochemical study. J Pathol *158:*213–217, 1989.

7

ULTRASTRUCTURAL DIAGNOSIS OF PITUITARY ADENOMAS AND HYPERPLASIAS

EVA HORVATH
KALMAN KOVACS

Electron microscopy (EM) has a pivotal role in the identification of adenohypophysial cell types (1) as well as in the morphological classification of pituitary adenomas (2). Immunohistochemistry (IH) is an invaluable technique in the routine investigation of pituitary lesions (3,4). Nevertheless, EM nearly always has an edge whenever differential diagnosis has to be made between entities with overlapping immunohistochemical profiles. Unfortunately, EM is an expensive and time-consuming technique and, especially in times of austerity, it is abandoned by some laboratories for the most cost-effective methods. However, it always should be kept in mind that specific morphological diagnosis may be crucial for selecting appropriate postoperative treatment. Therefore, it is highly recommended to preserve a piece of adenoma tissue in EM fixative and keep it refrigerated until the permanent sections are examined. If histology and IH do not provide unequivocal diagnosis, then the tissue should be processed and investigated either locally or at a larger reference center. We caution against the so-called "paraffin rescue" (reprocessing tissue already embedded in paraffin), which can be helpful only if specific diagnostic markers (such as filamentous structures) are preserved. Optimal tissue preservation is of paramount importance for reaching conclusive diagnosis. Cells of endocrine neoplasms possess similar constituents, and secretory granule sizes often overlap in various tumor types. The characteristic appearance of many endocrine tumors, including pituitary adenomas, is furnished by the many-fold patterns by which cellular components are arranged. These distinguishing configurations, such as size and shape of cells, nuclear morphology, quantity, morphology and distribution pattern of rough endoplasmic reticulum (RER) and Golgi membranes, can be reliably assessed only in well-preserved tissue samples.

In this chapter, the ultrastructural appearance of all known pituitary adenomas and hyperplastic lesions will be reviewed, with comments on diagnostic criteria and the need for EM in their diagnosis.

The classification of pituitary adenomas and their frequency, based on a large sample (1560 cases) of unselected surgical material, are shown in Table 7–1.

PROLACTIN (PRL)-PRODUCING ADENOMAS

PRL cell adenomas are the most common adenohypophysial neoplasms in both surgical and autopsy material (2). These tumors can

Table 7–1. Frequency of Pituitary Adenoma Types in Unselected Surgical Material

Adenoma Type	%
PRL-producing adenoma	27.0
GH-producing adenoma	13.4
PRL- and GH-producing adenoma	7.2
Corticotroph cell adenoma	10.2
Thyrotroph adenoma	1.0
Gonadotroph adenoma	9.2
Silent adenoma (subtypes 1, 2, 3)	5.2
Null cell adenoma–oncocytoma	25.6
Unclassified plurihormonal adenoma	1.2

be conclusively diagnosed clinically if a macroadenoma is associated with grossly elevated serum PRL levels (several hundred or over a thousand µg/L). In such a case, the pathologist can easily provide confirmation of clinical diagnosis by demonstrating PRL by IH. Even microadenomas displaying the characteristic Golgi pattern immunoreactivity for PRL in an overwhelming majority of tumor cells can be conclusively characterized and diagnosed without EM. On the other hand, extreme caution is advised when a large sellar lesion is associated with mild or moderate hyperprolactinemia (PRL less than 200 µg/L). Such

a mass could represent an unusual form of PRL cell adenoma associated with massive fibrosis or calcification (2,5). Often, however, different pathology is found. In older age groups, a null cell adenoma or oncocytoma impinging on the pituitary stalk is most likely to be responsible. In younger patients other tumor types, such as gonadotroph adenoma, any of the three silent adenomas, as well as thyrotroph or PRL cell hyperplasia or lymphocytic hypophysitis, may be the underlying disease process. We strongly advise to perform EM in such cases, since it could be the only way to provide specific diagnosis. We also wish to emphasize that to consider such lesions as PRL cell adenoma and treat them with dopamine agonists may hold serious consequences for the patient. Various primary and secondary neoplasms of non-pituitary origin (craniopharyngioma, meningioma, plasmacytoma, lymphoma, metastatic tumors) may also induce hyperprolactinemia.

Sparsely granulated PRL cell adenoma is the common form of PRL-secreting tumors. This neoplasm is endowed with highly characteristic EM features, showing little variation from one case to another (Fig. 7–1) (2,5,6).

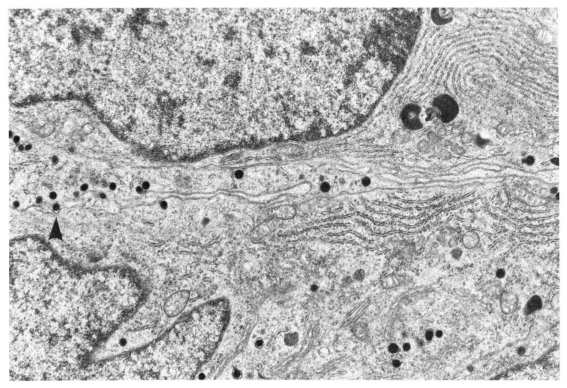

Figure 7–1. Electron micrograph showing characteristics of sparsely granulated PRL cell adenoma: abundant RER, prominent Golgi complex and "misplaced" exocytosis *(arrowhead)* (×10,400).

The polyhedral, often irregularly outlined cells possess a chiefly euchromatic, sometimes quite irregular nucleus with a large, dense nucleolus. About one half of the cytoplasm is occupied by masses of RER arranged in parallel cisternae or in concentric whirls (nebenkern). Within the other half of the cell, the dominant structure is the Golgi apparatus, which harbors several spherical and pleomorphic immature secretory granules within its sacculi. In highly active tumors the substantial majority of secretory granules may be seen within the Golgi region (Fig. 7–2), since the mature secretory granules are rapidly released. The form of discharge is granule extrusion (exocytosis), which is the single most important marker of the cell type and its tumors (7). The frequency of granule extrusions varies from one tumor to another, whereas their presence is constant. Extrusion of secretory granules occurs either at orthotopic sites (basal part of the cell) or along lateral cell membranes (misplaced exocytosis). The secretory granules are sparse in the cytoplasm and usually do not exceed 300 nm.

The mitochondria show regular features; oncocytic change is rare in this tumor type.

Densely granulated PRL cell adenoma is very rare (2,6). The middle-sized polyhedral cells of this tumor possess less prominent RER and Golgi membranes and significantly larger and more numerous secretory granules (Fig. 7–3). The secretory granules measure up to 700 nm, although most commonly they are in the 350 to 400 nm range. The extruded secretory granules may be difficult to detect within the tightly fitting membranous pits. Such granules often have an electron-dense but uneven, blotchy texture (Fig. 7–4).

PRL cell adenomas may exhibit calcification (8,9) or produce endocrine amyloid (10,11). The extent of both alterations is variable. If amyloid formation is microscopic, the fibrillar substance may be found only within dilated RER profiles of affected tumor cells (Figs. 7–5 and 7–6). In advanced forms extracellular masses are noted as well.

The ever-increasing use of dopamine agonist drugs in the medical treatment of PRL cell adenomas led to new problems in the

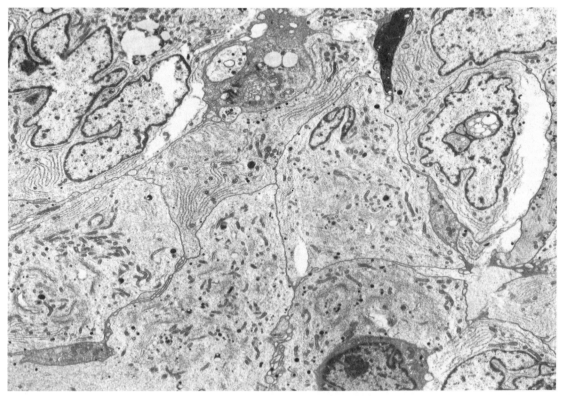

Figure 7–2. Highly active sparsely granulated PRL cell adenoma with extensively developed Golgi apparatus harboring nearly all of the secretory granules (×4200).

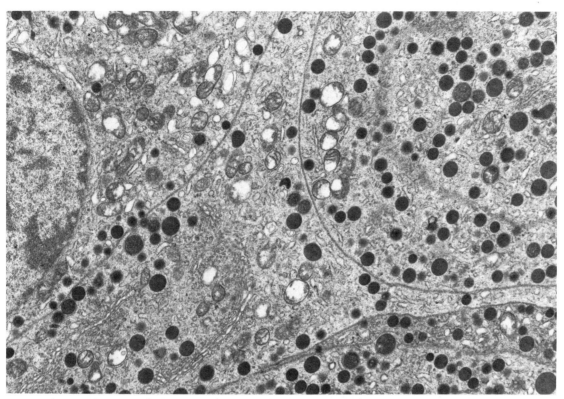

Figure 7–3. Densely granulated PRL cell adenoma. The secretory granules are in the range of GH granules, but pleomorphic immature granules in the Golgi sacculi and the uneven texture of some secretory granules are characteristic of PRL cells (×11,300).

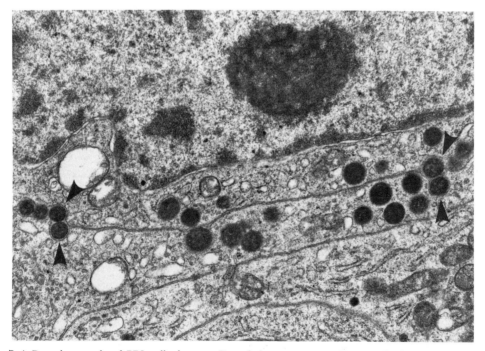

Figure 7–4. Densely granulated PRL cell adenoma. Extruded secretory granules *(arrowheads)* within tight membranous pits display uneven blotchy texture (×18,150).

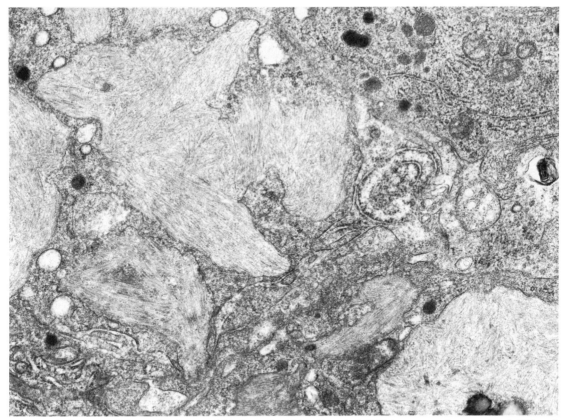

Figure 7–5. Intracellular endocrine amyloid formed within distended RER in a sparsely granulated PRL cell adenoma (×21,000).

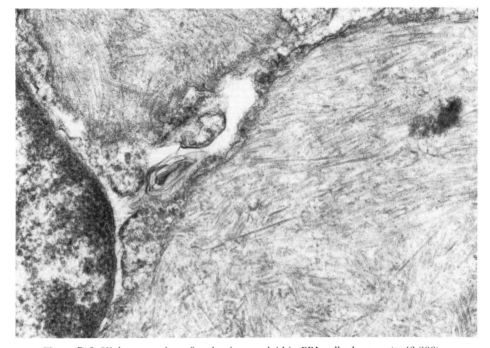

Figure 7–6. High-power view of endocrine amyloid in PRL cell adenoma (×43,800).

morphological diagnosis of these tumors. The remarkable uniformity seen in untreated PRL cell adenomas is turned into a striking variability by bromocriptine and other dopaminergic agents (12). The morphological effect of these drugs depends on the dose, length of treatment and responsiveness of tumor cells, which might be determined by their receptor status (13,14). The responsiveness of adenoma cells within one tumor may vary widely during dopamine agonist treatment, as well as following interruption of medication, resulting in unpredictability in the morphology of exposed PRL cell tumors (12).

Maximal functional suppression by dopamine agonists results in markedly increased cellularity due to involution of the entire tumor cell, especially the cytoplasm, RER and Golgi membranes (15–18). The nucleus be-

comes very irregular and heterochromatic (Fig. 7–7). Extrusions of the small secretory granules are still detectable. Such suppressed cells may have the appearance of null cells, and without the aid of granule extrusions as markers, their derivation cannot be ascertained. At this phase the tumor cells may cease to express the PRL gene as shown by *in situ* hybridization (19). Less complete inhibition by dopamine agonist is characterized by moderate loss of RER and Golgi membranes and/or an increase in lysosomal activity and crinophagy (uptake of secretory material by lysosomes). In these cells the suppressive effect of dopamine agonist is manifested through inhibition of PRL release (12). Owing to varying responsiveness within their cell population, morphological variability may be seen in some PRL cell adenomas.

Following cessation of dopamine agonist

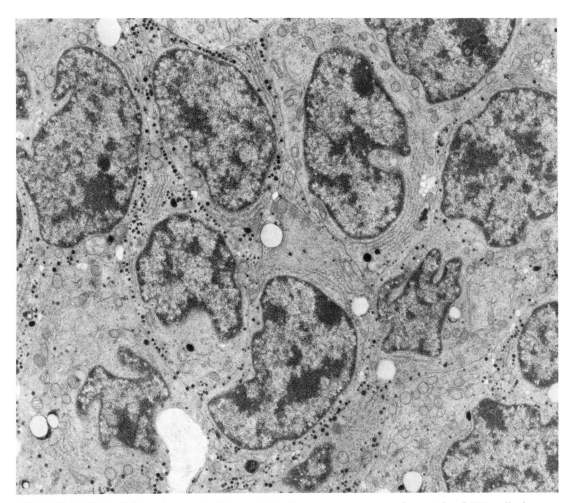

Figure 7–7. Effect of dopamine agonist (bromocriptine) treatment on a sparsely granulated PRL cell adenoma. Note the heterochromatic nucleus, reduction of cytoplasm and involution of RER and Golgi complex (×2400).

administration, the original morphology of adenoma cells is fully restored in many cases. The presence of profoundly suppressed cells in some PRL cell adenomas with a history of remote dopamine agonist exposure, however, strongly suggests that restitution may be incomplete (12,19).

In addition to cytological changes, sustained use of dopamine agonists may result in variable extents of fibrosis and calcification (2,6,20,21).

GROWTH HORMONE (GH)– PRODUCING ADENOMAS

After hyperprolactinemia and its sequelae, the second most common pituitary hypersecretory syndrome is acromegaly or, rarely, gigantism, most commonly caused by a GH-producing pituitary adenoma. In contrast to the morphologically uniform and usually monohormonal PRL cell adenomas, five distinct morphological entities may be found in cases of acromegaly. The most frequent types (approximately 70%) are the monomorphous densely and sparsely granulated GH cell adenomas; the bihormonal variants are less common. For the demonstration of GH production, IH is sufficient. However, EM is necessary to determine the morphological type. It should be noted that there are considerable differences in the biological behavior of the five types (22): the densely granulated GH cell adenoma and mammosomatotroph adenoma are likely to be slow growing and quiescent, whereas the sparsely granulated GH cell adenoma, mixed (GH cell–PRL cell) adenoma and acidophil stem cell adenoma grow faster and may be more difficult to treat. It should also be mentioned that acromegaly may rarely be caused by pituitary tumors other than GH cell adenoma (see "Silent Adenomas") and ectopic production of growth hormone releasing hormone (GHRH) (23). Ectopic production of GH itself is exceptionally rare (24).

Densely granulated GH cell adenomas (2,6,25–28) consist of middle-sized polyhedral or elongated cells with centrally placed, chiefly euchromatic nuclei (Fig. 7–8). The moderately or well-developed RER is usually detected as well-organized parallel cisternae at the periphery of cells. The prominent, spherical Golgi complex regularly harbors maturing secretory granules. The cytoplasmic stor-

age granules are chiefly spherical, evenly electron dense and range between 150 and 600 nm, most commonly measuring 350 to 500 nm. Secretory granules larger than 600 nm are likely to be irregular in shape. Some densely granulated GH cell tumors display an abnormality of secretory granule formation; crystallization of secretory material results in formation of odd, geometrically shaped "granules" (Fig. 7–9), sometimes measuring 2000 nm or more along their longest diameter. This phenomenon of unknown causation and significance appears to be specific for densely granulated GH cells and mammosomatotrophs.

The _sparsely granulated GH cell adenoma_ (2,6,25–28) represents an entirely different phenotype having little resemblance to the densely granulated variant and the GH cells found in the normal adenohypophysis (Fig. 7–10). The cells of this adenoma are rounded, polyhedral or irregular and often vary in size. The eccentric nuclei are flattened, crescent shaped, bilobed or multiple. They may also be markedly irregular. The RER may be abundant and well organized in some tumors and less prominent and dispersed in others. The Golgi sacculi are often enmeshed within or wrapped around the fibrous bodies. The latter are the highly conspicuous markers of this adenoma type. They are invariably located in the Golgi region on the concave side of the nucleus and are composed partly of type 2 filaments (a type of cytokeratin) (29) and partly of tubular smooth endoplasmic reticulum (SER). The fibrous bodies often trap various cytoplasmic constituents such as mitochondria, lysosomes and secretory granules. It is not uncommon to find centrioles and cilia, which may be supernumerary, in or around fibrous bodies. The secretory granules are small (less than 250 nm), sparse and of uncharacteristic appearance.

The sparsely granulated GH cell adenoma has two rare variants. One is a morphologically typical tumor with appropriately developed hormone synthetic machinery but unassociated with signs and symptoms of GH overproduction (30). As documented by _in situ_ hybridization and IH, a varying number of adenoma cells express the GH gene, but only a few cells display GH immunoreactivity. The reasons accounting for the clinical silence of these tumors are not understood. The other unusual variant is the association

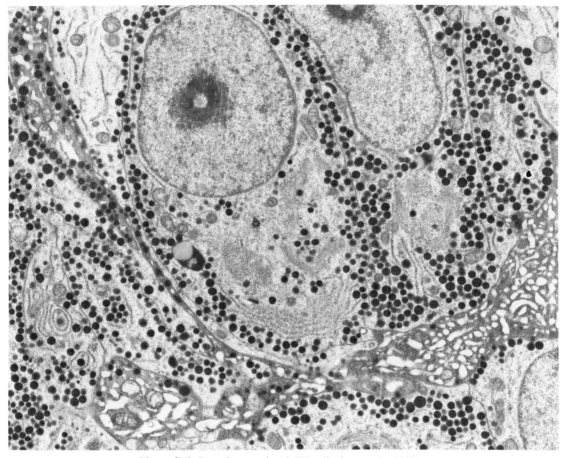

Figure 7–8. Densely granulated GH cell adenoma (×6400).

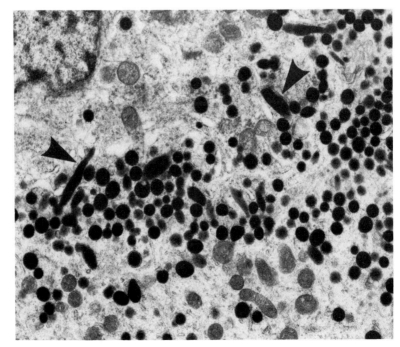

Figure 7–9. Elongated, odd-shaped secretory granules *(arrow-heads)* in a densely granulated GH cell adenoma (×12,200).

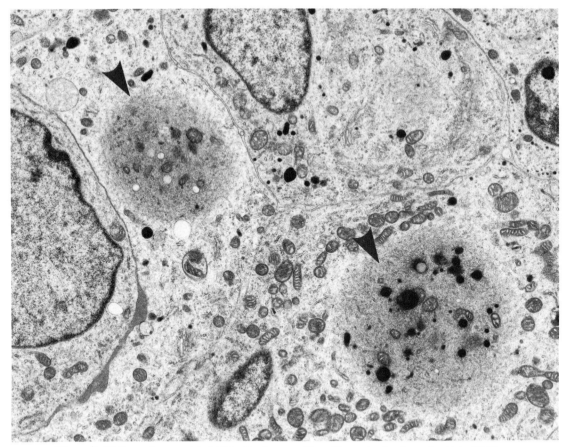

Figure 7–10. Sparsely granulated GH cell adenoma. Note fibrous bodies *(arrowheads)* (× 7900).

of a sparsely granulated GH cell adenoma with what is called "hypothalamic gangliocytoma" or "neuronal choristoma" (31–33). This rare sellar lesion may be interpreted in different ways, but no conclusive data are available concerning its histogenesis.

A poorly understood finding, occurring in some GH-producing adenomas, is the presence of tubulo-reticular aggregates in the capillary endothelium (34).

The effect of medical treatment with either dopamine agonists or somatostatin analogues on the ultrastructure of GH cell adenomas is much less spectacular than that seen in the PRL cell adenomas (35–38). The ultrastructural findings in GH cell adenomas range from no obvious change to lysosomal accumulation with or without discernible crinophagy, slight to moderate reduction of cell size and increase in size and number of secretory granules. Varying degrees of perivascular and interstitial fibrosis may also be noted.

Three of the five GH-producing adenomas also elaborate PRL. Among these, the most frequent is the bimorphous *mixed (GH cell– PRL cell) adenoma* consisting of two distinct morphological phenotypes having the description of both GH cells and PRL cells (Fig. 7–11) (39–41). These tumors are always associated with acromegaly, whereas the grade, and thus the manifestations, of hyperprolactinemia show considerable variations. In most of these tumors, densely granulated GH cells are combined with sparsely granulated PRL cells. The relative proportion and intratumoral distribution of GH- and PRL-producing components may vary considerably. In some cases bihormonal mammosomatotrophs may also be detectable.

The *mammosomatotroph adenoma* (42–44) is a primarily GH-producing tumor with mild or moderate elevation of serum PRL levels. It is monomorphous, consisting of one cell type (Fig. 7–12). In typical cases the adenoma cells are heavily granulated with large, often

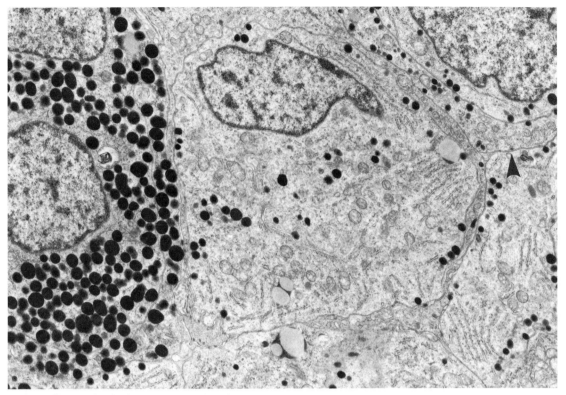

Figure 7–11. Mixed adenoma comprising densely granulated GH cells and sparsely granulated PRL cells. Note granule extrusion in PRL cell component *(arrowhead)* (×6700).

irregular secretory granules, which may measure up to 1500 nm. Geometrically shaped granules with a crystalline matrix may occur. Large, irregular secretory granules with a rarefied, mottled matrix are characteristic of the cell type. The most important marker is granule extrusion, which may have some unique features. Often, the extruded secretory granules are large and retain their electron density more than extruded secretory granules in PRL cell adenomas, which rapidly dissipate. In some cases, a narrow tube is formed by the limiting membrane of the secretory granule and the plasma membrane through which the secretory material is funnelled into the extracellular space (Fig. 7–13). This unique form of exocytosis is seen only in mammosomatotroph cells.

The *acidophil stem cell adenoma* (45) is a predominantly PRL-producing tumor with scant immunoreactivity for GH. Clinically it is associated with hyperprolactinemia and its sequelae, and signs and symptoms of acromegaly are only rarely associated with it. By EM, it is a monomorphous neoplasm comprising cells that possess markers of PRL cells

(exocytosis) and GH cells (SER and fibrous bodies), but have a distinct appearance of their own (Fig. 7–14). Probably the most distinctive feature of this tumor type is a diffuse, advanced oncocytic change consistently associated with a unique type of mitochondrial gigantism not seen in any other pituitary adenoma type. The adenoma cells might contain several enlarged mitochondria, often harboring electron-dense tubular structures of unknown origin and significance. However, there is usually only one giant form, the size of which comes close to that of the nucleus. These enormous structures retain the mitochondrial double membranes but contain fine granular substance instead of cristae. The giant mitochondria are easily recognized as clear cytoplasmic vacuoles by histology as well.

An additional feature in GH-producing tumors is a form of endocrine amyloid (2,6,11,46). In contrast to the amyloid substance of PRL cell adenomas, which is always detectable within adenoma cells, GH adenomas contain extracellular asteroid masses (Fig. 7–15) (46). Straight bundles of fibrillar

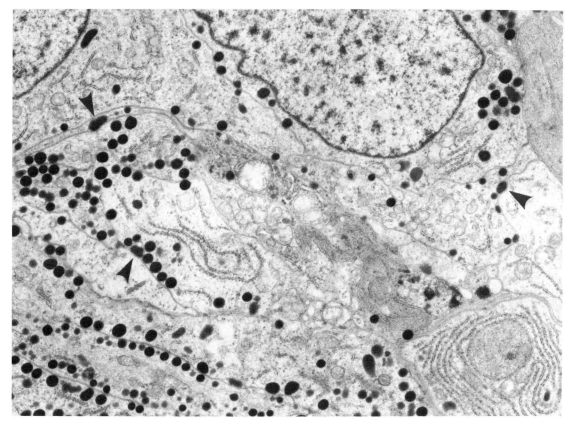

Figure 7–12. Mammosomatotroph cell adenoma. Note granule extrusions *(arrowheads)* distinguishing this tumor from densely granulated GH cell adenoma (×8100).

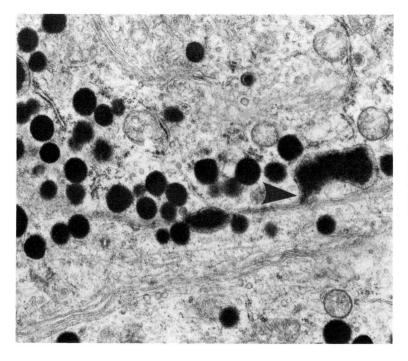

Figure 7–13. The content of large (1500 nm) secretory granule is funnelled into the extracellular space *(arrowhead)*. This type of exocytosis is typical of mammosomatotroph cell adenoma (×18,500).

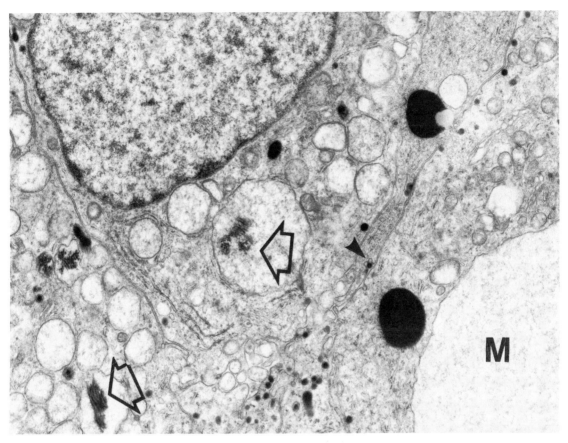

Figure 7–14. Ultrastructural appearance of acidophil stem cell adenoma. A generalized oncocytic change is associated with occurrence of giant mitochondria (M). Some moderately enlarged mitochondria harbor bundles of electron-dense tubular structures *(open arrows)*. The arrowhead marks granule extrusion (×12,000).

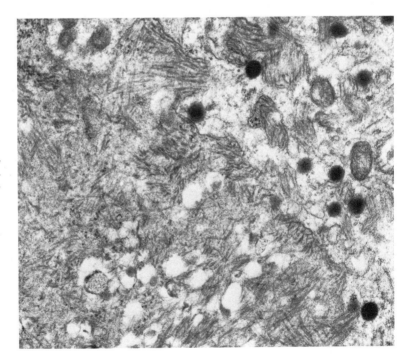

Figure 7–15. Predominantly extracellular endocrine amyloid in GH-producing adenoma (×19,700).

amyloid appear to originate from the tumor cells, but no fibrillar substance is detected intracellularly.

CORTICOTROPH CELL ADENOMA

Among pituitary lesions, those associated with Cushing's disease are the most challenging for clinicians and pathologists alike. While the overwhelming majority of lesions deriving from other cell types are autonomous adenomas, the pituitary pathology in cases of Cushing's disease is often equivocal. In a large majority of cases, a solitary adenoma appears to be responsible for the adrenocorticotropic hormone (ACTH) overproduction, whereas in about 15% of cases, non-neoplastic proliferation of corticotrophs or a combination of hyperplastic and neoplastic changes is found (2,6). It is a complicating factor that the adenomas are likely to be very small (a few millimeters in diameter) and poorly demarcated, making intraoperative sampling extremely difficult. For these reasons, surgeons may opt to perform resection of the median wedge, the most common site of corticotroph adenomas, or hemihypophysectomy or even total hypophysectomy if fertility is of no concern. It is essential to save and process every bit of tissue removed at surgery. Serial sectioning is often needed to define the underlying pathology.

The role of EM in pituitary Cushing's disease is two-fold: to recognize and classify adenoma tissue if present and to identify the type and functional state of non-tumorous adenohypophysial cells.

The EM features of the most common basophil adenoma are rather predictable (2,6,47,48) (Fig. 7–16). These tumors consist of middle-sized, elongated, angular cells, often arranged along vessels. The ovoid nucleus harbors a fairly prominent nucleolus localized close to the inner nuclear membrane. The slightly dilated RER is randomly distributed; the spherical Golgi apparatus harbors immature secretory granules, which often possess a halo around the electron-dense core. The secretory granules are nu-

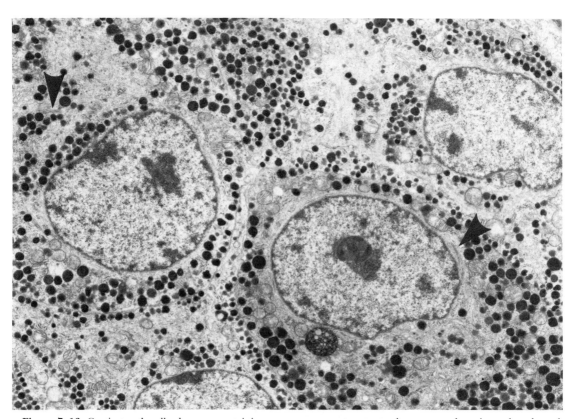

Figure 7–16. Corticotroph cell adenoma containing numerous secretory granules, among them irregular, dented and heart-shaped forms. Note type 1 filaments *(arrowheads)* (×6500).

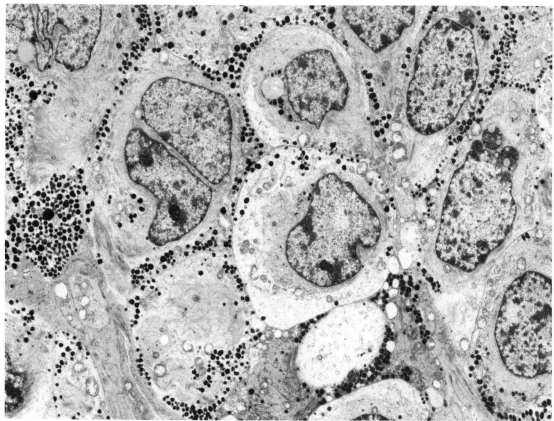

Figure 7–17. Corticotroph cell adenoma consisting of cells having characteristics of Crooke's cells. Marked perinuclear deposition of type 1 filaments and displacement of secretory granules to the cell periphery are evident (×4300).

merous and display distinctive morphology. They are spherical, dented, heart shaped or drop shaped and often exhibit varying electron density. The secretory granule size is fairly constant, in the range of 150 to 450 nm, with the majority being 300 to 350 nm. In addition to the secretory granule morphology, the other important and apparently specific morphological marker is the type 1 filament (2,6,49–51). A few bundles of these cytokeratin filaments are noted chiefly around the nucleus. Adenomas associated with Nelson's syndrome have similar ultrastructure but contain few or no type 1 filaments.

Excessive accumulation of type 1 filaments, known also as "Crooke's hyalinization," is the characteristic of the functionally suppressed non-tumorous corticotroph and is not expected to occur in adenomas. Nevertheless, a minority of corticotroph cell adenomas consist partly or entirely of adenoma cells that are morphologically indistinguishable from Crooke's cells (50,52,53). These cells display a massive, ring-like accumulation of filamentous substance occupying most of the cytoplasm and displacing other cytoplasmic constituents (Fig. 7–17). The size and morphology of secretory granules are similar to those seen in the typical tumors, but their number is reduced. The secretory granules are confined to the cell periphery and to the Golgi region.

The reason for the excessive accumulation of filamentous material is poorly understood. It is of note that Crooke's cell adenomas have no clinical correlate; they may be associated with florid Cushing's disease or a more subtle form of hypercorticism.

A rare form of corticotroph adenoma is chromophobic with scanty immunoreactivity for ACTH (2,6). Such tumors are usually macroadenomas at the time of diagnosis and are likely to be associated with a relatively mild form of Cushing's disease. By EM, only a minority of adenoma cells possess characteristic secretory granules and type 1 filaments. The rest of the cell population displays uncharacteristic features, including poorly developed membranous organelles and sparse, small secretory granules.

The non-neoplastic proliferation of corticotrophs will be discussed later (see "Pituitary Hyperplasia").

TUMORS OF GLYCOPROTEIN HORMONE–PRODUCING CELLS

While adenomas arising in GH, PRL or ACTH cells are well defined and easy to recognize, the tumors of the glycoprotein hormone cells are notoriously troublesome. There is a notion of uncertainty and unpredictability in the diagnostics of these lesions for a number of reasons. First, clinically they are often atypical or appear hormonally nonfunctioning. For instance, morphologically typical thyrotroph adenomas may be associated clinically with hyperthyroidism, hypothyroidism or euthyroidism. Similarly, morphologically recognizable gonadotroph adenomas in males may appear inactive biochemically. In females with gonadotroph adenoma, the serum levels of FSH and LH are likely to be normal for the woman's age. Second, immunohistochemical findings in glycoprotein hormone cell tumors are often capricious and inconsistent. Strong immunoreactivity for TSH, FSH or LH may be unassociated with elevated serum hormone levels and vice versa; negative IH results may be seen in cases with elevated TSH or gonadotropin levels. IH demonstrates the hormone that is stored in the cell. The relatively soluble glycoprotein hormones are subject to loss during tissue processing. It is not clear how neoplastic glycoprotein cells perform glycosylation, which influences solubility, or packaging of hormones into secretory granules, which is necessary for detectability by IH. Maybe *in situ* hybridization can provide more accurate information concerning the functional differentiation of adenoma cells. Third, EM documents features particular to all glycoprotein hormone tumors: polarity of cells and small secretory granules, most often displaying uneven distribution. Apart from these, glycoprotein hormone–producing tumors exhibit a wide spectrum of ultrastructure, from highly differentiated tumors with recognizable character of TSH or gonadotroph cells to the non-descript appearance of

null cell adenomas, apparently showing no consistent correlation with clinical or other morphological findings. Undoubtedly, further work is required to define this group of adenomas.

Thyrotroph cell adenoma (2,6,54–57) is the least common pituitary tumor type. In the majority of the cases EM documents well-differentiated tumors comprising moderately polar, angular cells resembling the shape of the normal thyrotroph (Fig. 7–18). The nuclei may be spherical or ovoid and uniform, although focal nuclear pleomorphism is often noted. The prominent RER may display mild, uniform dilation as seen in the normal active counterpart. The globoid Golgi apparatus is prominent with maturing secretory granules and numerous vesicles. In a few tumors, small, randomly located aggregates of SER and intermediate filaments are noted. In the majority of thyrotroph adenomas, the secretory granules are small (150 to 250 nm), sparse and form a single layer under the plasmalemma outlining the cell borders. A few tumors are more granular; in these, the secretory granules tend to be larger, measuring up to 400 nm. Notably, instead of spherical secretory granules, a minority of thyrotroph tumors possess rod-shaped and drop-shaped secretory granules. This duality is also detected in non-tumorous thyrotrophs, the reason for which is not known.

Thyrotroph adenomas may show less functional differentiation and thus less characteristic morphological appearance. It is also known that in some tumors, well-differentiated typical areas may alternate with parts resembling inactive null cells, underlining the importance of generous tissue sampling. It should be pointed out that there is no obvious correlation between thyroid function and ultrastructural appearance of thyrotroph adenomas.

GONADOTROPH ADENOMA

Gonadotroph adenomas' unique attribute is their sex-linked ultrastructural dichotomy (2,6,59–62). Gonadotroph adenomas in males do not have unusual features (2,6,58,60–64). They consist of middle-sized, moderately polar cells with uniform, chiefly euchromatic nuclei (Fig. 7–19). About 50% of these adenomas possess well-developed RER throughout and prominent Golgi complex endowed with regular appearance. The small (200 to

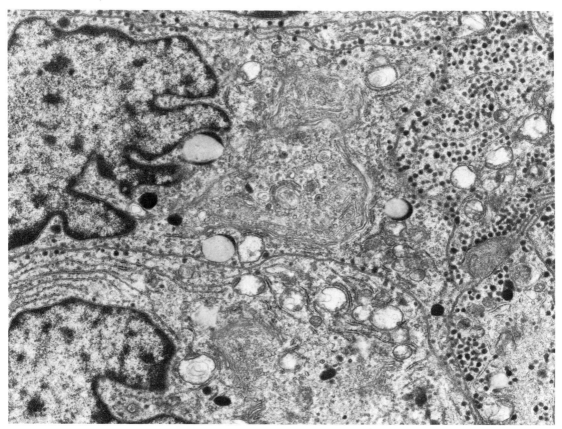

Figure 7–18. Thyrotroph cell adenoma associated with hyperthyroidism. The prominent Golgi complex contains numerous vesicles. The small secretory granules accumulate in cell processes (×11,900).

250 nm) secretory granules display markedly uneven distribution, being very sparse within the nuclear pole and quite numerous in the cell processes converging toward the basement membrane. Some adenomas contain a varying number of ovoid or polyhedral cells with larger (up to 450 nm) secretory granules resembling those of normal mature gonadotrophs (Fig. 7–20). The other 50% of gonadotroph adenomas in males display more variability, having better differentiated areas alternating with regions that reflect signs of inactivity similar to those seen in null cells. An important morphological marker in gonadotroph tumors, especially in men, is the frequent formation of follicles. They are easy to detect even by histology on periodic acid–Schiff (PAS)–stained section, owing to the bright PAS positivity of the follicular content. Follicles are rare in other pituitary tumor types, especially in other "chromophobic" adenomas. A significant feature is oncocytic transformation, seen in as many as 50% of male-type gonadotroph adenomas.

A significant majority (about 70%) of gonadotroph adenomas in women exhibit a rather monotonous ultrastructure (59,60,62). These are comprised of closely apposed, markedly polar cells with long, attenuated cytoplasmic processes. The uniform, ovoid nuclei are euchromatic. The cytoplasmic organelles, especially the delicate network of well-developed, slightly dilated RER, display rather low electron density compared to other adenoma types. The most recognizable structure of adenoma cells is the honeycomb Golgi complex, the result of a vacuolar transformation of the conventional Golgi apparatus (Figs. 7–21 and 7–22). Depending on the plane of sectioning, one to three clusters of evenly sized spheres are seen containing low-density proteinaceous substance but usually not forming secretory granules. The honeycomb Golgi complex is specific for gonadotroph adenoma in females. The frequency of the structure varies; they are most numerous (close to 100% of adenoma cells) in tumors in young women, whereas their presence is

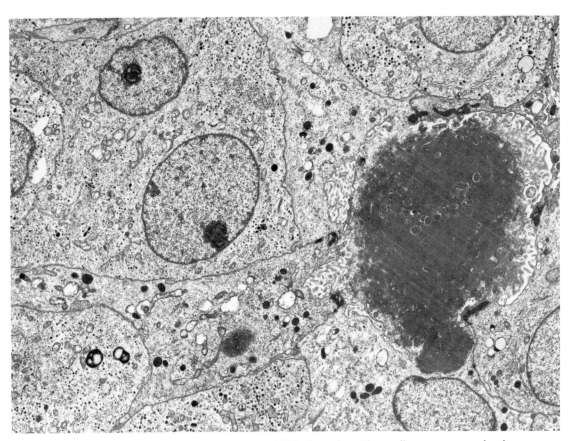

Figure 7–19. Gonadotroph adenoma, male type with follicle formation. The small secretory granules show uneven distribution (×4600).

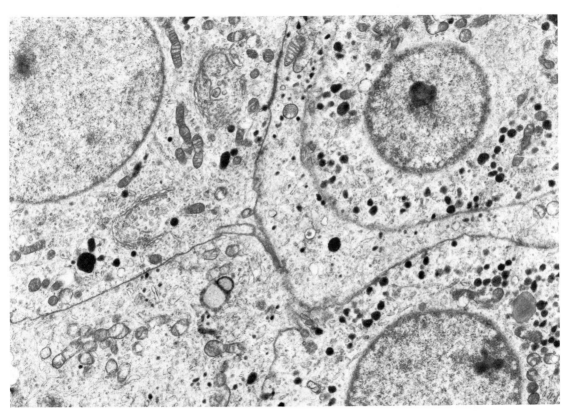

Figure 7–20. Gonadotroph adenoma, male type. In addition to small granule cells, ovoid cells with larger secretory granules, similar to those of normal mature gonadotrophs, also occur (×9100).

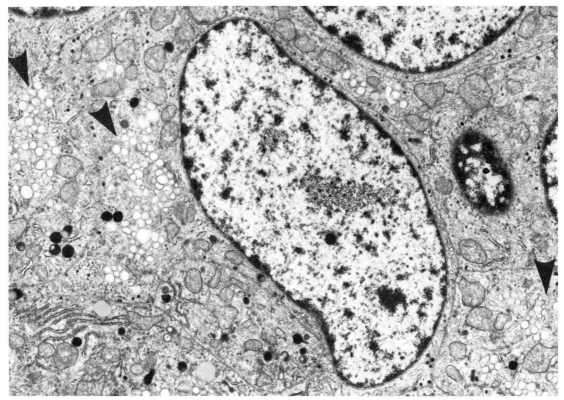

Figure 7–21. Gonadotroph adenoma, female type. Vacuolar transformation of Golgi complexes (honeycomb Golgi complex) *(arrowheads)* is evident (×9100).

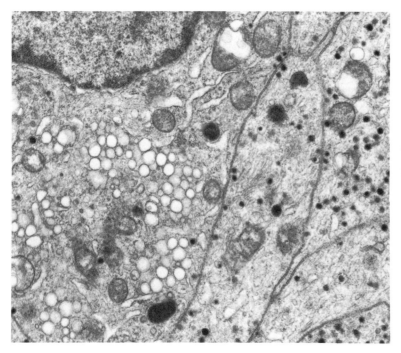

Figure 7–22. High-power view of a honeycomb Golgi complex. Note almost total absence of immature secretory granules (×16,250).

less striking in elderly females. The secretory granules are uniformly small (around 150 nm), and they accumulate within the long cytoplasmic processes.

The well-differentiated ultrastructure alternates with less developed areas with EM signs of low secretory activity in almost 20% of tumors. Finally, a small minority (approximately 10%) of gonadotroph adenomas in women represent an unusual variant (60). These tumors consist partly or entirely of cells having a striking resemblance to normal gonadotrophs (Fig. 7–23). The adenoma cells are polyhedral, exhibiting little polarity. The RER is generally well developed, often showing dilation, the degree of which varies from one cell to another. In some cells, the morphology of expanded RER may be indistinguishable from that seen in stimulated, non-tumorous gonadotrophs (gonadal deficiency cells, castration cells). The Golgi apparatus is prominent but displays no vacuolar transformation. The secretory granules measure up to 500 nm and are spherical or slightly irregular, having ruffled limiting membranes and

varying electron density as observed in the non-tumorous counterpart.

We wish to call attention to a little-known structure that may be present in gonadotroph adenomas, especially in those of men. The so-called "light body," a structure of unknown origin and significance, is assumed to denote gonadotroph differentiation (65) (Fig. 7–24). In our experience, light bodies are rarely detected in other tumor types, and if seen, they may be used as gonadotroph markers.

CLINICALLY NON-FUNCTIONING ADENOMAS: NULL CELL ADENOMA AND ONCOCYTOMA

Clinically non-functioning tumors represent pituitary neoplasms that are unassociated with the overproduction of any known pituitary hormone and possess no immunohistochemical and ultrastructural marker that would conclusively indicate their cellular derivation (2,6,66). Being the most common

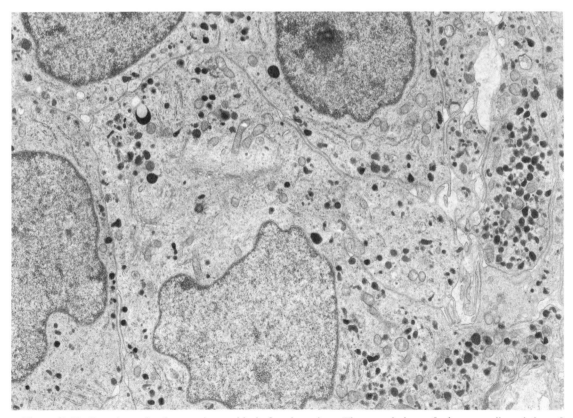

Figure 7–23. Gonadotroph adenoma in an elderly female patient. The morphology of adenoma cells and that of the secretory granules are similar to those seen in normal gonadotrophs (×8200).

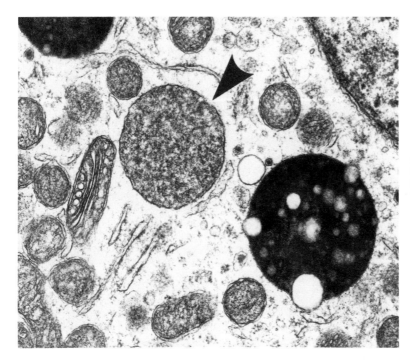

Figure 7–24. "Light body" *(arrowhead)* in a gonadotroph adenoma of a man. The origin and significance of the structure are unclear (×29,900).

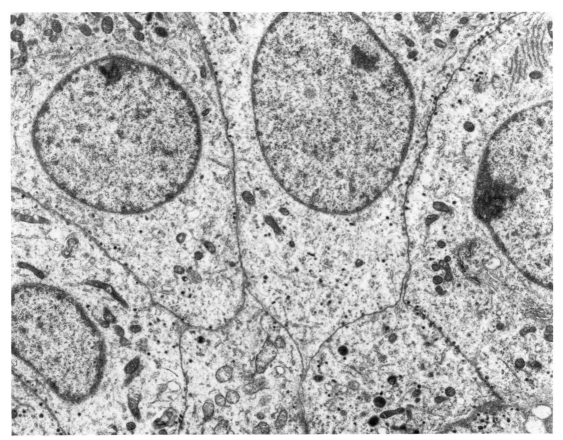

Figure 7–25. Null cell adenoma having undeveloped RER and Golgi membranes and a few small secretory granules (×6500).

types in older age groups, these adenomas account for as many as 25% of tumors in surgical material. It appears that a substantial number of these adenomas show some degree of glycoprotein hormone differentiation (66–69), whereas a minority express the genes for GH, PRL or ACTH (70). Thus, this large group of tumors is probably heterogeneous but displays similar morphological features owing to very low hormonal activity. It is noteworthy that there is an overlap between the gonadotroph adenoma and the null cell adenoma/oncocytoma group, and in some cases, it is difficult to draw the line between these entities (71).

By EM, *null cell adenomas* (2,6,66,72) consist of rather small, polyhedral cells with irregular, kidney-shaped or deeply cleaved nuclei. They harbor profiles of poorly developed RER and Golgi membranes in their cytoplasm as well as sparse and small (less than 250 nm) secretory granules (Fig. 7–25). The secretory granules may be spherical, rod shaped, drop shaped or haloed and often exhibit variable electron densities. The number, size and morphology of mitochondria are within normal limits in the majority of cells, but scattered oncocytic change may be present in many null cell adenomas.

Pituitary oncocytoma is regarded as the oncocytic form of null cell adenoma (2,6,72). Owing to undue accumulation of mitochondria, the adenoma cells are somewhat larger than those of null cell adenoma and tend to be polyhedral or rounded with no polarity. Otherwise, the morphology and quantity of other cellular constituents are similar to those observed in non-oncocytic null cell adenomas (Fig. 7–26).

SILENT ADENOMAS

Not to be confused with tumors of the clinically non-functioning null cell adenoma/oncocytoma group, silent adenomas are pituitary neoplasms unassociated with recognizable endocrine hypersecretory syndrome but possessing well-differentiated, distinctive ultrastructure. The three types of silent adenomas encountered in classification studies cannot be related to any of the known cell types, and we assume that they derive from yet uncharacterized adenohypophysial cells.

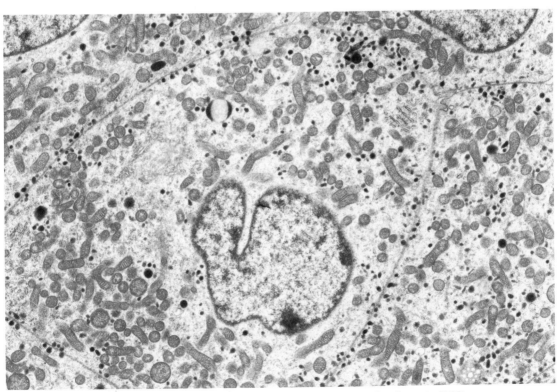

Figure 7–26. Pituitary oncocytoma displaying mitochondrial abundance (×7700).

In all probability, these postulated cell types secrete their own hormonally active substances, but presently neither their hormones nor their target tissues are known. Therefore, EM is an indispensable tool for recognition, especially of subtype 2 and subtype 3 adenomas.

Silent adenoma, subtype 1 (2,6,73–75), is morphologically indistinguishable from basophil adenomas associated with Cushing's disease (Fig. 7–27). These tumors strongly express the proopiomelanocortin (POMC) gene (76). Because of their apparent clinical silence, the tumors are diagnosed at the macroadenoma stage. In 40% of our cases, this adenoma type becomes manifest by an acute hemorrhagic event. This unusual bleeding tendency is unexplained.

Since the ultrastructure of the tumor is essentially similar to that of a corticotroph adenoma, it can be recognized only if the clinical history of the patient is known. The POMC-producing posterior lobe basophils, which show great morphological, including ultrastructural, similarities to corticotrophs, may serve as the parent cell of this adenoma type.

Silent adenoma, subtype 2 (2,6,74), occurs chiefly in men. This tumor is also POMC-producing, but the expression of POMC gene is less frequent (76), and by EM, the ultrastructural similarity to corticotrophs is less conspicuous. These tumors consist of polyhedral, angular cells with somewhat irregular, centrally placed nuclei (Fig. 7–28). The well-developed, randomly distributed RER and the fairly prominent Golgi complex possess no unusual features. The secretory granules, present in fair numbers, are evenly distributed. They occur in various shapes such as spherical, irregular, dented and drop-shaped forms. The secretory granules measure up to 400 nm, most commonly 250 to 300 nm, along their longest diameter. The morphology of secretory granules is reminiscent of that of corticotroph secretory granules, but silent adenoma, subtype 2, secretory granules are smaller. Type 1 filaments, regular constituents of corticotroph and silent "corticotroph" subtype 1 adenomas, are not detectable in subtype 2 tumors.

The silent adenoma, subtype 3 (2,3,74,77), is likely to be discovered before reaching macroadenoma stage, especially in women. The

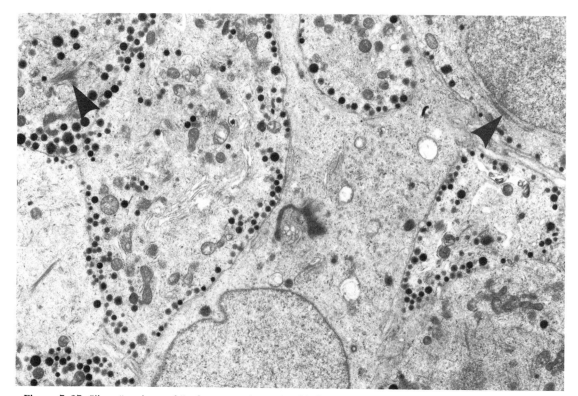

Figure 7–27. Silent "corticotroph" adenoma, subtype 1, with features similar to those of corticotroph adenomas. Bundles of type 1 filaments are also present *(arrowheads)* (×7800).

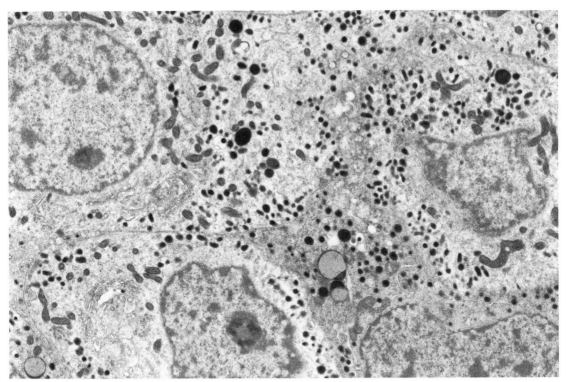

Figure 7–28. Silent "corticotroph" adenoma, subtype 2. The polyhedral adenoma cells contain evenly distributed, often drop-shaped or rod-shaped secretory granules (×8100).

tumor is quite consistently associated with low-grade hyperprolactinemia as well as amenorrhea, oligomenorrhea and galactorrhea. It appears that the source of excess PRL is the non-tumorous adenohypophysis, but the mechanism of hyperprolactinemia is unknown at present. In men, hyperprolactinemia may also be present, and in a few cases, acromegaly may develop, presumably as a consequence of plurihormonal differentiation of the tumor. To our knowledge, this is the only situation in which a pituitary tumor other than a GH cell adenoma induces acromegaly.

EM detects tumors displaying all characteristics of glycoprotein hormone differentiation (Fig. 7–29). The larger than average cells exhibit marked polarity. The large, sometimes pleomorphic nuclei harbor prominent nucleoli and, in the majority of tumors, prominent nuclear inclusions (spheridia) (Fig. 7–30). The ample cytoplasm is packed with abundant RER, sometimes masses of SER and extensive, multifocal Golgi apparatus. The sparse secretory granules are spherical and usually measure around 200 nm. The secretory granules show uneven distri-

bution, being more numerous in cell processes. Groups of mitochondria are often displaced by proliferating endoplasmic reticulum. In several tumors, rich plexiform interdigitations of neighboring plasma membranes are prominent.

PITUITARY HYPERPLASIA

Owing to the lack of established diagnostic criteria, the existence of pituitary hyperplasia as a morphological entity was in doubt for many years. Before the introduction of immunohistochemistry, the reliable diagnosis of non-neoplastic proliferation of pituitary cell types was often problematic, even when the entire gland was available for morphological study. The recognition of hyperplasia in surgical material may still be difficult for a number of reasons, such as the regional distribution of some of the pituitary cell types and the fragmented nature of surgical specimens. It also has to be stressed that hyperplasia has no ultrastructural criteria. However, an experienced electron microscopist familiar with the EM appearance of pituitary cell types in

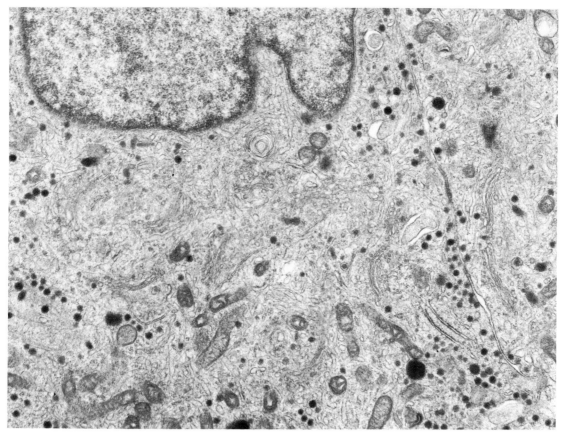

Figure 7–29. Silent adenoma, subtype 3. Note extensively developed Golgi complex and small, uniform secretory granules (×13,000).

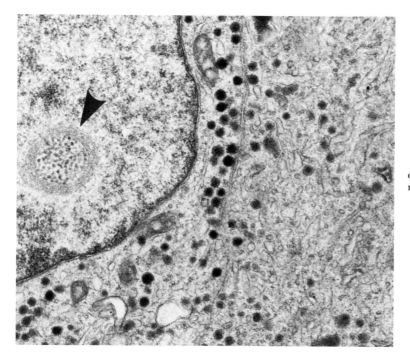

Figure 7–30. Nuclear spheridium *(arrowhead)* in silent adenoma, subtype 3 (×17,200).

various functional states can recognize it if the change is sufficiently pronounced (2,6,78,79). Depending on its degree, pituitary hyperplasia may be dispersed, nodular or diffuse. In dispersed hyperplasia, there is a slight numerical increase of a cell type with normal morphology that does not lead to noticeable changes in tissue architecture. The chance of recognizing this form in an EM specimen is slim. In *nodular hyperplasia,* there is a marked increase in the number of cells within well-circumscribed foci associated with enlargement of the affected pituitary acini. In the nodular form, the morphology of cell types may be different from the normofunctional state. *Diffuse hyperplasia* is marked, advanced hyperplasia, possibly including both dispersed and nodular forms, potentially leading to enlargement of the gland and thus local symptoms.

GH Cell Hyperplasia. A rare cause of acromegaly is GH cell hyperplasia (80) secondary to ectopic production of GHRH secreted by some endocrine tumors of the pancreas, bronchi, or adrenal medulla. A few

such pituitaries have been investigated with EM in the past. Owing to increased awareness of the syndrome, as well as improved detection and removal of the GHRH-producing tumors, clinical cure of the acromegaly with regression of the pituitary lesion is the most likely outcome. Based on the primarily light microscopic studies of a limited number of cases, GHRH-induced GH cell hyperplasia is an intensely acidophilic lesion displaying immunoreactivity for GH or, in some cases, GH and PRL. The pituitary acini in the lateral wings are expanded, containing a larger than normal number of cells. The limited EM experience detected densely granulated GH cells with large secretory granules and an unusually prominent Golgi complex (Fig. 7–31).

The idiopathic form of GH cell hyperplasia leading to childhood gigantism appears to have a different morphological equivalent (81,82). In the two cases observed so far, the enlarged pituitaries contained a hyperplastic lesion comprised of all morphological variants of the acidophil cell line producing GH

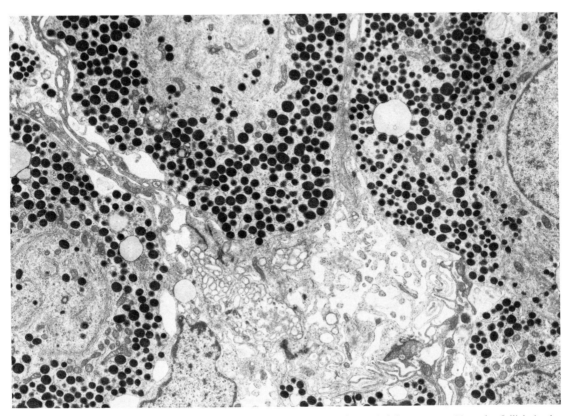

Figure 7–31. GH cell hyperplasia. The GH cells possess large, prominent Golgi apparatus. Note the follicle in the center of the acinus (×5800).

and/or PRL. Many of the cells are chromophobic with masses of RER and only a few small secretory granules. In our experience, the ultrastructural appearance of cells in these unusual hyperplasias does not necessarily reflect their hormone content. Thus, cell identification has to rely on immunoelectron microscopy. The hyperplasia seen in a case of McCune-Albright syndrome was bihormonal as well (83).

PRL Cell Hyperplasia. In addition to the physiological PRL cell hyperplasia during pregnancy and lactation (84), the non-neoplastic proliferation of PRL cells as an accompaniment to various suprasellar space-occupying lesions (e.g., craniopharyngioma, Rathke's cleft cyst, meningioma, sarcoidosis) or to lesions of adenohypophysial origin (corticotroph cell adenoma, TSH cell hyperplasia) is not uncommon (2,6,85,86). Suprasellar masses may cause PRL cell hyperplasia by impinging on the pituitary stalk and blocking or hindering the transport of hypothalamic PRL-inhibiting factors, chiefly dopamine. On the other hand, the cause of PRL cell prolif-

eration is unexplained in cases of Cushing's disease and TSH hyperplasia, especially because PRL cell hyperplasia is not a consistent concomitant of these conditions.

The idiopathic form of PRL cell hyperplasia occurring as a single pathologic lesion in the pituitary and resulting in clinical manifestations of hyperprolactinemia is exceedingly rare (87).

The EM appearance of PRL cell hyperplasia is very similar in all cases (87). The enlarged acini are filled mostly with large, chiefly sparsely granulated PRL cells (Fig. 7–32). The hyperplastic cells reflect signs of enhanced secretory activity such as extensively developed, well-organized RER and large, conspicuous Golgi apparatus harboring numerous spherical or irregular immature secretory granules. The cytoplasmic storage granules are often very sparse, and therefore, granule extrusions may also be infrequent. In a few specimens, we have also encountered a component consisting of hyperplastic, densely granulated PRL cells (Fig. 7–33). At this point, it is not clear whether a

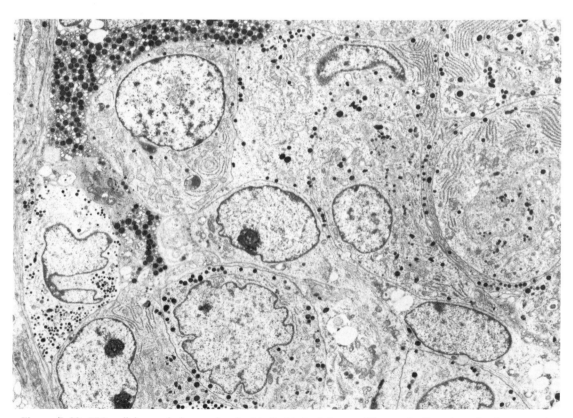

Figure 7–32. PRL cell hyperplasia associated with Rathke's cleft cyst. The markedly enlarged acinus contains predominantly stimulated PRL cells (×3400).

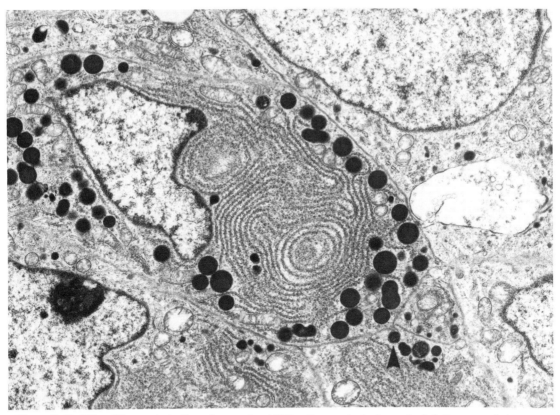

Figure 7–33. PRL cell hyperplasia. Densely granulated PRL cells may also be intermingled. Note extruded secretory granule with uneven matrix *(arrowhead)* (×8800).

densely granulated contingent is always part of the lesion or whether its presence depends on the endocrine milieu within which the hyperplasia develops (e.g., stimulation vs. lack of inhibition).

Corticotroph Hyperplasia. Corticotroph hyperplasia is perhaps the most controversial topic in contemporary pituitary pathology. The role of hyperplasia in the causation of Cushing's disease and even the existence of hyperplasia are hotly debated subjects. It appears that in about 15% of cases, the underlying cause of pituitary-dependent Cushing's disease is not an autonomous adenoma but hyperplasia or a combination of hyperplastic and neoplastic changes (88–92). The condition is notoriously difficult to diagnose in fragmented surgical material. In mild dispersed hyperplasia, the corticotrophs are large and exhibit Crooke's hyaline change. Because of lack of significant changes in tissue architecture, this form may not be recognized in surgical specimens, especially in small EM samples. Most often, the dispersed form coexists with nodular hyperpla-

sia consisting of relatively small, uniform corticotrophs with no significant Crooke's hyalinization within enlarged acini (Fig. 7–34). Diffuse, advanced hyperplasia, characterized by a profusion of proliferating corticotrophs throughout the anterior lobe, is a rare cause of Cushing's disease (93). To our knowledge, no EM study of corticotroph hyperplasia secondary to ectopic corticotroph-releasing hormone production has been performed. Such hyperplasia can be massive leading to enlargement of the gland.

Thyrotroph Hyperplasia. Thyrotroph hyperplasia (2,6,85,94) occurs in patients with long-standing primary hypothyroidism; it may lead to marked enlargement of the pituitary and cause local symptoms. Hyperprolactinemia, amenorrhea and galactorrhea may be associated with the condition, thus mimicking PRL-producing adenoma, for which some of the patients undergo pituitary surgery. Such lesions represent nodular or nodular-diffuse thyrotroph hyperplasia, sometimes also associated with PRL cell hyperplasia. By EM, the hyperplastic thyrotrophs have

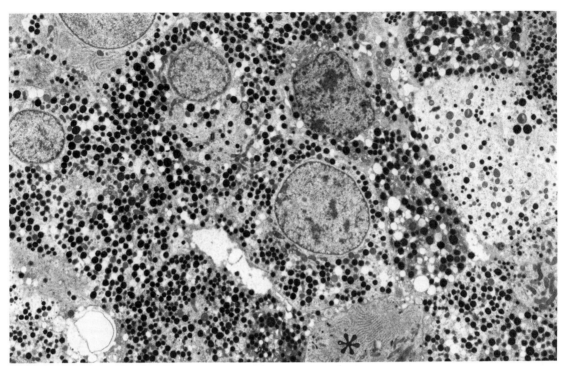

Figure 7–34. Corticotroph cell hyperplasia. The enlarged acinus consists chiefly of relatively small corticotrophs with few type 1 filaments. Part of a stimulated PRL cell is shown *(asterisk)*. PRL cell hyperplasia was also present in this case (×3500).

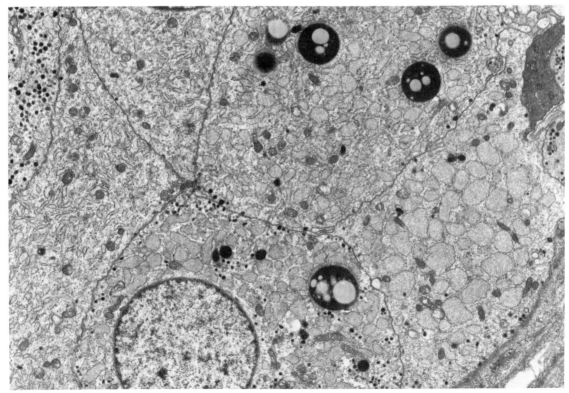

Figure 7–35. Thyrotroph hyperplasia associated with hypothyroidism. Note the typical thyroid deficiency cells with abundant, dilated RER; small, sparse secretory granules and large, dense lysosomes (×6100).

the appearance of so-called "thyroidectomy" or "thyroid deficiency" cells (Fig. 7–35). The large, rounded or polyhedral cells possess a spherical euchromatic nucleus; abundant, dilated RER with low-density proteinaceous content; and prominent Golgi apparatus with numerous vesicles. The degree of dilation of the RER is uniform within the same cell but varies widely from one cell to another. The small (around 250 nm) secretory granules may be quite numerous in the basal portion of the cytoplasm of cells, which show only mild dilation of the RER. With the progression of the thyroidectomy changes, however, the number of secretory granules shows a gradual decline, explaining the often weak thyroid-stimulating hormone–immunoreactivity of these cells.

Gonadotroph Hyperplasia. Gonadotroph hyperplasia is extremely rare and has not yet been reported in surgical material. Unless it is massive, gonadotroph hyperplasia is difficult to recognize, even in autopsy material, since the normal range of gonadotrophs is not established in the human gland. In laboratory animals, the profound stimulation of gonadotrophs due to ablation of gonads results in the enlargement of the cells, progressive proliferation and dilation of RER, prominence of the ring-shaped Golgi apparatus and gradual reduction in the number of secretory granules (gonadectomy cells, castration cells) (1). As incidental findings, gonadectomy cells are also noted in the adenohypophysis of ovariectomized or orchidectomized patients and of postmenopausal women (1). However, a marked enlargement of the gland, similar to that seen in hypothyroidism, is not known to occur.

Acknowledgments

This work was supported in part by grant MA-6349 of the Medical Research Council of Canada. The excellent technical assistance of Mrs. D. Lietz and the invaluable secretarial help of Ms. L. Horvath are gratefully acknowledged.

REFERENCES

1. Horvath E, Kovacs K. Fine structural cytology of the adenohypophysis in rat and man. J Electr Micr Tech 8:401–432, 1988.
2. Kovacs K, Horvath E. Tumors of the pituitary gland. In: Hartmann NH (ed) Atlas of Tumor Pathology. Fascicle XXI. 2nd Series. Washington, DC, Armed Forces Institute of Pathology, 1986, pp 1–264.
3. Kovacs K, Horvath E, Ryan N. Immunocytology of the human pituitary. In: DeLellis RA (ed). Diagnostic Immunohistochemistry. New York, Masson, 1981, pp 17–35.
4. Heitz PU, Landolt AM, Zenklusen HR, Kasper M, Reubi JC, Oberholzer M, Roth J. Immunocytochemistry of pituitary tumors. J Histochem Cytochem 35:1005–1011, 1987.
5. Horvath E, Kovacs K. Pathology of prolactin cell adenomas of the human pituitary. Semin Diagn Pathol 3:4–17, 1986.
6. Horvath E, Kovacs K. The adenohypophysis. In: Kovacs K, Asa SL (eds). Functional Endocrine Pathology. Boston, Blackwell Scientific, 1991, pp 245–281.
7. Horvath E, Kovacs K. Misplaced exocytosis: Distinct ultrastructural feature in some pituitary adenomas. Arch Pathol 97:221–224, 1974.
8. Landolt AM, Rothenbuhler V. Pituitary adenoma calcification. Arch Pathol Lab Med 101:22–27, 1977.
9. Rilliet B, Mohr G, Robert F, Hardy J. Calcification in pituitary adenomas. Surg Neurol 15:249–255, 1981.
10. Saitoh Y, Mori H, Matsumoto K, Ushio Y, Hayakawa T, Mori S, Arita N, Mogami H. Accumulation of amyloid in pituitary adenomas. Acta Neuropathol (Berl) 67:87–92, 1985.
11. Landolt AM, Kleihues P, Heitz PU. Amyloid deposits in pituitary adenomas. Arch Pathol Lab Med 111:453–458, 1987.
12. Horvath E, Kovacs K, Killinger DW, Gonzalez J, Smythe HS. Diverse ultrastructural response to dopamine agonist's medication in human pituitary prolactin cell adenomas. In: Hoshino K (ed). Prolactin Gene Family and Its Receptors. Amsterdam, Elsevier Science, 1988, pp 307–311.
13. Bression D, Brandi AM, Martres MP, Nousbarin A, Cesselin F, Peillon F. Dopaminergic receptors in human prolactin-secreting adenomas: A quantitative study. J Clin Endocrinol Metab 51:1037–1043, 1980.
14. Koga M, Nakao H, Arao M, Sato B, Noma K, Morimoto Y, Kishimoto S, Mori S, Nozumi T. Demonstration of specific dopamine receptors on human pituitary adenomas. Acta Endocrinol 114:595–602, 1987.
15. Tindall GT, Kovacs K, Horvath E, Thorner MO. Human prolactin-producing adenomas and bromocriptine: A histological, immunocytochemical, ultrastructural and morphometric study. J Clin Endocrinol Metab 55:1178–1183, 1982.
16. Bassetti M, Spada A, Pezzo G, Giannattasio G. Bromocriptine treatment reduces the cell size in human macroprolactinomas: A morphometric study. J Clin Endocrinol Metab 58:268–273, 1984.
17. Saitoh Y, Mori S, Arita N, Hagakawa T, Mogani H, Matsumoto K, Mori H. Cytosuppressive effect of bromocriptine on human prolactinomas: Stereological analysis of ultrastructural alterations with special reference to secretory granules. Cancer Res 46:1507–1512, 1986.
18. Schottke H, Saeger W, Ludecke DK, Caselitz J. Ultrastructural morphometry of prolactin-secreting adenomas treated with dopamine agonists. Pathol Res Pract 181:280–290, 1986.
19. Kovacs K, Stefaneanu L, Horvath E, Lloyd RV, Lancranjan I, Buchfelder M, Fahlbusch R. Effect of dopamine agonist medication on prolactin-produc-

ing pituitary adenomas. A morphologic study including immunocytochemistry, electron microscopy and in situ hybridization. Virchows Arch Pathol Anat 418:439–446, 1991.

20. Landolt AM, Osterwalder V. Perivascular fibrosis in prolactinomas: Is it increased by bromocriptine? J Clin Endocrinol Metab 58:1179–1183, 1984.

21. Esiri MM, Bevan JS, Burke CW, Adams CBT. Effect of bromocriptine treatment on the fibrous tissue component of prolactin-secreting and nonfunctioning macroadenomas of the pituitary gland. J Clin Endocrinol Metab 63:383–388, 1986.

22. Killinger DW, Gonzalez J, Horvath E, Kovacs K, Smyth HS. Correlation between preoperative testing and tumour morphology in acromegaly. In: Lamberts SWJ (ed). Sandostatin R in the Treatment of Acromegaly. Berlin, Springer, 1988, pp 9–16.

23. Thorner MO, Frohman LA, Leong DA, Thominet J, Downs T, Hellmann P, Chitwood J, Vaughan JM, Vale W. Extrahypothalamic growth hormone-releasing factor (GRF) secretion is a rare cause of acromegaly: Plasma GRF levels in 177 acromegalic patients. J Clin Endocrinol Metab 59:846–849, 1984.

24. Melmed S, Ezrin C, Kovacs K, Goodman RS, Frohman LA. Acromegaly due to secretion of growth hormone by an ectopic pancreatic islet cell tumor. N Engl J Med 312:9–17, 1985.

25. Trouillas J, Girod C, Lheritier M, Claustrat B, Dubois MP. Morphological and biological relationships in 31 human pituitary adenomas with acromegaly. Virchows Arch Pathol Anat 389:127–142, 1980.

26. Kovacs K, Horvath E. Pathology of growth hormone-producing tumors of the human pituitary. Semin Diagn Pathol 3:18–33, 1986.

27. Scheithauer BW, Kovacs K, Randall RV, Horvath E, Laws ER Jr. Pathology of excessive production of growth hormone. Clin Endocrinol Metab 15:655–681, 1986.

28. Saeger W, Rubenach-Gerz K, Caselitz J, Ludecke DK. Electron microscopical morphometry of GH-producing pituitary adenomas in comparison with normal GH cells. Virchows Arch Pathol Anat 411:467–472, 1987.

29. Neumann PE, Goldman JE, Horoupian DS, Hess MA. Fibrous bodies in growth hormone-secreting adenomas contain cytokeratin filaments. Arch Pathol Lab Med 109:505–508, 1985.

30. Kovacs K, Lloyd RV, Horvath E, Asa SL, Stefaneanu L, Killinger DW, Smyth HS. Silent somatotroph adenomas of the human pituitary. A morphologic study of three cases including immunocytochemistry, electron microscopy, in vitro examination and in situ hybridization. Am J Pathol 134:345–353, 1989.

31. Asa SL, Scheithauer BW, Bilbao JM, Horvath E, Ryan N, Kovacs K, Randall RV, Laws ER Jr, Singer W, Linfoot JA, Thorner MO, Vale W. A case for hypothalamic acromegaly: A clinicopathological study of six patients with hypothalamic gangliocytomas producing growth hormone-releasing factor. J Clin Endocrinol Metab 58:796–803, 1984.

32. Kamel OW, Horoupian DS, Silverberg GD. Mixed gangliocytoma adenoma: A distinct neuroendocrine tumor of the pituitary fossa. Hum Pathol 20:1198–1203, 1989.

33. Li JY, Racadot O, Kujas M, Kouadri M, Peillon F, Racadot J. Immunocytochemistry of four mixed adenomas and intrasellar gangliocytomas associated with different clinical syndromes: Acromegaly,

amenorrhea-galactorrhea, Cushing's disease and isolated tumoral syndrome. Acta Neuropath 77:320–328, 1989.

34. Landolt AM, Ryffel U, Hosbach HU, Wyler R. Ultrastructure of tubular inclusions in endothelial cells of pituitary tumors associated with acromegaly. Virchows Arch Pathol Anat 370:129–140, 1976.

35. George SR, Kovacs K, Asa SL, Horvath E, Cross EG, Burrow GN. Effect of SMS 201-995, a long-acting somatostatin analog, on the secretion and morphology of a pituitary growth hormone cell adenoma. Clin Endocrinol 26:395–405, 1987.

36. Landolt AM, Osterwalder V, Stuckmann G. Preoperative treatment of acromegaly with SMS 201-995: Surgical and pathological observations. In: Ludecke DK, Tolis G (eds). Growth Hormone, Growth Factors, and Acromegaly. New York, Raven, 1987, pp 229–244.

37. Barkan AL, Lloyd RV, Chandler WF, Hatfield MK, Gebarski SS, Kelch RP, Beitins IZ. Preoperative treatment of acromegaly with long-acting somatostatin analog SMS 201-995: Shrinkage of invasive pituitary macroadenomas and improved surgical remission rate. J Clin Endocrinol Metab 67:1040–1048, 1988.

38. Beckers A, Stevenaert A, Kovacs K, Horvath E, Bastings E, Hennen G. The treatment of acromegaly with SMS 201-995. Adv Biosci 69:227–228, 1988.

39. Guyda H, Robert F, Colle E, Hardy J. Histologic, ultrastructural, and hormonal characterization of a pituitary tumor secreting both hGH and prolactin. J Clin Endocrinol Metab 36:531–547, 1973.

40. Corenblum B, Sirek AMT, Horvath E, Kovacs K, Ezrin C. Human mixed somatotrophic and lactotrophic pituitary adenomas. J Clin Endocrinol Metab 42:857–863, 1976.

41. Bassetti M, Spada A, Arosio M, Vallar L, Brina M, Giannattasio G. Morphological studies on mixed growth hormone (GH)- and prolactin (PRL)-secreting human pituitary adenomas. Coexistence of GH and PRL in the same secretory granule. J Clin Endocrinol Metab 62:1093–1100, 1986.

42. Horvath E, Kovacs K, Killinger DW, Smyth HS, Weiss MH, Ezrin C. Mammosomatotroph cell adenoma of the human pituitary: A morphologic entity. Virchows Arch Pathol Anat 398:277–289, 1983.

43. Felix IA, Horvath E, Kovacs K, Smyth HS, Killinger DW, Vale J. Mammosomatotroph adenoma of the pituitary associated with gigantism and hyperprolactinemia. A morphological study including immunoelectron microscopy. Acta Neuropathol (Berl) 71:76–82, 1986.

44. Beckers A, Courtoy R, Stevenaert A, Boniver J, Closset J, Frankenne F, Reznik M, Hennen G. Mammosomatotrophs in human pituitary adenomas as revealed by electron microscopic double gold immunostaining method. Acta Endocrinol (Kbh) 118:503–512, 1988.

45. Horvath E, Kovacs K, Singer W, Smyth HS, Killinger DW, Ezrin C, Weiss MH. Acidophil stem cell adenoma of the human pituitary: Clinico-pathological analysis of 15 cases. Cancer 47:761–771, 1981.

46. Mori H, Mori S, Saitoh Y, Moriwaki K, Iida S, Matsumoto K. Growth hormone-producing pituitary adenoma with crystal-like amyloid immunohistochemically positive for growth hormone. Cancer 55:96–102, 1985.

47. Saeger W. Morphology of ACTH-producing pituitary tumors. In: Fahlbusch R, Werder KV (eds).

Treatment of Pituitary Adenomas. Stuttgart, Thieme, 1978, pp 122–130.

48. Robert F, Hardy J. Human corticotroph cell adenomas. Semin Diagn Pathol 3:34–41, 1986.

49. Neumann PE, Horoupian DS, Goldman JE, Hess MA. Cytoplasmic filaments of Crooke's hyaline change belong to the cytokeratin class. An immunocytochemical and ultrastructural study. Am J Pathol 116:214–222, 1984.

50. Horvath E, Kovacs K. Pituitary and adrenal pathology in Cushing's disease/syndrome. In: Ludecke DK, Chrousos GP, Tolis G (eds). ACTH, Cushing's Syndrome and Other Hypercortisolemic States. New York, Raven, 1990, pp 137–145.

51. Halliday WC, Asa SL, Kovacs K, Scheithauer BW. Intermediate filaments in the human pituitary gland: An immunohistochemical study. Can J Neurol Sci 17:131–136, 1990.

52. Horvath E, Kovacs K, Josse R. Pituitary corticotroph cell adenoma with marked abundance of microfilaments. Ultrastruct Pathol 5:249–255, 1983.

53. Felix IA, Horvath E, Kovacs K. Massive Crooke's hyalinization in corticotroph cell adenomas of the human pituitary. A histological, immunocytological and electron microscopic study of three cases. Acta Neurochir (Wien) 58:235–243, 1982.

54. Afrasiabi A, Valenta L, Gwinup GA. A TSH-secreting pituitary tumour causing hyperthyroidism: Presentation of a case and review of the literature. Acta Endocrinol (Kbh) 92:448–454, 1979.

55. Katz MS, Gregerman RI, Horvath E, Kovacs K, Ezrin C. Thyrotroph cell adenoma of the human pituitary gland associated with primary hypothyroidism: Clinical and morphological features. Acta Endocrinol (Khb) 95:41–48, 1980.

56. Saeger W, Ludecke DK. Pituitary adenomas with hyperfunction of TSH. Frequency, histological classification, immunocytochemistry and ultrastructure. Virchows Arch Pathol Anat 394:255–267, 1982.

57. Girod C, Trouillas J, Claustrat B. The human thyrotropic adenoma: Pathologic diagnosis in five cases and critical review of the literature. Semin Diagn Pathol 3:58–68, 1986.

58. Kovacs K, Horvath E, Van Loon GR, Rewcastle NB, Ezrin C, Rosenbloom AA. Pituitary adenomas associated with elevated blood follicle-stimulating hormone levels. A histologic, immunocytologic and electron microscopic study of two cases. Fertil Steril 29:622–628, 1978.

59. Kovacs K, Horvath E, Rewcastle NB, Ezrin C. Gonadotroph cell adenoma of the human pituitary in woman with long-standing hypogonadism. Arch Gynaecol 299:57–65, 1980.

60. Horvath E, Kovacs K. Gonadotroph adenomas of the human pituitary: Sex-related fine structural dichotomy. A histologic, immunocytochemical and electron microscopic study of 30 tumors. Am J Pathol 117:429–440, 1984.

61. Murray IC, McComb DJ, Horvath E, Kovacs K. Morphometric evidence of sexual dimorphism in the ultrastructure of gonadotroph adenomas of human pituitary. Ultrastruct Pathol 8:49–56, 1985.

62. Kontogeorgos G, Horvath E, Kovacs K. Sex-linked ultrastructural dichotomy of gonadotroph adenomas of the human pituitary. An electron microscopic analysis of 145 tumors. Ultrastruct Pathol 14:475–482, 1990.

63. Trouillas J, Girod C, Sassolas G, Claustrat B, Lheritier M, Dubois MP, Goutelle A. Human pituitary gonadotropic adenoma: Histological, immunocytochemical, ultrastructural and hormonal studies in 8 cases. J Pathol 135:315–336, 1981.

64. Trouillas J, Girod C, Sassolas G, Claustrat B. The human gonadotropic adenoma: Pathologic diagnosis and hormonal correlations in 26 tumors. Semin Diagn Pathol 3:42–57, 1986.

65. Holck S, Albrechtsen R, Weever UM. Laminin in the anterior pituitary gland of the rat. Laminin in the gonadotrophic cells correlates with their functional state. Lab Invest 56:481–488, 1987.

66. Kovacs K, Horvath E, Ryan N, Ezrin C. Null cell adenoma of the human pituitary. Virchows Arch Pathol Anat 387:165–174, 1980.

67. Jameson JL, Klibanski A, Black P McL, Zervas NT, Lindell CM, Hsu DW, Ridgway EC, Habener JF. Glycoprotein hormone genes are expressed in clinically nonfunctioning pituitary adenomas. J Clin Invest 80:1472–1478, 1987.

68. Kovacs K, Asa SL, Horvath E, Ryan N, Singer W, Killinger DW, Smyth HS, Scheithauer BW, Ebersold MJ. Null cell adenomas of the pituitary: Attempts to resolve their cytogenesis. In: Lechago J, Kameya T (eds). Endocrine Pathology Update. Philadelphia, Field and Wood Publishers, 1990, pp 17–31.

69. Yamada S, Asa SL, Kovacs K, Muller P, Smyth HS. Analysis of hormone secretion by clinically nonfunctioning human pituitary adenomas using the reverse hemolytic plaque assay. J Clin Endocrinol Metab 68:73–80, 1989.

70. Sakurai T, Seo H, Yamamoto N, Nagaya T, Nakane T, Kuwayama A, Kageyama N, Matsui M. Detection of mRNA of prolactin and ACTH in clinically nonfunctioning pituitary adenomas. J Neurosurg 69:653–659, 1988.

71. Asa SL, Gerrie BM, Singer W, Horvath E, Kovacs K, Smyth HS. Gonadotropin secretion in vitro by human pituitary null cell adenomas and oncocytomas. J Clin Endocrinol Metab 62:1011–1019, 1986.

72. Yamada S, Asa SL, Kovacs K. Oncocytomas and null cell adenomas of the human pituitary: Morphometric and in vitro functional comparison. Virchows Arch Pathol Anat 413:333–339, 1988.

73. Kovacs K, Horvath E, Bayley TA, Hassaram ST, Ezrin E. Silent corticotroph cell adenoma with lysosomal accumulation and crinophagy: A distinct clinicopathologic entity. Am J Med 64:492–499, 1978.

74. Horvath E, Kovacs K, Killinger DW, Smyth HS, Platts ME, Singer W. Silent corticotropic adenomas of the human pituitary gland: A histologic, immunocytologic and ultrastructural study. Am J Pathol 98:617–638, 1980.

75. Serri O, Robert F, Pelletier G, Beauregard H, Hardy J. Hyperprolactinemia associated with clinically silent adenomas: Endocrinologic and pathologic studies; a report of two cases. Fertil Steril 47:792–796, 1987.

76. Lloyd RV, Fields K, Jin L, Horvath E, Kovacs K. Analysis of endocrine active and clinically silent corticotropic adenomas by in situ hybridization. Am J Pathol 137:479–488, 1990.

77. Horvath E, Kovacs K, Smyth HS, Killinger DW, Scheithauer BW, Randall R, Laws ER Jr, Singer W. A novel type of pituitary adenoma: Morphological features and clinical correlations. J Clin Endocrinol Metab 66:1111–1118, 1988.

78. Saeger W, Ludecke DK. Pituitary hyperplasia. Definition, light and electron microscopic structures and

significance in surgical specimens. Virchows Arch Pathol Anat *399:*277–287, 1983.

79. Horvath E. Pituitary hyperplasia. Path Res Pract *183:*623–625, 1988.

80. Thorner MO, Perryman RL, Cronin MJ, Rogol AD, Draznin M, Johanson A, Vale W, Horvath E, Kovacs K. Somatotroph hyperplasia. J Clin Invest *70:*965–977, 1982.

81. Moran A, Asa SL, Kovacs K, Horvath E, Singer W, Sagman U, Reubi JC, Wilson C, Larson R, Pescovitz OH. Gigantism due to pituitary mammosomatotroph hyperplasia. N Engl J Med *323:*322–326, 1990.

82. Zimmerman D, Young WF Jr, Ebersold MJ, Whitaker MD, Scheithauer BW, Kovacs K, Downs TR, Frohman LA. Gigantism due to growth hormone-releasing hormone (GRH) excess and pituitary hyperplasia with adenomatous transformation. Proc Endocr Soc Abstract No. 1581, p. 426, 1991.

83. Kovacs K, Horvath E, Thorner MO, Rogol AD. Mammosomatotroph hyperplasia associated with acromegaly and hyperprolactinemia in a patient with the McCune-Albright syndrome. A histologic, immunocytologic and ultrastructural study of the surgically-removed adenohypophysis. Virchows Arch Pathol Anat *403:*77–86, 1984.

84. Scheithauer BW, Sano T, Kovacs KT, Young WF Jr, Ryan N, Randall RV. The pituitary gland in pregnancy: A clinicopathologic and immunohistochemical study of 69 cases. Mayo Clin Proc *65:*461–474, 1990.

85. Pioro EP, Scheithauer BW, Laws ER Jr, Randall RV, Kovacs K, Horvath E. Combined thyrotroph and lactotroph cell hyperplasia simulating prolactin-secreting pituitary adenoma in long-standing primary hypothyroidism. Surg Neurol *29:*218–226, 1988.

86. Wowra B, Peiffer J. An immunoperoxidase study of a human pituitary adenoma associated with Cushing's syndrome. Pathol Res Pract *178:*349–354, 1984.

87. Jay V, Kovacs K, Horvath E, Lloyd RV, Smyth HS. Idiopathic prolactin cell hyperplasia of the pituitary mimicking prolactin cell adenoma. A morphologic study including immunocytochemistry, electron microscopy and *in situ* hybridization. Acta Neuropathol (Wien) *82:*147–151, 1991.

88. Lamberts SWJ, Stefanko SZ, DeLange SA, Fermin H, Van der Vijver JCM, Weber RFA, DeJong FH. Failure of clinical remission after trans-sphenoidal removal of a microadenoma in a patient with Cushing's disease: Multiple hyperplastic and adenomatous cell nests in surrounding pituitary tissue. J Clin Endocrinol Metab *50:*793–795, 1980.

89. McNicol AM. Patterns of corticotropic cells in the adult human pituitary in Cushing's disease. Diagn Histopathol *4:*335–341, 1981.

90. McKeever PE, Koppelman MC, Metcalf D, Quindlen E, Kornblith PL, Strott CA, Howard R, Smith BH. Refractory Cushing's disease caused by multinodular ACTH-cell hyperplasia. J Neuropathol Expt Neurol *41:*490–499, 1982.

91. Lloyd RV, Chandler WF, McKeever PE, Schteingart DE. The spectrum of ACTH-producing pituitary lesions. Am J Surg Pathol *10:*618–626, 1986.

92. Young WF Jr, Scheithauer BW, Gharib H, Laws ER Jr, Carpenter PC. Cushing's syndrome due to primary multinodular corticotrope hyperplasia. Mayo Clin Proc *63:*256–262, 1988.

93. Schnall AM, Kovacs K, Brodkey JS, Pearson OH. Pituitary Cushing's disease without adenoma. Acta Endocrinol (Kbh) *94:*297–303, 1980.

94. Khalil A, Kovacs K, Sima AAF, Burrow GN, Horvath E. Pituitary thyrotroph hyperplasia mimicking prolactin-secreting adenoma. J Endocrinol Invest *7:*399–404, 1984.

Chapter

8

MOLECULAR BIOLOGICAL ANALYSIS OF PITUITARY DISORDERS

Ricardo V. Lloyd

Advances in recombinant DNA technology have contributed immensely to the study and diagnosis of pituitary disorders. A wide variety of molecular biological analyses have been used in the study of pituitary diseases; these include Southern and Northern analyses of DNA and RNA, respectively. Some of the techniques that have had the greatest impact in molecular diagnostic pathology include *in situ* hybridization and the polymerase chain reaction (PCR) for amplification and analysis of DNA and RNA.

HYBRIDIZATION METHODS

Various hybridization techniques for the study of endocrine tissues have been described. During nucleic acid hybridization, complementary sequences of bases form hydrogen bonds resulting in stable complexes or hybrids. If one of the nucleic acid strands is used as a probe and labeled with radioactive or nonradioactive materials, the hybridization product can be readily detected by various methods. The most commonly used hybridization methods include (1) solution hybridization, in which the association of nucleic acids in a liquid state is analyzed; (2) filter hybridization, such as Southern and Northern blots, in which the DNA and RNA are immobilized to an inert support such as nitrocellulose or nylon membrane and reacted with the probe (1–3) and (3) *in situ*

hybridization (ISH), which relies on the hybridization reaction occurring in cytological or histological preparations (Fig. 8–1) (4–7).

For morphologists, there are many advantages of using ISH for the study of pituitary gene expression. Because the probe hybridizes to the mRNAs fixed *in situ* within cells, the relationship of cells expressing specific gene products to other cells can be readily detected. A combination of ISH analysis and immunochemistry can localize both the transcribed gene product or mRNA and the translated protein product in the same cell.

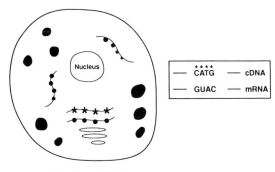

Pituitary Cell

Figure 8–1. Schematic diagram showing the localization of specific messenger RNA in a pituitary cell by *in situ* hybridization. The cDNA probe can be labeled with a radioactive or a nonradioactive detection system. The specific subtypes of mRNAs are localized in the cytoplasm. This localization is dependent on the specificity of the probe.

TISSUE PREPARATION AND PROCESSING FOR ISH

Many analytical studies have been done to optimize tissue processing, including fixation and storage, for nucleic acid preservation (7,8). Nucleic acids are better preserved in frozen tissue sections than in paraffin-embedded tissues. After fixation in liquid nitrogen, tissues can be stored at $-70°C$ for more than 1 year with good preservation of RNA. Dehydration is decreased if the specimens are embedded before freezing. Formalin-fixed, paraffin-embedded tissues provide satisfactory results for ISH to localize DNA and RNA (9–11). The signal detected in localizing mRNA is less intense in paraffin sections compared with that detected in frozen tissue sections. Archival material has been used successfully to localize mRNA after 10 or more years of storage (9). The studies by Singer *et al.* (7) have shown that paraformaldehyde is an excellent fixative for preserving mRNA, although adequate signals can be obtained from tissue fixed with other cross-linking fixatives such as glutaraldehyde. Relatively poor RNA preservation is obtained with acetic acid/ethanol and related fixatives.

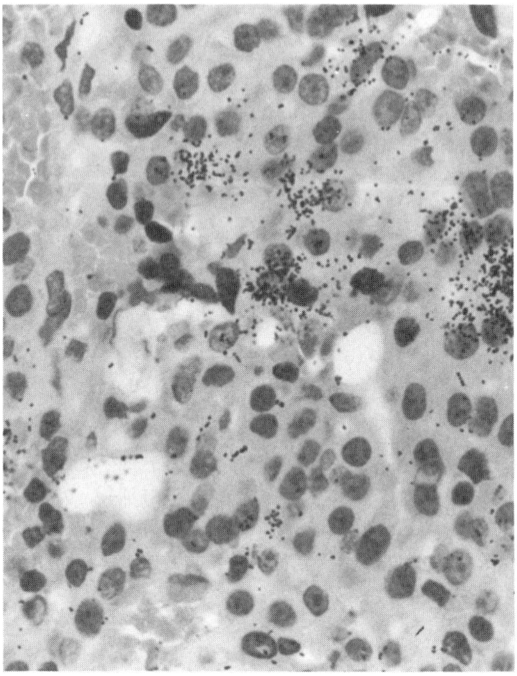

Figure 8–2. *In situ* hybridization localizing PRL mRNA in the normal pituitary with a ^{35}S-labeled oligonucleotide probe. After autoradiography, the cells with PRL mRNA are represented by the black silver grains over specific cells ($\times 350$).

PROBES

The types of probes commonly available for hybridization studies include cDNA and cRNA probes (12,13). Synthetic oligonucleotide cDNA and cRNA probes generated by automated synthesizers are commonly used (14–16). Oligonucleotide probes probably penetrate into cells more readily and produce excellent hybridization signals (Fig. 8–2). A major advantage of oligonucleotide probes is that once a specific gene has been cloned and sequenced, large amounts of the probe can be synthesized and the same reagent used for many experiments.

Complementary RNA probes, or riboprobes, are frequently used for ISH studies also (13,17). These cRNA, or antisense, probes form stable hybrids with cellular RNA. In addition, the background signal or nonspecific binding can be reduced with the use of the enzyme ribonuclease (RNase) A, which digests single-stranded, but not double-stranded, RNA hybrids. The corresponding sense probe represents the ideal control when using asymmetric riboprobes.

SIGNAL DETECTION

Probes can be linked to radioactive or nonradioactive signal detectors to localize the nucleic acid hybrids after hybridization. Radioactive signal detectors include ^{32}P-, ^{35}S-, ^{125}I-, and ^{3}H-labeled nucleotides. Biotinylated probes are the most popular nonradioactive ones, although mercurated, fluorescent-labeled, and other nonradioactive probes have also been described (18–24). Radioactive probes are very sensitive, and experimental results with these probes can be readily quantified. Disadvantages of radioactive probes include the hazards associated with radioactive materials, the long period of signal development, and the need for autoradiographic supplies and a darkroom. The relatively short half-life of some radionuclides, such as ^{32}P, presents a significant problem with probe stability.

Biotinylated and other nonradioactive probes are ideally suited for the diagnostic pathology laboratory because of their long shelf lives and excellent resolution in tissue sections (Fig. 8–3). One disadvantage of bio-

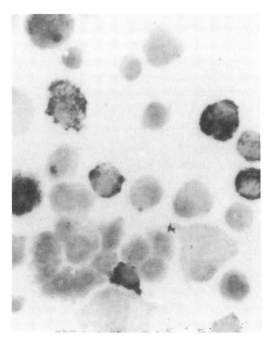

Figure 8–3. *In situ* hybridization localizing GH mRNA in cultured pituitary cells using a biotinylated oligonucleotide probe. After hybridization, the positive signal is detected by reacting the tissues with alkaline phosphatase followed by nitroblue tetrazolium and 5-bromo-4-chloro-3-indolylphosphate (×350).

tinylated and other nonradioactive probes remains the lower degree of sensitivity compared with radioactive signal detectors. To localize mRNA present in low abundance, i.e., few copy numbers of mRNA per cell, radioactive probes remain the method of choice. With newer developments to enhance the detection system, such as the use of photobiotinylated probes (18) and silver enhancement, the sensitivity of these nonradioactive techniques should continue to improve.

CONTROLS NECESSARY FOR *IN SITU* HYBRIDIZATION STUDIES

Numerous controlled studies should be performed routinely with ISH analyses. These can include (1) pretreatment of cells or tissues with RNase or DNase where appropriate, which should abate the hybridization signal; (2) substitution of an irrelevant nucleic acid probe that does not bind the target nucleic acid of interest; (3) Northern or Southern blot analysis to characterize the molecular sizes of the nucleic acid of interest; (4) localization of the translated protein prod-

uct along with the transcribed RNA product in the same tissue section; and (5) use of a sense probe when using riboprobes or oligonucleotide probes.

PITFALLS IN THE INTERPRETATION OF *IN SITU* HYBRIDIZATION STUDIES

The technical difficulties involved in performing ISH may lead to problems with false-negative and false-positive results. RNase contamination can diminish or even abolish the hybridization signal when an RNA probe is used or detection of tissue RNA is attempted. Ensuring RNase-free conditions, including the use of gloves during the ISH procedure, can help to decrease such problems. Contamination of enzymes or other reagents with nucleases that may degrade the probe or tissue nucleic acids can be avoided by using high-quality reagents.

The specificity of the probes must be rigorously evaluated, especially when using short oligonucleotides as probes. Each individual probe must be evaluated to learn about its specificity. The use of high-stringency (elevated temperatures or low-salt concentration) conditions for hybridization and during posthybridization washing helps to reduce cross-hybridization.

Positive and negative chemography (the creation of reduced crystals in the emulsion or the removal of latent images by chemicals present in the specimen during autoradiography) may occur with the use of radioactive probes. The presence of endogenous biotin, which appears to be more abundant in frozen tissue sections than in paraffin sections (e.g., kidney and liver), can lead to false-positive interpretations with the use of biotinylated probes. Likewise, endogenous alkaline phosphatase can also lead to false-positive interpretations when using alkaline phosphatase methods for signal detection. Levamisole can aid in reducing endogenous alkaline phosphatase in some tissues (25).

APPLICATIONS OF *IN SITU* HYBRIDIZATION

Use of Broad-Spectrum Probes

Many broad-spectrum neuroendocrine markers can be identified with specific antibodies

(26). These include chromogranins, synaptophysin, protein 7B2, neuron-specific enolase, and protein gene product 9.5 (PGP 9.5). Many of these are present in the pituitary gland. With advances in molecular endocrine biology, the cDNA clones and derived mRNA and protein sequences for many hormone gene products have been analyzed. Such studies have shown that there is usually one mRNA species that may be processed into various protein products. Examples include the mRNA for proopiomelanocortin that is processed into adrenocorticotropic hormone (ACTH), β-endorphin, melanocyte-stimulating hormone, lipotropins, and several other biologically active peptides (27).

The chromogranins are a complex family of proteins, with the predominant forms known as chromogranin A and B and secretogranin II. Chromogranin A is an important marker in diagnostic pathology (30,31). For diagnostic purposes, ISH can be used to detect the intact mRNA for chromogranin A that contains the sequence for both pancreastatin and betagranin. This mRNA is present in most endocrine tissues with secretory granules, including anterior pituitary cells and tumors. For experimental and analytical purposes, specific antibodies against various fragments of the chromogranins or nucleic acid probes for specific chromogranins can be extremely useful.

Oncogene and Growth Factor Expression in the Pituitary

Analysis of oncogenes and growth factors in the pituitary gland remains largely a research tool but has provided new information about the regulation of pituitary cells. The stimulation of specific oncogene products by hypothalamic releasing hormones has been analyzed in the rat model. For example, growth hormone releasing hormone (GHRH) has been shown to induce c-*fos* expression in cultured primary pituitary cells (32). These studies showed that the mitogenic effect of GHRH was mediated through rapid induction of c-*fos* mRNA synthesis. The GH_3 tumor cell line has also been used to examine regulation of oncogene expression. Thyrotropin releasing hormone stimulated c-*fos* mRNA in GH_3/B_6 tumor cells (33), while the somatostatin analogue octreotide inhibited cell pro-

liferation as well as c-*myc* and c-*fos* mRNA levels (33).

The role of growth factors in the regulation of human pituitary cell growth and differentiation has been analyzed by various investigators (35–42). Growth factors are polypeptide molecules that can stimulate cell proliferation and modulate cell differentiation. Growth factors that have been found to be expressed in the pituitary gland include epidermal growth factor (EGF), transforming growth factor (TGF), thyroid hormone–inducible growth factor, insulin-like growth factors (IGF I and IGF II), chrondrocyte growth factor, mammary cell growth factor, folliculo-stellate–derived growth factor, nerve growth factor (NGF), adrenal growth factor and fibroblast growth factor (FGF).

EGF receptors have been found in human pituitary cells (36). While EGF binding was readily detected in normal human pituitary tissues, it was not present in any of the 22 adenomas analyzed in one study. The reason for the lack of EGF binding in adenomas was not apparent in this study, but the possibility of an altered c-*erb*-B proto-oncogene, which normally encodes the wild type EGF receptor, has been proposed as a reason to account for the attenuated EGF binding (35,36). Basic fibroblast growth factor (bFGF), which is an angiogenic factor and a mitogen for many mesoderm-derived cells, has been localized in the bovine pituitary gland (37). In an analysis of bFGF in human pituitaries, Silverlight *et al.* found immunoreactive bFGF in normal pituitary gland tissues, but 41 adenomas that were examined contained less FGF than normal tissues (38). These investigators found that FGF inhibited growth of cultured human pituitary adenoma cells and postulated that the reduction in bFGF in many pituitary tumors may favor the stimulation of pituitary growth (39).

IGFs have been studied extensively in the pituitary by hybridization analyses (40–42). The IGFs are highly homologous with proinsulin and share metabolic properties with insulin, including growth stimulation and metabolic effects. While the physiological functions of IGF II in adult tissues are unknown, IGF I, or somatomedin C, has been found in normal rat and neoplastic rat pituitary tumor cells. IGF I appears to participate in endocrine and paracrine pathways in the regulation of growth hormone (GH). IGF I in the pituitary may also be under the control of GH (42).

Hybridization Studies of the Pituitary

Analysis and characterization of the normal human pituitary gland by *in situ* and Northern hybridization have relied on the use of autopsy tissues (see Fig. 8–2). Some studies have shown that there is no significant degradation of abundant RNAs such as those for pituitary hormones within the first 8 hours post mortem (43). Analysis of GH- and prolactin (PRL)-producing adenomas has shown that tumors from patients with a clinical diagnosis of acromegaly frequently express PRL mRNA, in addition to GH mRNA, whereas tumors from most patients with a clinical diagnosis of prolactinoma have only PRL mRNA in the tumors (43). These observations fit with other studies using transgenic mice that have shown that GH cells in the developing fetus are precursors for most PRL cells (44), suggesting that the PRL cell represents the final stage of differentiation of acidophil cells in the anterior pituitary. ISH studies of some acidophilic pituitary tumors from patients without acromegaly have helped to characterize a silent GH-producing adenoma subtype. Although these tumors contain some immunoreactive GH as well as the mRNA for this hormone, there is only a minimal serum elevation of GH, and these patients do not have acromegaly (45).

ACTH-producing adenomas have been studied by ISH by various investigators (46, 47). Clinically active adenomas consistently express the mRNA for proopiomelanocortin (POMC) as determined by ISH and Northern analysis. However, there were significant differences in POMC mRNA expression in the subtypes of silent corticotroph adenomas. Subtype 1 neoplasms are morphologically and ultrastructurally similar to adenomas associated with Cushing's disease and Nelson's syndrome, but patients do not have ACTH or cortisol excess. POMC mRNA was readily detected in paraffin sections in this subtype of tumors. The subtype 2 tumor, which has smaller secretory granules than the type 1 or clinically active tumors, and subtype 3 tumors, which are more varied, did not usually have significant levels of POMC mRNA, thus suggesting decreased expression of POMC gene products (46). Northern hybridization analysis on one silent adenoma showed that the size of the POMC mRNA was similar to that of the clinically active tumor (47).

Other clinically silent adenomas, including null cell adenomas, have been studied with molecular biological techniques by various investigators. Clinically non-functional tumors often contain proteins and gene products for FSH and LH and for other pituitary hormones (48–53). Although immunohistochemistry can readily detect protein and glycoprotein hormone products, in some cases the mRNA may be detected when very little immunoreactive protein is present, as in one study of clinically non-functional adenomas that had PRL and ACTH mRNA, even though these hormones were not detected by immunohistochemistry (52). A hybridization analysis of null cell adenomas, oncocytomas and gonadotroph adenomas showed a striking similarity with respect to gene products for glycoprotein hormone expression in the null cell and gonadotroph adenomas. Few oncocytomas expressed the mRNAs for glycoprotein hormones. Interestingly, all three groups of tumors expressed the mRNA for chromogranin A, which is the principal secretory granule protein in many pituitary cells (53).

Southern Blot Hybridization

DNA analysis by Southern blot hybridization is commonly used to analyze inherited patterns of specific genes and to detect gene deletion. Analysis has shown that GH deficiency, which is associated with dwarfism, may be related to numerous causes. In some rare conditions, deletion of the GH gene can occur as an inherited condition and is known as isolated GH deficiency type 1A (54,55). Patients often have clinical features of GH deficiency and anti-GH antibodies in the serum. Southern hybridization analysis of families with GH deficiency type 1A often reveals that parents may have only one copy of one GH1 gene with only fragments of the GH1 functional GH gene and the variant GH gene (GH2), which has various mutations that impair normal gene function. If the parents are heterozygotes, the offspring may have only the mutated defective GH gene (54,55). This use of DNA from blood leukocytes with restriction enzyme digestion and Southern hybridization analysis can readily lead to the characterization of the pattern of GH deficiency in this subset of individuals.

CLONAL ORIGIN OF PITUITARY ADENOMAS

Molecular analysis has been used to investigate the clonality of pituitary adenomas.

Restriction fragment length polymorphism (RFLP) and allelic X-chromosome inactivation are the two most commonly used methods of analysis in these investigations (56–58). Clonal analysis by X-chromosome inactivation relies on the Lyon hypothesis, which states that in females, there is inactivation of either the maternal or paternal X chromosome as a random process that occurs during early embryogenesis. Progeny cells will retain the X-inactivated pattern of their progenitor cells. This activation of genes on the X chromosome is associated with methylation changes of cytosine nucleotides that can be stably transmitted to progeny cells. RFLP analysis relies on the digestion of DNA by specific endonucleases. X-linked loci such as the phosphoglycerate kinase (PGK) and hypoxanthine phosphoribosyl transferase (HPRT) genes are used to compare X-inactivation patterns from patients' control blood leukocytes with those from their pituitary adenomas. The polymorphic rates of PGK and HPRT are 27% and 31%, respectively. After digestion with the endonucleases, the relative proportion of active maternal and paternal X-linked alleles can be determined by DNA hybridization and autoradiography. Cells with a monoclonal origin have identical X-inactivation patterns with only one band after digestion with a methylation-sensitive enzyme such as *Hpa* II, while polyclonal tissues with random and balanced X-inactivation patterns have two bands after *Hpa* II digestion, and the bands have reduced intensity because the maternal and paternal alleles are equally represented.

In one analysis of three pituitary tumors, including a mixed PRL cell–GH cell adenoma, one adenoma producing gonadotropin hormones and a third tumor without immunoreactive hormones, all three adenomas were monoclonal in origin. In another study by Herman *et al.* (58), 3 of 3 GH adenomas, 4 of 4 prolactin adenomas, 3 of 4 corticotroph adenomas, a gonadotroph adenoma and a nonsecretory adenoma were all monoclonal. Polyclonal adenomas included a plurihormonal adenoma and one corticotroph adenoma, which also contained normal pituitary tissues. Monoclonal X inactivation has also been found in six clinically nonfunctioning pituitary tumors analyzed by Alexander *et al.* (56). These studies all indicate that a somatic cell mutation precedes clonal expansion of proliferating neoplastic cells

and suggest that these mutations may play a role in the development of pituitary tumors.

MOLECULAR BIOLOGICAL ANALYSIS BY TARGET AMPLIFICATION

The use of DNA amplification by the PCR has had a profound impact in diagnostic and investigative pathology, including studies of the pituitary gland. With the PCR reaction, small amounts of DNA present in a sample can be amplified up to a million-fold, and the final reaction product can be analyzed by Southern hybridization and ethidium bromide staining methods (59,60). The target DNA can be isolated from cells, or DNA can be generated from isolated RNA by reverse transcriptase. Primers, or short fragments of oligonucleotides of about 20 bases, complementary to the known DNA sequence, are synthesized and added to the target DNA sample with DNA polymerase such as heat-stable Taq DNA polymerase isolated from the thermophilic bacterium *Thermus aquaticus.* The primers hybridize to the target and provide a starting point for the polymerase to begin synthesizing a second strand of DNA. After synthesis is completed, the DNA is heated to denature the two strands, then cooled to allow re-annealing of the primers. Repeat of the PCR cycle for 20 to 25 cycles results in a specific target sequence that is greatly amplified and can be readily detected by the conventional Southern technique. Because of the sensitivity of the technique, cross-hybridization and general contamination with other DNAs must be carefully avoided.

PCR analysis has been applied to the study of pituitary adenomas. For example, analyses have shown that some GH-secreting pituitary adenomas contain mutant forms of the α-chain of the guanine nucleotide–binding protein, G_s, which stabilizes the protein in the active conformation by inhibiting its intrinsic guanosine triphosphatase (GTPase) activity (61,62). Patients with this mutation often have hypersecretory activity with densely granulated cells containing prominent rough endoplasmic reticulum and Golgi complexes. These tumors were also smaller than those without the mutations, and further analyses suggest that this size difference may be due to the increased sensitivity of these tumors to inhibitory agents such as somatostatin and dopamine, which may counteract the expression of the activating mutation (62).

Landis *et al.* used the PCR technique to characterize the G$_s$ mutant proteins in GH adenomas and found that point mutations occurred at two critical sites, arginine 201 and glycine 227 (63,64). G$_s$ mutations were present in 40% of 25 GH tumors. Patients with the mutations in their adenomas had smaller tumors at the time of surgery and lower serum GH levels (63). In an analysis of a larger group of pituitary adenomas, the mutation was seen only in GH tumors and not in PRL, thyroid-stimulating hormone (TSH), ACTH or clinically nonfunctional adenomas (64). These and other studies have suggested that the G$_s$ mutation in GH pituitary adenomas may arise from a shared oncogenic mechanism (61–64).

● ● ●

The use of molecular biological techniques in the analysis of pituitary adenomas is in its infancy, and with continued developments in molecular techniques and applications to the study of the pituitary gland, a great increase in the understanding of pituitary biology can be anticipated.

REFERENCES

1. Alwine JC, Kemp DJ, Parker BA, Reiser J, Renart J, Stark GR, Wahl GM. Detection of specific RNAs or specific fragments of DNA by fractionation in gels and transfer to diazobenzyloxymethyl paper. Methods Enzymol 68:220–242, 1979.
2. Thomas PS. Hybridization of denatured RNA and small DNA fragments transferred to nitrocellulose. Proc Natl Acad Sci USA 77:5201–5205, 1980.
3. Southern EM. Detection of specific sequences among DNA fragments separated by gel electrophoresis. J Mol Biol 98:503–517, 1975.
4. Gee CE, Roberts JL. *In situ* hybridization histochemistry; a technique for the study of gene expression in single cells. DNA 2:157–163, 1983.
5. Lawrence JB, Singer RH. Quantitative analysis of *in situ* hybridization methods for the detection of actin gene expression. Nucleic Acids Res 13:1777–1799, 1985.
6. Wilcox JN, Gee CE, Roberts JL. *In situ* cDNA:mRNA hybridization: Development of a technique to measure mRNA levels in individual cells. Methods Enzymol 124:510–533, 1986.
7. Singer RH, Lawrence JB, Villnave C. Optimization of *in situ* hybridization using isotopic and non-isotopic detection methods. Biotechniques 4:230–259, 1986.
8. Lloyd RV, Cano M, Landefeld TD. The effects of estrogens on tumor growth and on prolactin and growth hormone mRNA expression in rat pituitary tissues. Am J Pathol 133:397–406, 1988.
9. Hankin RC, Lloyd RV. Detection of messenger RNA in routinely processed tissue sections with biotinylated oligonucleotide probes. Am J Clin Pathol 92:166–171, 1989.
10. Lloyd RV, Iacangelo A, Eiden LE, Cano M, Jin L, Grimes M. Chromogranin A and B messenger ribonucleic acids in pituitary and other normal and neoplastic human endocrine tissues. Lab Invest 60:548–556, 1989.
11. Morley DJ, Hodes ME. *In situ* localization of amylase mRNA and protein: An investigation of amylase gene activity in normal human parotid gland. J Histochem Cytochem 35:9–14, 1987.
12. Coghlan JP, Aldred P, Haralambidis J, Niall HD, Penschow JD, Tregear GW. Hybridization histochemistry. Anal Biochem 149:1–28, 1985.
13. Cox KH, De Leon DV, Angerer LM, Angerer RC. Detection of mRNAs in sea urchin embryos by *in situ* hybridization using asymmetric RNA probes. Dev Biol 101:485–502, 1984.
14. Lewis ME, Sherman TG, Watson SJ. *In situ* hybridization histochemistry with synthetic oligonucleotides: Strategies and methods. Peptides 6(suppl 2):75–87, 1985.
15. Lewis ME, Sherman TG, Burke S, Akil H, Davis LG, Arentzen R, Watson SJ. Detection of proopiomelanocortin mRNA by *in situ* hybridization with an oligonucleotide probe. Proc Natl Acad Sci USA 83:5419–5423, 1986.
16. Lloyd RV. Analysis of human pituitary tumors by *in situ* hybridization. Pathol Res Pract 183:558–560, 1988.
17. Hoefler H, Childers H, Montminy MR, Lechan RM, Goodman RH, Wofle HJ. *In situ* hybridization methods for the detection of somatostatin mRNA in tissue sections using antisense RNA probes. Histochem J 18:597–604, 1986.
18. Childs GV, Lloyd JM, Unabia G, Gharib SD, Wierman ME, Chin WW. Detection of luteinizing hormone beta messenger ribonucleic acid (RNA) in individual gonadotropes after castration: Use of a new *in situ* hybridization method with a photobiotinylated complementary RNA probe. Mol Endocrinol 1:926–932, 1987.
19. Chu BC, Orgel LE. Detection of specific DNA sequences with short biotin-labeled probes. DNA 4:327–331, 1985.
20. Hofler H, Putz B, Ruhri C, Wirnsberger G, Klimpfinger M, Smolle J. Simultaneous localization of calcitonin mRNA and peptide in a medullary thyroid carcinoma. Virchows Arch (B) 54:144–151, 1987.
21. Hopman AH, Wiegant J, Van Duijn P. A new hybridocytochemical method based on mercurated nucleic acid probes and sulfhydryl-hapten ligands. I. Stability of the mercury-sulfhydryl bond and influence of the ligand structure on immunochemical detection of the hapten. Histochemistry 84:169–178, 1986.
22. Hopman AH, Wiegant J, Raap AK, Landegent JE, van der Ploeg M, van Duijn P. Bi-color detection of two target DNAs by non-radioactive *in situ* hybridization. Histochemistry 85:1–4, 1986.
23. Singer RH, Ward DC. Actin gene expression visualized in a chicken muscle tissue culture by using *in situ* hybridization with a biotinated nucleotide analog. Proc Natl Acad Sci USA 79:7331–7335, 1982.

24. Varndell IM, Polak JM, Sikri KL, Minth CD, Bloom SR, Dixon JE. Visualization of messenger RNA directing peptide synthesis by *in situ* hybridization using a novel single-stranded cDNA probe: Potential for the investigation of gene expression and endocrine cell activity. Histochemistry *81*:597–601, 1984.

25. Larsson L-I, Christensen T, Dalboge H. Detection of proopiomelanocortin mRNA by *in situ* hybridization using a biotinylated oligodeoxynucleotide probe and avidin-alkaline phosphatase histochemistry. Histochemistry *89*:109–116, 1988.

26. Bishop AE, Power RF, Polak JM. Markers for neuroendocrine differentiation. Pathol Res Pract *183*:119–128, 1988.

27. Nakanishi S, Inoue A, Kita T, Nakamura M, Chang AC, Cohen SN, Numa S. Nucleotide sequence of cloned cDNA for bovine corticotropin–beta-lipotropin precursor. Nature *278*:423–427, 1979.

28. Hagn C, Schmid KW, Fischer-Colbrie R, Winkler H. Chromogranin A, B and C in human adrenal medulla and endocrine tissues. Lab Invest *55*:405–411, 1986.

29. Helman LJ, Gazdar AF, Park J-G, Cohen PS, Cotelingam JD, Israel MA. Chromogranin A expression in normal and malignant human tissues. J Clin Invest *82*:686–690, 1988.

30. Lloyd RV, Wilson BS. Specific endocrine tissue marker defined by a monoclonal antibody. Science *222*:628–630, 1983.

31. O'Connor DT, Deftos LJ. Secretion of chromogranin A by peptide-producing endocrine neoplasms. N Engl J Med *314*:1145–1151, 1986.

32. Billestrup N, Mitchell RL, Vale W, Verma IM. Growth hormone-releasing factor induces c-*fos* expression in cultured primary pituitary cells. Mol Endocrinol *1*:300–305, 1987.

33. Weisman AS, Tixier-Vidal A, Gourdji D. Thyrotropin-releasing hormone increases the levels of c-*fos* and β-actin mRNA in GH3/B6 pituitary tumor cells. In Vitro Cell Dev Biol *23*:585–590, 1987.

34. Pelicci G, Pagliacci MC, Lanfroncone L, Pelicci PG, Grigromi F, Nicoletti I. Inhibitory effects of the somatostatin analog octreotide on rat pituitary tumor cell (GH3) proliferation *in vitro*. J Endocrinol Invest *13*:657–662, 1990.

35. Ezzat S, Melmed S. The role of growth factors in the pituitary. J Endocrinol Invest *13*:691–698, 1990.

36. Birman P, Michard M, Li JY, Peillon F, Bression D. Epidermal growth factor–binding sites, present in normal human and rat pituitaries, are absent in human pituitary adenomas. J Clin Endocrinol Metab *65*:275–281, 1987.

37. Grothe C, Unsicker K. Immunocytochemical localization of basic fibroblast growth factor in bovine adrenal gland, ovary and pituitary. J Histochem Cytochem *37*:1877–1883, 1989.

38. Silverlight JJ, Prysor-Jones RA, Jenkins JS. Basic fibroblast growth factor in human pituitary tumours. Clin Endocrinol *32*:669–676, 1990.

39. Prysor-Jones RA, Silverlight JJ, Jenkins JS. Oestradiol, vasoactive intestinal peptide and fibroblast growth factor in the growth of human pituitary tumor cells *in vitro*. J Endocrinol *120*:171–177, 1989.

40. Lund PK, Moats-Staats BM, Hynes MA, Simmons JG, D'Ercole AJ, Jansen M, Van Wyk JJ. Somatomedin-C/insulin-like growth factor I and insulin-like growth factor II mRNAs in rat fetal and adult tissues. J Biol Chem *261*:14539–14544, 1986.

41. Murphy LJ, Bell GI, Friesen HG. Tissue distribution of insulin-like growth factor I and II messenger ribonucleic acid in the adult rat. Endocrinology *120*:1279–1282, 1987.

42. Fagin JA, Pixley S, Slanina S, Ong J, Melmed S. Insulin-like growth factor I gene expression in GH3 rat pituitary cells: Messenger ribonucleic acid content, immunocytochemistry, and secretion. Endocrinology *120*:2037–2043, 1987.

43. Lloyd RV, Cano M, Chandler WF, Barkan AL, Horvath E, Kovacs K. Human growth hormone and prolactin secreting pituitary adenomas analyzed by *in situ* hybridization. Am J Pathol *134*:605–613, 1989.

44. Borrelli E, Heyman RA, Arias C, Sawchenko PE, Evans RM. Transgenic mice with inducible dwarfism. Nature *339*:538–541, 1989.

45. Kovacs K, Lloyd RV, Horvath E, Asa SL, Stefaneanu L, Killinger DW, Smythe HS. Silent somatotroph adenomas of the human pituitary. A morphologic study of three cases including immunocytochemistry, electron microscopy, *in vitro* examination and *in situ* hybridization. Am J Pathol *134*:345–353, 1989.

46. Lloyd RV, Fields K, Jin L, Horvath E, Kovacs K. Analysis of endocrine active and clinically silent corticotropic adenomas by *in situ* hybridization. Am J Pathol *137*:479–488, 1990.

47. Nagaya T, Seo H, Kuwayama A, Sakurai T, Tsukamoto N, Nakane T, Sugita K, Matsui N. Pro-opiomelanocortin gene expression in silent corticotroph-cell adenoma and Cushing's disease. J Neurosurg *72*:262–267, 1990.

48. Black PM, Hsu DW, Klibanski A, Kliman B, Jameson JL, Ridgeway EC, Hedley-Whyte ET, Zervas NT. Hormone production in clinically non-functioning pituitary adenomas. J Neurosurg *66*:244–250, 1987.

49. Jameson JL, Lindell CM, Habener JF. Gonadotropin and thyrotropin α- and β-subunit gene expression in normal and neoplastic tissues characterized using specific messenger ribonucleic acid hybridization probes. J Clin Endocrinol Metab *64*:319–327, 1987.

50. Jameson JL, Lindell CM, Hsu DW, Habener JF, Ridgway EC. Expression of chorionic gonadotropin-β–like messenger ribonucleic acid in an α-subunit–secreting pituitary adenoma. J Clin Endocrinol Metab *62*:1271–1278, 1986.

51. Sakurai TM, Seo H, Yamamoto N, Nagaya T, Nakane T, Kuwayama A, Kageyama N, Matsui N. Detection of mRNA of prolactin and ACTH in clinically nonfunctioning pituitary adenomas. J Neurosurg *69*:653–659, 1988.

52. Jameson JL, Klibanski A, Black PM, Zervas NT, Lindell CM, Hsu DW, Ridgway EC, Habener JF. Glycoprotein hormone genes are expressed in clinically nonfunctioning pituitary adenomas. J Clin Invest *80*:1472–1478, 1987.

53. Lloyd RV, Jin L, Fields K, Chandler WF, Horvath E, Stefaneanu L, Kovacs K. Analysis of pituitary hormones and chromogranin A mRNAs in null cell adenomas, oncocytomas and gonadotroph adenomas by *in situ* hybridization. Am J Pathol *139*:553–564, 1991.

54. Jameson JL, Arnold A. Clinical review 5: Recombinant DNA strategies for determining the molecular basis of endocrine disorders. J Clin Endocrinol Metab *70*:301–307, 1990.

55. Vnencak-Jones CL, Phillips JA, Chen EY, Seeburg PH. Molecular basis of human growth hormone gene deletions. Proc Natl Acad Sci USA *85*:5615–5619, 1988.

56. Alexander JM, Biller BMK, Bikkal H, Zervas NT, Arnold A, Klibanski A. Clinically nonfunctioning pituitary tumors are monoclonal in origin. J Clin Invest 86:336–340, 1990.

57. Jacoby LB, Hedley-Whyte T, Pulaski K, Seizinger BR, Martuza RL. Clonal origin of pituitary adenomas. J Neurosurg 73:731–735, 1990.

58. Herman V, Fagin J, Gonsky R, Kovacs K, Melmed S. Clonal origin of pituitary adenomas. J Clin Endocrinol Metab 71:1427–1433, 1990.

59. Saiki RK, Scharf S, Faloona F, Mullis KB, Horn GT, Erlich HA, Arnheim N. Enzymatic amplification of beta-globin genomic sequences and restriction site analysis for diagnosis of sickle cell anemia. Science 230:1350–1354, 1985.

60. Saiki RK, Gelfand DH, Stoffel S, Scharf SJ, Higuchi R, Horn GT, Mullis KB, Erlich HA. Primer-directed enzymatic amplification of DNA with a thermostable DNA polymerase. Science 239:487–491, 1988.

61. Landis CA, Masters SB, Spada A, Pace AM, Bourne HR, Vallar L. GTPase inhibiting mutations activate the α chain of GS and stimulate adenylyl cyclase in human pituitary tumors. Nature 340:692–696, 1989.

62. Spada A, Arosio M, Bochicchio D, Bazzoni N, Vallar L, Bassetti M, Faglia G. Clinical, biochemical and morphological correlates in patients bearing growth hormone-secreting pituitary tumors with or without constitutively active adenylyl cyclase. J Clin Endocrinol Metab 71:1421–1426, 1990.

63. Landis CA, Harsh G, Lyons J, Davis RL, McCormick F, Bourne HR. Clinical characteristics of acromegalic patients whose pituitary tumors contain mutant Gs protein. J Clin Endocrinol Metab 71:1416–1420, 1990.

64. Lyons J, Landis CA, Harsch G, Vallar L, Grunewald K, Feichtinger H, Duh QY, Clark OH, Kawasaki E, Bourne HR, McCormick F. Two G protein oncogenes in human endocrine tumors. Science 249:655–659, 1990.

9

TISSUE CULTURE IN THE DIAGNOSIS AND STUDY OF PITUITARY ADENOMAS

Sylvia L. Asa

Tissue culture provides a method for studying the behavior of cells, tissues or organs independent of the organism from which they derive (1). It enables precise control of the cell environment with defined chemical, neural or hormonal influences; manipulation of those factors allows documentation of the physiological conditions required for cell survival and function and provides a method of analyzing intracellular activities as well as interactions among cells or between the cells and their environment. Tissue culture studies have contributed significantly to the understanding of pituitary physiology and pathology. Numerous studies have documented hormone synthesis *in vitro*, stimulation or inhibition of hormone secretion, ligand binding, postreceptor events, drug and hormone actions and responses to alteration in the hormonal environment; they have also identified regulators of cell growth, differentiation and proliferation. The technique is ideal to analyze these aspects of pituitary cells, given an accurate understanding of the nutritional requirements of cells in culture.

The techniques of tissue culture require considerable expertise. In particular, studies of pituitary adenomas are limited by small quantities of tissue, entailing significant work and relatively high cost to maintain the artificial environment for small yield. The risk of contamination must always be considered; viral transformation of cultures is always a possibility. The major disadvantages of *in vitro* cultures arise from differences between the *in vitro* and *in vivo* environments. Removal of cells from an intact organism alters cellular homeostasis. Short-term primary cultures may be heterogeneous and unstable. The isolation of clonal populations ensures homogeneity, but continuous cell lines are subject to chromosome instability as well; moreover, cell strains and cell lines have increased growth fraction but tend to lose specific phenotypic traits. The fact that a piece of tissue was obtained from a specific organ does not guarantee that a cell line developed from it performs the function of that tissue. Dedifferentiation is often observed *in vitro*, and a prime consideration is overgrowth of fibroblasts, which have a selective advantage *in vitro*. True dedifferentiation of specialized cells does occur, and manipulation of the artificial environment may alter the dedifferentiation process.

TECHNIQUES OF CULTURE

The term "tissue culture" encompasses many types of preparations, each with its own advantages and disadvantages. "Organ culture" refers to three-dimensional cultures of intact fragments of tissues that retain some or all of their native histological features. This technique has been used most widely to study embryonic differentiation and was initially applied to demonstrate hormone synthesis and secretion (2–4). Organ cultures of hemipituitaries played a major role in the isolation and identification of several hypothalamic adenohypophysiotropic hormones (5). The size of the cultures restricts nutrition and respiration and limits survival and growth. To overcome this, "primary explant cultures" were developed; a fragment of tissue is allowed to attach to a substrate, and cells migrate out from the tissue in the plane of the substrate (Fig. 9–1). This technique has also been used to study embryology (6, 7). The phenomenon of contact inhibition, common to most non-neoplastic tissues, limits cell proliferation to the periphery of the explant. The specimens in both of these techniques cannot be propagated; reproducibility and quantitation are exceedingly difficult.

Dispersion of cells allows more precise quantitation and equal viability for all cells (8–10). Cells may be dispersed by enzymatic or mechanical disaggregation techniques (see later discussion). Disaggregated cells may be grown as "monolayer cell cultures" (Fig. 9–

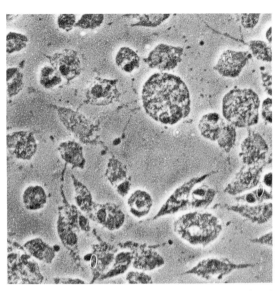

Figure 9–2. Dispersed cells of a densely granulated somatotroph adenoma grow in monolayer culture attached to a collagen-coated plastic well. Note the elongated shape of some of the cells. (Phase contrast microscopy; ×400)

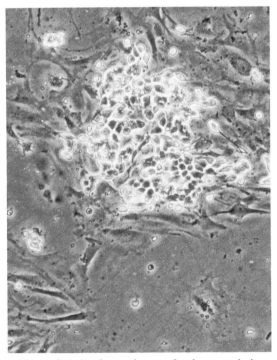

Figure 9–1. Explant cultures of a human pituitary lactotroph adenoma. Fragments of tumor tissue are attached to a plastic culture well, and cells migrate out in the plane of the dish; many of these are flattened, elongated fibroblasts, whereas the rounded epithelial cells remain in clusters. (Phase contrast microscopy; ×150)

2) attached to a solid substrate (11) or as "suspension cell cultures" that grow as floaters in a medium (12). They may be reaggregated or grown in a matrix to create a three-dimensional structure known as "histotypic culture" or as "aggregate suspensions" (Fig. 9–3) (13, 14). "Continuous perifusion" is useful for studies of hormone secretion dynamics, since it offers the advantage of documenting pulsatile secretion and the time course of responses to pulsatile or prolonged exposures to test substances (15–18). This system also avoids the accumulation of proteolytic enzymes or hormones, which may, by short-loop feedback mechanisms, affect relevant cellular processes. Its disadvantages include the small number of simultaneous tests, which precludes testing of numerous substances or concentrations; the difficulty in obtaining consistent dose-related responses; and the large number of samples in any given experiment.

Tissue disaggregation may be mechanical or enzymatic. The former, which involves slicing, pressing tissue fragments through sieves of gradually reduced mesh, forcing cells through a syringe and needle or repeated pipetting, is a fast and inexpensive technique but may cause extensive cell damage and loss. Enzymatic dispersion yields a higher number of cells. The various enzymes used include

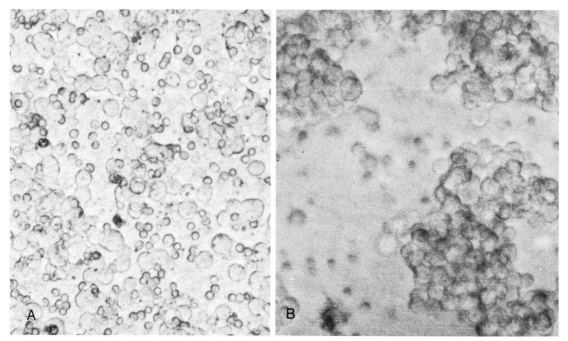

Figure 9–3. Reaggregate cultures of a pituitary somatotroph adenoma. A, Dispersed cells remain separate 2 hours after plating onto an extracellular matrix. B, Within 24 hours *in vitro*, the same cells reaggregate into small clumps. (Phase contrast microscopy; ×300)

trypsin, collagenase, elastase, hyaluronidase, pronase or deoxyribonuclease (DNase). Trypsin and pronase give the most complete disaggregation but may damage cells, particularly cell membranes and surface receptors. Collagenase is less harmful but may result in incomplete disaggregation.

The prime objective of tissue culture techniques is to maintain viability of cells in a specified environment with aseptic techniques. Successful culturing depends on stable conditions of the environment. These vary with the choice of substrate, medium, gas phase and temperature.

Substrates are generally adhesive surfaces. Glass is the traditional vessel; it is inexpensive and readily washed and sterilized for re-use, but sterile plastics have provided a number of distinct advantages in that they are permeable to oxygen and carbon dioxide and may be adjusted to the needs of the investigator. For example, some plastics are well suited for sectioning in histological or ultrastructural studies of cultured cells. Others are available as beads to act as microcarriers for anchorage-dependent cells in suspension. Attachment to natural substrates may alter cell morphology and function, for example, by simulating basement membrane and indicat-

ing polarity for epithelial cells. Generally, treatment of vessels with collagen, fibronectin, polylysine or laminin improves plating efficiency and growth of many cell types. Some investigators use confluent monolayers of an appropriate cell type, so-called "extracellular matrix" (ECM) (19). In some instances, three-dimensional matrices, such as collagen gel, cellulose sponge or Gelfoam, or nonadhesive substrates, such as agar (12), agarose or Methocell are used to study specific cell types. Another method uses perfused microcapillary bundles, which allow diffusion of nutrients or dissolved substances to permeate cells, analogous to intact tissue (20).

Medium requirements vary with species and cell type as well as with the laboratory environment and investigator. Many defined media have been established, and the selection of the medium is empirical (21). Most cells require supplementation of the medium with serum. The search for highly defined media has led to attempts to avoid serum addition and substitute it with specific proteins, electrolytes, polypeptide growth factors and hormones (22).

The significant constituents of the *gaseous environment in vitro* are oxygen (O_2) and carbon dioxide (CO_2); most cultures require up to 95% O_2. Carbon dioxide maintains the acid-base equilibrium of culture media, and the CO_2 tension is therefore critical for viability of cultures. The optimum *temperature* for human cells *in vitro* is 37°C. Cultured cells can survive for up to several days at 4°C when necessary, but they cannot tolerate temperatures near 39°C for more than a few hours and die rapidly at 40°C or higher.

Primary cultures are heterogeneous, and investigators have sought to clone cells of a single type to develop a homogeneous cell strain. Cultures derived from non-neoplastic tissues survive only a limited number of generations, and thus *cloning* has been most successful to isolate transformed cells or variants to form continuous cell lines.

Other techniques of *cell separation* have been used to obtain enriched subpopulations for culture. Most methods have a high yield but less purity than cloning. Cells can be separated based on size, density (13), surface charge, surface chemistry or antigenicity (23), light scatter or fluorescence emission. These techniques have been useful in separating the cell types of the nontumorous adenohypophysis. The use of *flow cytometry* also allows separation based on differences in DNA, RNA, protein, enzyme activity or specific antigens. Although this has been used extensively to characterize cell populations, sterile collection of cells with similar properties is an expensive proposition with limited yield.

Morphological characterization of cells in culture must be applied to verify that cultures are representative of the tissue of origin. Most conventional morphological techniques can be applied to cells in culture. Phase-contrast microscopy is the simplest and fastest method of studying cultured cells; it allows characterization of their shape and size, but these are not definitive identifying features, since they vary with the plasticity of cells in different culture conditions. Stained preparations of fixed cultures can be made using virtually any conventional technique. Cells can be grown on regular glass microscopic slides, or cytologic specimens can be prepared from cell suspensions by smearing, centrifugation or filtration. Conventional histochemical techniques, immunocytochemical methods (Fig. 9–4) and *in situ* hybridization can be applied to define features of cell differentiation.

Cell morphology can also be analyzed by

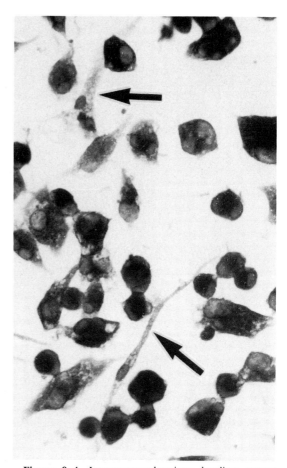

Figure 9–4. Immunocytochemistry localizes strong GH reactivity in the cytoplasm of cells from a densely granulated somatotroph adenoma cultured *in situ* on a glass chamber-slide. Elongated fibroblasts *(arrows)* are negative. (Avidin-biotin-peroxidase complex technique; ×450)

electron microscopy (Fig. 9–5 and 9–6). This can be performed on cells grown on specific substrates that facilitate fixation and embedding *in situ* (24–26); alternatively, cultured cells can be suspended and centrifuged into pellets for fixation and embedding.

Cells studied *in vitro* can be analyzed individually using the *reverse hemolytic plaque assay*. The original hemolytic plaque assay was developed for the detection of immunoglobulin secretion by individual lymphocytes; the method was adapted to assess antigen secretion by individual cells in culture, and this adaptation was named the "reverse hemolytic plaque assay" (27, 28). In this type of study, protein A–coated erythrocytes are coincubated with potential antigen-secreting cells; antigen secreted by the cells diffuses into the

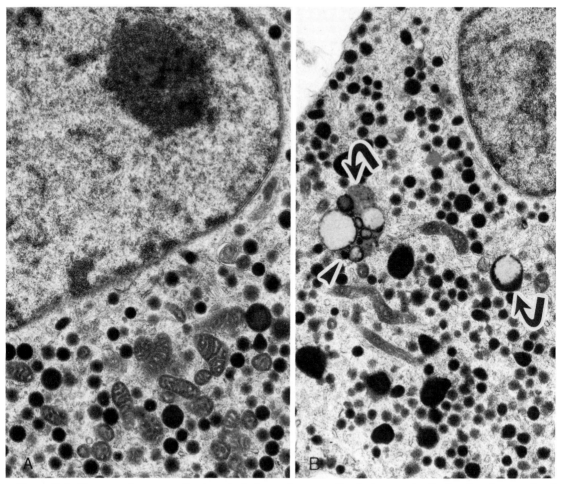

Figure 9–5. Electron microscopy of cultured pituitary adenoma cells. *A,* A control cell of a densely granulated somatotroph adenoma *in vitro* has numerous large, electron-dense secretory granules almost completely occupying the cytoplasm (×14,900). *B,* After incubation in somatostatin, a densely granulated cell from the same adenoma has several prominent lysosomes *(arrows)*; one contains dense structures resembling secretory granules *(arrowhead),* suggestive of crinophagy (×14,900). (From Asa SL, Felix I, Kovacs K, Ramyar L. Effects of somatostatin on somatotroph adenomas of the human pituitary; an in vitro functional and morphological study. Endocr Pathol *1*:228–235, 1990. Reprinted by permission of Blackwell Scientific Publications.)

lawn of red blood cells, and addition of specific antibody and complement causes hemolysis of erythrocytes surrounding secretory cells, resulting in clear areas of lysis known as "plaques" (Fig. 9–7). The localization of a plaque allows identification of an individual cell secreting the antigen recognized by the specific antibody utilized in the study. This assay permits qualitative assessment of mixed cell populations and quantitation of amounts of hormone released by individual cells, since plaque size is proportional to the amount of hormone that diffuses around a given cell. Because the cells remain viable, the technique can be applied sequen-

tially in the analysis of individual cells to measure variations in hormonal activity over time or to identify cells that secrete more than one substance (27–29). It can also be combined with immunocytochemistry (30, 31), electron microscopy (32), autoradiography or *in situ* hybridization.

Application of these sophisticated methods can provide information about cell function and growth as well as regulation of those activities. This is the most frequent objective of tissue culture studies in the diagnosis and study of pituitary adenomas. These techniques have been applied to characterize cells in primary culture and clonal cell lines, to

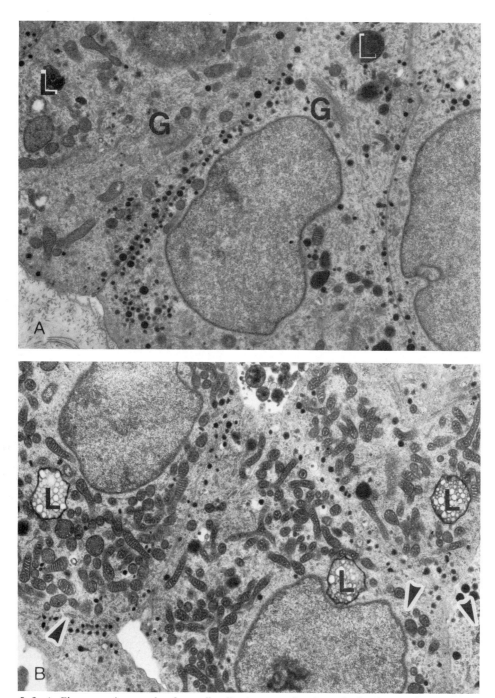

Figure 9–6. *A,* Electron micrograph of a null cell adenoma after 2 weeks in tissue culture. The tumor has morphological features similar to those of the surgically resected tissue. The rough endoplasmic reticulum is scant, and lysosomes (L), Golgi regions (G) and small secretory granules are seen ($\times 10,200$). *B,* Electron micrograph of an oncocytoma after 3 weeks *in vitro.* The tumor cells maintain their morphological characteristics; the cytoplasm is filled with numerous mitochondria, small numbers of secretory granules, a few rough endoplasmic reticulum profiles *(arrowheads)* and lysosomes (L) ($\times 10,200$). (From Asa SL, Gerrie BM, Singer W, Horvath E, Kovacs K, Smyth HS. Gonadotropin secretion *in vitro* by human pituitary null cell adenomas and oncocytomas. J Clin Endocrinol Metab *62*:1011–1019, 1986, © by the Endocrine Society.)

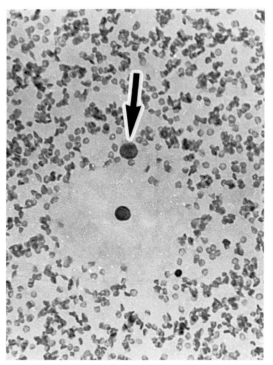

Figure 9–7. The reverse hemolytic plaque assay identifies two cells from a null cell adenoma that release β-FSH and make "plaques," clear areas with only the ghosts of erythrocytes; another cell *(arrow)* is not surrounded by a plaque, indicating that it did not release that hormone during this experiment (×450).

demonstrate production of hormones and other substances and to expand structure-function correlations by identifying morphological alterations that may be attributed to specific regulatory substances that could have pathogenetic or therapeutic implications. This chapter will be limited to a review of human pituitary adenomas in primary culture; data on normal physiology, animal-derived tissues and cell lines are beyond the scope of this work and will be restricted to those areas of major importance that have not as yet been applied to human pathology.

TISSUE CULTURE STUDIES OF PITUITARY ADENOMAS

The first studies of pituitary tumors in culture concentrated on the documentation of hormone release by tumor cells (33–37). These studies confirmed good correlation between hormone release *in vitro* and the clinical and biochemical features of hormone excess *in vivo*. In some cases, release of hor-

mones *in vitro* correlated better with the hormone profile *in vivo* than immunohistochemistry (38).

One of the principal applications of tissue culture is the study of regulation of cell function. Isolation of the cell from the complex hormonal milieu *in vivo* allows detailed examination of cellular responses to specific substances. Pituitary adenomas have been shown to respond to numerous regulatory substances, including hypothalamic hypophysiotropic hormones, products of target organs, various neurotransmitters and other hypothalamic peptides, as well as cytokines and growth factors. Some of the substances that regulate hormone production have diagnostic and/or therapeutic value; others may play pathogenetic roles in tumor development.

Somatotroph Adenomas

Characterization of growth hormone (GH) release by somatotroph adenomas has been shown to be similar in both densely granulated and sparsely granulated tumors (39). However, the use of the reverse hemolytic plaque assay has shown that GH secretion by individual somatotrophs is highly variable both within and between adenomas; the percentage of active GH-secreting cells among adenomas associated with acromegaly is extremely heterogeneous (40), and within a single adenoma, the amount of GH released differs among individual pituitary adenoma cells (32). The ultrastructural appearance of individual cells correlates with the hormone release; larger plaques are formed by cells with fewer secretory granules and well-developed rough endoplasmic reticulum and Golgi regions (32).

A significant proportion of somatotroph adenomas is known to release α subunit of glycoprotein hormones *in vitro* (41–43). Parallel response of GH and α subunit release to stimulation by growth hormone releasing hormone (GHRH) is consistent with production of both hormones by the same cell (41).

The majority of somatotroph adenomas respond to stimulation by GHRH (39–41, 44–52). In short-term incubations, densely granulated tumors release more GH in response to the stimulus than do sparsely granulated ones (49), probably reflecting the amount of stored hormone; in the reverse hemolytic plaque assay, GHRH had no preferential effect on any subpopulation of adenoma cells (40). In contrast, during long-term exposure to GHRH, the two morphological variants of somatotroph adenomas respond equally, and there is ultrastructural evidence of increased hormone synthesis as well as release (39), a finding that was confirmed by the documentation of increased levels of GH mRNA (52). Unlike nontumorous adenohypophysial cells (53) or hyperplastic pituitaries in patients with tumors secreting GHRH (54), which are desensitized by persistent GHRH exposure and show down-regulation of GHRH binding sites, there is no desensitization following continuous GHRH stimulation of adenomas (39, 50); this had led to the suggestion that continuous hormonal stimulation may play a role in the pathogenesis of these tumors. The evidence that GHRH is involved in tumorigenesis was strengthened by the finding that it causes proliferation of GH-containing cells from the nontumorous rat pituitary *in vitro* (55), confirming its direct role in the development of hyperplasia in patients with tumors secreting GHRH (56) and in mice transgenic for GHRH (57); the transgenic mice go on to develop pituitary adenomas (58). However, the proliferative effect of GHRH on somatotroph adenomas has not been verified.

Thyrotropin releasing hormone (TRH) has also been shown to stimulate GH release by some somatotroph adenomas (40, 48, 59, 60). The response is thought to correlate with the presence of functional TRH receptors in this subpopulation of somatotroph adenomas (61). Vasoactive intestinal polypeptide (VIP), another putative prolactin-releasing substance, also can directly stimulate GH release by some adenomas; the effect is additive to that of GHRH (48, 62).

A role for corticosteroids in the maintenance of GH secretion has also been demonstrated *in vitro* (63, 64); they prevent rapid decline of hormone release and extend the functional abilities of cultured cells for weeks to months. Some have found that dexamethasone enhances the stimulatory effect of GHRH (63), whereas others have reported partial or complete inhibition of this response by cortisol (64).

Somatostatin-induced inhibition of GH secretion by somatotroph adenomas has been documented *in vitro* (2, 47, 48, 60, 62, 65, 66). The inhibition seems to affect the most actively secreting cells, shown in the reverse hemolytic plaque assay by reduction of

plaque size and shift in the GH plaque area frequency distributions toward smaller plaques, but it has no effect on the overall percentage of plaque-forming cells (40). Morphological as well as molecular correlates have been established using ultrastructural analysis (67) and Northern blot analysis of GH mRNA (51, 52) in cultured somatotroph adenoma cells incubated with somatostatin. These studies have shown that somatostatin does not reduce GH mRNA or alter the organelles involved in hormone synthesis, such as endoplasmic reticulum and Golgi complexes, parallel to the inhibition of hormone release that it induces. Instead, there is an accumulation of lysosomes (see Fig. 9–5), suggesting that inhibition of hormone release is accompanied by lysosomal degradation of stored hormone (67). The interaction of somatostatin and GHRH on somatotroph adenoma cells has been investigated *in vitro* (47); somatostatin is able to completely overcome GHRH-induced GH release.

Several studies have also indicated that dopamine and its agonists such as bromocriptine are able to inhibit GH release from some pituitary somatotroph adenomas (48, 59, 62, 65, 66, 68–70), indicating the presence of dopamine receptors in these tumors. Dopamine effectively inhibits GHRH-mediated GH release (62).

Careful study of the secretory activity of GH-producing adenomas *in vitro* identified a group of tumors with high basal secretion and no appreciable response to GHRH stimulation. This led to the identification of mutations in the stimulating guanine nucleotide–binding (G_s) proteins that result in autonomous adenylate cyclase activity in these adenomas (71).

Lactotroph Adenomas

Production of prolactin (PRL) by lactotroph adenomas was documented *in vitro* (38, 72, 73); in some cases, the hormone release *in vitro* was more sensitive for detection of PRL production than immunohistochemical localization of that hormone (38).

In cultures of PRL-secreting rat pituitary tumors, estrogen directly stimulates hormone production (74). Application of this information to humans is controversial, and the role of estrogen in the pathogenesis of human prolactinomas is unclear; some have found that estrogen stimulates both hormone secretion and DNA synthesis by these tumors (75), and tamoxifen, an antiestrogen, inhibits colony formation of PRL-producing pituitary adenomas in soft agar (12). Cultured normal human pituitary cells are more sensitive to dopamine inhibition of PRL release after preincubation with estradiol; in contrast, prolactinoma cells become insensitive to bromocriptine inhibition after similar pretreatment (74, 76), and the sensitivity can be restored by tamoxifen (74).

TRH stimulates PRL secretion from adenoma cells in a dose-dependent manner in some tumors (59, 77), despite the blunted PRL response to this substance found *in vivo* in patients bearing such tumors. In some cases, TRH responsiveness is dependent on the presence of dopamine (76).

VIP has been implicated as a PRL-releasing factor and has been shown to directly stimulate PRL release by prolactinomas in culture (78, 79). At a given concentration of VIP, the effect is greater on cells derived from microadenomas than on those derived from macroadenomas (78). The potential role of VIP in promoting growth of prolactinomas was suggested by the documentation of cell proliferation by these tumors *in vitro* during incubation with VIP (75).

Studies of lactotroph adenomas in culture have clarified the mechanism of bromocriptine inhibition of hormone synthesis and secretion as a direct effect on the cells of lactotroph adenomas (12, 48, 68–70, 76, 78, 80–82). In contrast to the response to VIP, cells from macroadenomas respond more than those from microadenomas (78). The ability to study morphological changes *in vitro* after varying durations of exposure to dopamine or its agonists led to the finding that cell shrinkage and involution of synthetic organelles occur rapidly, whereas loss of secretory granules is slower, and in the early phases of exposure, lysosomes may play a role in degradation of stored hormone (80, 82). Altered microtubule structure was also found after incubation of rat prolactinoma cells with bromocriptine (83). Bromocriptine was also shown to inhibit the growth of PRL-secreting adenomas in soft agar (12).

Endogenous opiates, especially β-endorphin, are thought to participate in the regulation of PRL release. The direct stimulatory effect of opioid ligands on prolactinoma cells was revealed in culture; they modulate the inhibitory effect of dopamine on PRL release by these tumors (84). Somatostatin also can inhibit PRL release by some human pituitary prolactinomas (81).

Both gonadotropin releasing hormone (GnRH) and GnRH-associated peptide (GAP) are thought to inhibit PRL secretion from nontumorous adenohypophysis, but neither has had its effect substantiated in studies of lactotroph adenomas *in vitro* (85, 86), suggesting that their action may be mediated by paracrine factors present in the nontumorous pituitary.

Bihormonal GH- and PRL-secreting Adenomas

The existence of cells secreting both GH and PRL was initially suggested by Goluboff and Ezrin, who observed that the increase in PRL-containing cells during pregnancy is accompanied by a reduction in the number of GH-containing cells (87). Secretion of these two hormones by adenomas was proven using tissue culture methods (35, 48, 59, 60, 68, 88–92). Morphological studies identified at least three distinct adenomas that produce these hormones: the bimorphous mixed somatotroph-lactotroph adenomas composed of two mature cell types, the monomorphous mammosomatotroph adenomas and the monomorphous acidophil stem cell adenomas (93). The difference in hormone release between mammosomatotroph tumors and acidophil stem cell adenomas was also shown in culture; the former release much greater amounts of GH, correlating well with the clinical presentation of acromegaly in patients with these lesions, whereas the latter release greater amounts of PRL, again consistent with the clinical presentation of these tumors, which mimic prolactinomas (94).

The existence of individual cells capable of producing both hormones was ultimately proven by the reverse hemolytic plaque assay in the nontumorous human pituitary and in human pituitary adenomas (30); this study applied methodology used to establish the presence of mammosomatotrophs in the rodent pituitary (29, 95). The role of bihormonal mammosomatotrophs as stem cells of the acidophil cell line was strongly indicated by studies of the human and rodent fetal gland (96–98) in which mammosomatotrophs are identified at early stages of gestation, antedating the development of mature lactotrophs (97). The importance of this potential precursor cell was emphasized by the recognition that mammosomatotroph hyperplasia is a cause of gigantism in young children (99); this insight may lead to a better understanding of the high incidence of mammosomatotroph adenomas in young patients with gigantism.

Differences in the production of GH and PRL may be regulated by changes in the hormonal environment; the addition of cortisol preferentially increases release of GH while decreasing secretion of PRL (90).

Tumors producing GH and PRL respond somewhat differently than pure somatotroph or lactotroph adenomas to some hypothalamic stimuli. Release of both GH and PRL is stimulated by GHRH (45, 48, 100), TRH (48, 59, 101) or VIP (48) and is inhibited by somatostatin (45, 48, 68, 100) or dopaminergic agents (48, 59, 101). In a study with structure-function correlations, parallel responses of GH and PRL were found in mammosomatotroph adenomas but not among bimorphous mixed adenomas; interestingly, acidophil stem cell adenomas, which release greater quantities of PRL, respond to GHRH with a greater proportional increase in GH secretion, and neither hormone's release is inhibited by bromocriptine (94).

Corticotroph Adenomas

Production of proopiomelanocortin (POMC)-derived peptides by corticotroph adenomas has been studied *in vitro*. In most cases, the pattern of secretion of adrenocorticotropic hormone (ACTH) and its related peptides by tumor cells in culture is similar to that of the normal pituitary (102, 103); however, abnormal POMC processing has been reported to produce high-molecular-weight ACTH-like peptides that can cause Cushing's disease (104).

Abnormal hormonal regulation of ACTH release by corticotrophs has long been speculated to play a role in the pathogenesis of corticotroph adenomas associated with Cushing's or Nelson's syndromes (105). Tissue culture studies have documented variability in the responsiveness of these tumors to stimulation by corticotropin releasing hormone (CRH); some have not found any response to stimulation (106), but the majority of functioning corticotroph tumors are stimulated to a variable degree by that substance (107–116). There is no evidence of desensitization of the adenoma cells during long-term exposure to CRH (115). Morphological studies have indicated that CRH causes cell flattening and extension of cytoplasmic processes (114). Ultrastructural examination after chronic stimulation *in vitro* suggests that CRH stimulates ACTH synthesis as well as release (116), consistent with the effects on mRNA levels in cultured cells (117).

Hormone release by corticotroph adenomas can be stimulated by arginine vasopressin (AVP), also implicated as a physiological ACTH-releasing substance (109, 112, 118–121); the effects of CRH and AVP are synergistic (109, 112). VIP is also a potent ACTH secretagogue with direct effects on tumor cells (119); the action of VIP is additive to that of AVP. There are reports of anomalous stimulation by TRH, not known to affect nontumorous corticotrophs (120, 122), as well as by oxytocin, substance P and metenkephalin (120).

Although some have suggested that these tumors have absent or reduced suppression of ACTH release by physiological levels of cortisol and have implicated this as a pathogenetic factor (118, 123), most corticotroph adenomas appear to be sensitive to feedback inhibition by corticosteroids (111, 116, 117, 119, 124); they undergo rounding up of shape in culture (114) and develop filament accumulations similar to but less marked than those of Crooke's hyalinization, seen in nontumorous cells after chronic exposure to corticosteroids (116). Interestingly, the cells do not show involution of the rough endoplasmic reticulum or Golgi complex (116); the reason for this is not known. Comparatively, the sensitivity of normal cells to dexamethasone suppression of POMC mRNA levels *in vitro* is much greater than that of adenomatous corticotrophs (117). The suppressive effects of corticosteroids attenuate the stimulation of CRH (112), VIP (119) or hypothalamic extract (118).

Cyproheptadine, thought to act centrally in reducing ACTH (105), also has a direct inhibitory effect on ACTH release *in vitro* (108, 122). Some corticotroph adenomas are subject to direct inhibition by dopaminergic agents (122, 125), reserpine (108), somatostatin (120) or ketoconazole (126).

Cytokines are novel regulators of adenohypophysial cell function (127, 128). Interleukin-1β directly stimulates ACTH release from cultured cells of corticotroph adenomas, as do thymosin fraction 5, interferon-γ and granulocyte colony–stimulating factor (129).

Thyrotroph Adenomas

Structure-function correlations in TSH-secreting adenomas have been strengthened using tissue culture analysis of tumors that are morphologically highly characterized. Tumors secreting only TSH are generally monomorphous adenomas with typical ultrastructural and immunocytochemical features of thyrotrophs (130–135). Variable amounts of free α and β subunits are also released (131, 133, 135).

Regulation of TSH production by thyrotroph adenomas *in vitro* has been studied in only a limited fashion. Some tumors respond to stimulation by TRH with release of TSH and α subunit (131, 135), whereas others do not (130). They may be inhibited by dopamine (131, 133), which suppresses release of intact TSH or β-TSH more than of α subunit (133); however, the dopaminergic resistance typical of some of these tumors may be due to altered or absent dopamine receptors (135). Somatostatin also exerts a direct inhibitory action as documented *in vitro*, rather than only the direct effect thought to act via the hypothalamus by reducing TRH; again the inhibition is more marked on the release of intact TSH than α subunit (133).

Gonadotroph Adenomas

Secretion of large amounts of gonadotropins, predominantly follicle-stimulating hormone (FSH), is found *in vitro* in tumors from patients with gonadotroph adenomas detected clinically (136–139); the amounts are much greater than those released by tumors that are not associated with elevated gonadotropin levels *in vivo* (31, 140). Impaired biological activity of these tumors may, in some cases, be due to secretion of uncombined α and β subunits of the gonadotropins (138, 141).

Gonadotroph adenomas are known to show variable responses to stimulation by GnRH or its agonists (139, 141–143). The morphological alterations after chronic stimulation suggest that GnRH stimulates both synthesis and release of hormone (139); this is consistent with the finding of increased hormone release into culture media as well as increased cell content of gonadotropins (142). The anticipated desensitizing effect of chronic GnRH stimulation is not observed,

suggesting that for these tumors also, as for somatotroph or corticotroph adenomas, sustained stimulation may play a pathogenetic role (143).

Variable effects of gonadal steroids on gonadotroph adenomas include paradoxical stimulation and modulation of the response to GnRH (139, 141). These tumors may respond to stimulation with TRH with increased hormone synthesis and release, established by the same morphological and biochemical means (138, 141–143). Bromocriptine inhibits hormone synthesis and/or release by some gonadotroph adenomas *in vitro* (142, 144).

Chromogranin A is produced by gonadotrophs, and GnRH has been found to regulate not only the synthesis and secretion of gonadotropic hormones but also chromogranin mRNA in these tumors *in vitro* (145). Curiously, GnRH stimulates the synthesis of chromogranin A (145).

Clinically Nonfunctioning Adenomas

Among the large group of clinically nonfunctioning tumors, the majority release small amounts of hormones in culture, predominantly glycoprotein hormones and their subunits (33, 36, 37, 146, 147). However, the development of sophisticated morphological techniques in association with tissue culture analysis led to a much broader understanding of structure-function correlations in these neoplasms. The concept of silent adenomas was developed for tumors that show morphological features of cell differentiation but are not associated with clinical or biochemical evidence of hormone excess; studies of hormone production and regulation *in vitro* can clarify the reasons for the lack of clinical detection of tumor function or differentiation.

The application of careful morphological classification, culture techniques and *in situ* hybridization elucidated the existence of *silent somatotroph adenomas*, which have the morphological features of sparsely granulated somatotroph adenomas and are capable of producing and releasing GH (148). In tissue culture, these tumors initially release small quantities of GH, significantly less than those seen in endocrinologically active somatotroph adenomas. After several days in culture, GH release increases, suggesting the possibility that GH secretion may have been suppressed *in vivo* (148).

Another group of silent tumors, *silent corticotroph adenomas*, is composed of cells that resemble well-differentiated corticotrophs, contain immunoreactivity for several POMC-derived peptides (93) and produce POMC mRNA (149). Tissue culture studies have revealed that these cells do release a substance with ACTH-like immunoreactivity, but specific analysis of ACTH 1–39 reveals only small amounts in culture media. This suggests that the tumors may be secreting biologically inactive POMC-derived peptides, such as a high-molecular-weight ACTH (150) or ACTH linked to the joining peptide that connects it to the POMC N-terminal fragment (151). Other possibilities include cleavage of ACTH into a melanocyte-stimulating hormone (MSH) or corticotropin-like intermediate lobe peptide (CLIP), which would support the proposed intermediate lobe differentiation of these adenomas.

The largest group of clinically silent but morphologically differentiated tumors is composed of *silent gonadotroph adenomas.* These tumors not infrequently present as mass lesions that do not give rise to detectable hormone excess *in vivo*. They may contain variable degrees of positivity for gonadotroph hormones and/or their subunits and may have characteristic ultrastructural features of gonadotrophs. *In vitro*, these tumors usually release FSH, luteinizing hormone (LH) and α subunit; however, the quantities are much lower than those released by tumors that give rise to detectable hormone excess *in vivo* (31, 140).

Approximately 25% of surgically removed pituitary adenomas do not have the characteristic morphological features of any recognized adenohypophysial cell type. The cells making up these tumors, classified as *null cell adenomas*, contain the organelles required for hormone synthesis and release (see Fig. 9–6A); a subgroup of these tumors, the *oncocytomas*, contain, in addition, large numbers of spherulated mitochondria (see Fig. 9–6B). Tissue culture analysis of these tumors has shown that they also release primarily intact gonadotropins and/or their subunits *in vitro* (140, 152). The levels of hormone release are generally low but not unlike those found in cultures of silent gonadotroph adenomas or in cultures of nontumorous adenohypophysis, in which only 5% to 10% of the cells are

gonadotrophs. The reasons for the low level of hormone release are unknown. Studies using the reverse hemolytic plaque assay (see Fig. 9–7) have shown that only a small percentage of tumor cells are actively releasing hormone at any given time, and the amount of hormone released as quantitated by the size of plaques is exceedingly low (31). Again, the results using this technique resemble those in silent gonadotroph adenomas in the same system (31).

Clinically nonfunctioning adenomas, primarily the null cell adenomas and oncocytomas, show responsiveness of gonadotropin release *in vitro* to GnRH and TRH (142, 144, 147, 153–155). GnRH also increases chromogranin B mRNA but not that of chromogranin A in these tumors (145). Like gonadotroph adenomas, they have variable responsiveness to inhibition by gonadal steroids (153, 154). In addition, null cell adenomas and oncocytomas may show unusual responses to stimulation by other hypothalamic hypophysiotropic hormones, including GHRH and CRH (145, 153, 154); incubation with these substances can affect gonadotropin release but does not appear to stimulate release of the appropriate target adenohypophysial hormone.

Gonadotropin release by clinically nonfunctioning tumors may be suppressed *in vitro* by bromocriptine (142, 144, 156); α subunit mRNA levels are reduced in parallel with the secretion (157). This has led to the suggestion that bromocriptine may be a useful therapeutic agent for the treatment of these tumors, but it remains to be seen whether it reduces their size in the way that it causes shrinkage of lactotroph adenomas.

Unclassified Plurihormonal Adenomas

The plurihormonal nature of pituitary adenomas has been recognized with increasing frequency since the 1980s (158). In this sphere as well, tissue culture studies have played an important role. The documentation of α subunit production and release by somatotroph tumors was corroborated *in vitro* (41, 42). The common occurrence of GH and PRL cosecretion, discussed earlier, indicates a common embryology of those two hormones. Gonadotrophs are known to synthesize and release both FSH and LH; gonadotroph adenomas, as well as null cell adenomas and oncocytomas, produce both hormones and their subunits and are therefore, by definition, plurihormonal.

Various other combinations of hormones are more rarely produced by unclassified plurihormonal adenomas. Production of TSH and PRL was shown *in vitro* by a tumor with the ultrastructural morphology of thyrotrophs (159); release of TSH, α subunit and PRL was suppressed by bromocriptine or triiodothyronine (T_3); however, only PRL responded to TRH stimulation.

Release of TSH, α subunit and GH by pituitary tumors has been documented in tissue culture (134, 160–164). Only a few of these rare tumors have been studied, and the reports offer conflicting data; their significance remains uncertain. Some TSH- and GH-producing tumors are monomorphous, suggesting production of all three substances by a single cell type (134, 161, 162). In culture, one such tumor, composed of monomorphous thyrotroph-like cells, responded to TRH with increased release of both TSH and GH, but other substances, such as the TRH precursor, TRH-glycine, T_3, dexamethasone, GnRH and somatostatin, induced differential alterations in the release of TSH and GH (162). Bimorphous tumors may produce the same combination of hormones (134, 163, 164); in one, although ultrastructural immunocytology revealed the presence of GH and TSH in the same cells, each of those hormones responded differently to somatostatin, bromocriptine or TRH (163). In another bimorphous tumor producing GH, TSH and α subunit, GHRH, TRH or GnRH stimulated release of all three hormones, whereas dexamethasone inhibited TSH while stimulating GH release (164). These data, although difficult to reconcile, may shed light on the regulation of differentiated cell function in adenohypophysial cells.

The very rare occurrence of plurihormonality in corticotroph adenomas has also been documented by immunohistochemistry and confirmed *in vitro* where POMC-derived peptides and gonadotropins were produced by a monomorphic cell type and showed parallel response to stimulation and inhibition; this was shown to be true for both functioning corticotroph adenomas giving rise to Cushing's disease (165) and a silent corticotroph adenoma (166).

PRODUCTION OF OTHER HORMONES BY PITUITARY ADENOMAS

Substances other than the classic adenohypophysial hormones are produced and released by pituitary tumor cells in culture. Chromogranins are produced *in vitro* by some pituitary adenomas (145, 167). Hypothalamic hormones are also entering into the spectrum of pituitary products; the implications of this are tantalizing, since these substances are thought to regulate adenohypophysial cell function, and if they are produced there, they may have paracrine or even autocrine effects. Large amounts of GHRH and somatostatin have been measured in the media of perifused normal pituitaries and GH-secreting adenomas (168). TRH and GnRH are released by pituitary cells maintained in culture for a prolonged period (169); TRH has also been shown to be released by human pituitary adenoma cells of several types, and the increasing content over time suggests synthesis by those cells (170). TRH stimulates release of somatostatin, and somatostatin stimulates release of GHRH by nontumorous cells, but both have opposite effects on adenomatous cells (168); dopamine can stimulate release of TRH from nontumorous cells and from tumors producing GH or PRL, but not from clinically nonfunctioning adenomas (170). These data suggest that differences in hypothalamic hormone production between normal and adenomatous cells may have paracrine or autocrine effects that play a role in the pathogenesis of the neoplasms. VIP has also been shown to be synthesized and released by pituitary cells *in vitro*; studies have shown that VIP production by adenohypophysial cells in culture is stimulated by TRH as well as by GHRH, but not by CRH or GnRH (171); VIP production has not yet been studied in adenomas.

CYTOKINES IN THE ANTERIOR PITUITARY

Cytokines are also known to be produced by cells within the pituitary. Studies using reaggregate cultures have shown that the presence of folliculo-stellate cells is essential for the production of interleukin-6 (172);

application of this information to the study of pituitary adenomas remains to be established, but it is known that interleukin-6 may play a role in the regulation of anterior pituitary hormone release (173). Other cytokines, including interleukin-1β and interleukin-2, tumor necrosis factor α (TNF-α), interferon-γ, thymosin and granulocyte colony-stimulating factor, play a direct role in pituitary regulation as demonstrated *in vitro* (129, 174, 175); the ongoing advances in the field of neuroendocrinimmunology are rapidly expanding the understanding of immune system–pituitary interactions (127, 128) and will no doubt have application in future studies of pituitary adenomas *in vitro*.

GROWTH FACTORS IN THE ANTERIOR PITUITARY

A large number of growth factors have been identified in adenohypophysial cells (176, 177). Some of these are known to be released by pituitary cells *in vitro* (178). They may modulate function as well as cell growth in pituitary adenomas.

Hypothalamic peptides, discussed earlier, may act as growth factors; GHRH is known to stimulate proliferation of nontumorous GH-containing cells *in vitro*, and evidence for its role in somatotroph and mammosomatotroph proliferation *in vivo* is accumulating (56–58). Similarly, CRH has been reported to stimulate corticotroph proliferation *in vivo* (179), but a direct effect *in vitro* has not been identified. VIP has a growth-stimulating effect on prolactinomas *in vitro* (75).

Insulin-like growth factor (IGF)-I may be produced by pituitary cells and is thought to be secreted by the rat tumor GH_3 cell line (180). IGF-I reduces basal and stimulated GH secretion and GH mRNA in pituitary adenomas (181, 182).

Epidermal growth factor (EGF), reported to be localized in pituitary cells (183), stimulates GH release *in vitro* (184). It may have important paracrine or autocrine effects in the regulation of adenohypophysial cell growth; EGF binding sites are present on normal adenohypophysial cells but are absent in pituitary tumors (185), and this alteration, if substantiated, may provide information about tumorigenic mutations in the EGF receptor.

Transforming growth factor α (TGF-α) is se-creted by adenohypophysial cells in culture (178). Its role in regulating secretion and/or proliferation in the same or neighboring pituitary cells is uncertain. Members of the *TGF-β family,* including *inhibins* and *activins,* regulate the release of gonadotropins (186) and may be produced by pituitary cells (187), but this has not as yet been shown *in vitro* or confirmed by analysis of mRNA.

Fibroblast growth factor (FGF) is abundant in the pituitary and plays a role in the regulation of PRL and TSH release (188–190). It is also highly mitogenic (189).

Other factors have been identified using tissue culture methods. Incubation of rabbit articular cartilage chondrocytes in pituitary-conditioned media revealed pituitary-derived factors that stimulated growth of those cells (191); similar substances are produced by pituitary adenomas of several types (192). A number of others, including ovarian growth factor, adipocyte growth factor and pituitary mammary growth factor, have been implicated from pituitary cell cultures (176). Pituitary adenomas have been reported to produce autocrine or paracrine substances that stimulate adenohypophysial cell replication *in vitro* (193).

PARACRINE INTERACTIONS IN THE PITUITARY

Tissue culture studies have led to the novel concept of paracrine regulation of pituitary cells. Suspensions of rat pituitary cells, especially enriched in subpopulations of gonadotrophs and lactotrophs, were found to reaggregate into tissue-like configurations with viable and functional characteristics (13). Selection of gonadotroph-poor populations altered the dynamics of PRL release and responses to GnRH, providing evidence for a gonadotroph-derived paracrine substance that activates lactotrophs (194). Gonadotroph-rich aggregates are a source of angiotensin I–like immunoreactivity which, after conversion to angiotensin II, can stimulate PRL release (14). Angiotensin II is therefore a potential paracrine PRL-releasing substance regulated by GnRH. Incubation of MtT/W15 and MtT/F4 cells with S-100 protein increases PRL secretion *in vitro*, suggesting that folliculo-stellate cells may exert paracrine effects that regulate the release of that hormone (195). There is also evidence for paracrine inhibition of GH and PRL in GH_3 cells (196), and T_3 is thought to stimulate growth of the GH-producing cell line via an autocrine factor (197). A number of other substances such as gastrin, cholecystokinin, galanin, neuropeptide Y, neurotensin, bombesin and opioids are being investigated *in vitro* to establish the nature of their putative paracrine role in adenohypophysial regulation.

CONCLUSION

This chapter has attempted to summarize the most important results obtained by tissue culture techniques that have furthered our understanding of the cytogenesis, regulation and pathogenesis of pituitary adenomas. This invaluable methodology, applied in conjunction with other investigative tools, can expand our knowledge greatly. The study of function as well as structure will prevent us from committing errors as, for example, Sherlock Holmes did when he "had come to an entirely erroneous conclusion, which shows . . . how dangerous it always is to reason from insufficient data."

REFERENCES

1. Asa SL. *In vitro* culture techniques. In: Kovacs K, Asa SL (eds). Functional Endocrine Pathology. Boston, Blackwell Scientific, 1991, pp 109–123.
2. Peillon F, Gourmelen M, Donnadieu M, Brandi A, Sevaux D, Pham Huu, Trung MT. Organ culture of human somatotrophic pituitary adenomas; ultrastructure and growth hormone production. Acta Endocrinol (Copenh) *79*:217–229, 1975.
3. Groom GV, Groom MA, Cooke ID, Boyns AR. The secretion of immuno-reactive luteinizing hormone and follicle-stimulating hormone by the human foetal pituitary in organ culture. J Endocrinol *49*:335–344, 1971.
4. Bégeot M, Li JY, Dubois MP, Dubois PM. Organ culture of the anterior pituitary in a synthetic medium. An immunocytochemical study. Acta Endocrinol (Copenh) *102*:35–41, 1983.
5. Guillemin R, Rosenberg B. Humoral hypothalamic control of anterior pituitary: A study with combined tissue cultures. Endocrinology *57*:599–607, 1955.
6. Siler-Khodr TM, Morgenstern LL, Greenwood FC. Hormone synthesis and release from human fetal adenohypophyses *in vitro*. J Clin Endocrinol Metab *39*:891–905, 1974.
7. Goodyer CG, Hall CStG, Guyda H, Robert F, Giroud CJP. Human fetal pituitary in culture; hormone secretion and response to somatostatin, luteinizing hormone releasing factor, thyrotropin releasing factor and dibutyryl cyclic AMP. J Clin Endocrinol Metab *45*:73–85, 1977.
8. Vale W, Grant G, Amoss M, Blackwell R, Guillemin R. Culture of enzymatically dispersed anterior pituitary cells; functional validation of a method. Endocrinology *91*:562–572, 1972.
9. Melmed S, Odenheimer D, Carlson HE, Hershman JM. Establishment of functional human pituitary tumor cell cultures. In Vitro Cell Dev Biol *18*:35–42, 1982.
10. Asa SL. In vitro studies of human pituitary adenomas. Pathol Res Pract *183*:561–564, 1988.
11. Ben-Jonathan N, Peleg E, Hoefer MT. Optimization of culture conditions for short-term pituitary cell culture. Methods Enzymol *103*:249–257, 1983.
12. Arafah BM, Wilhite BL, Rainieri J, Brodkey JS, Pearson OH. Inhibitory action of bromocriptine and tamoxifen on the growth of human pituitary tumors in soft agar. J Clin Endocrinol Metab *57*:986–992, 1983.
13. van der Schueren B, Denef C, Cassiman J-J. Ultrastructural and functional characteristics of rat pituitary cell aggregates. Endocrinology *110*:513–523, 1982.
14. Denef C. Paracrine interaction in anterior pituitary. In: MacLeod RM, Thorner MO, Scapagnini U (eds). Prolactin, Basic and Clinical Correlates. Padova, Italy, Liviana Press, 1985, pp 53–57.
15. Evans WS, Cronin MJ, Thorner MO. Continuous perifusion of dispersed anterior pituitary cells; technical aspects. Methods Enzymol *103*:294–305, 1983.
16. Negro-Vilar A, Culler MD. Computer-controlled perifusion system for neuroendocrine tissues; development and applications. Methods Enzymol *124*:67–79, 1986.
17. Badger TM. Perifusion of anterior pituitary cells; release of gonadotropins and somatotropins. Methods Enzymol *124*:79–90, 1986.
18. Rasmussen DD. In vitro perifusion of human hypothalamic and pituitary tissue. Methods Enzymol *168*:206–218, 1989.
19. Weiner RI, Bethea CL, Jaquet P, Ramsdell JS, Gospodarowicz DJ. Culture of dispersed anterior pituitary cells on extracellular matrix. Methods Enzymol *103*:287–293, 1983.
20. Knazek RA, Kohler PO, Gullino PM. Hormone production by cells grown in vitro on artificial capillaries. Exp Cell Res *84*:251–254, 1974.
21. Cronin MJ, Weiss J, Rogol AD, Baertschi AJ. Response of anterior pituitary cells to culture media. Endocr Res *13*:85–95, 1987.
22. Hayashi I, Sato GH. Replacement of serum by hormones permits growth of cells in a defined medium. Nature *259*:132–134, 1976.
23. Wynick D, Bloom SR. Magnetic bead separation of anterior pituitary cells. Neuroendocrinology *52*:560–565, 1990.
24. Kawamoto K, Hirano A, Herz F. Simplified in situ preparation of cultured cell monolayers for electron microscopy. J Histochem Cytochem *28*:178–180, 1980.
25. Kuhn H. A simple method for the preparation of cell cultures for ultrastructural investigation. J Histochem Cytochem *29*:84–86, 1981.
26. Ballou RJ, Simpson WG. Technical method. A convenient method for in situ processing of cultured cells for cytochemical localization by electron microscopy. J Pathol *147*:223–226, 1985.
27. Smith PF, Luque EH, Neill JD. Detection and measurement of secretion from individual neu-

roendocrine cells using a reverse hemolytic plaque assay. Methods Enzymol *124*:443–465, 1986.

28. Neill JD, Smith PF, Luque EH, Munoz de Toro M, Nagy G, Mulchahey JJ. Detection and measurement of hormone secretion from individual pituitary cells. Recent Prog Horm Res *43*:175–229, 1987.

29. Frawley LS, Boockfor FR, Hoeffler JP. Identification by plaque assays of a pituitary cell type that secretes both growth hormone and prolactin. Endocrinology *116*:734–737, 1985.

30. Lloyd RV, Anagnostou D, Cano M, Barkan AL, Chandler WF. Analysis of mammosomatotropic cells in normal and neoplastic human pituitary tissues by the reverse hemolytic plaque assay and immunocytochemistry. J Clin Endocrinol Metab 66:1103–1110, 1988.

31. Yamada S, Asa SL, Kovacs K, Muller P, Smyth HS. Analysis of hormone secretion by clinically nonfunctioning human pituitary adenomas using the reverse hemolytic plaque assay. J Clin Endocrinol Metab *68*:73–80, 1989.

32. Yamada S, Aiba T, Hattori A, Suzuki T, Asa SL, Kovacs K. Reverse hemolytic plaque assay. Electron microscopic observation of plaque-forming single adenoma cells in GH producing adenomas. Pathol Res Pract *187*:546–551, 1991.

33. Kohler PO, Bridson WE, Rayford PL, Kohler SE. Hormone production by human pituitary adenomas in culture. Metabolism *18*:782–788, 1969.

34. Batzdorf U, Gold V, Matthews N, Brown J. Human growth hormone in cultures of human pituitary tumors. J Neurosurg *34*:741–748, 1971.

35. Guyda H, Robert F, Colle E, Hardy J. Histologic, ultrastructural, and hormonal characterization of a pituitary tumor secreting both hGH and prolactin. J Clin Endocrinol Metab *36*:531–547, 1973.

36. Beitins IZ, Lipson LG, McArthur JW. Immunoreactive luteinizing hormone, follicle stimulating hormone and their subunits in tissue culture media from normal and adenomatous, human pituitary fragments. J Clin Endocrinol Metab *45*:1271–1280, 1977.

37. Lipson LG, Beitins IZ, Kornblith PD, McArthur JW, Friesen HG, Kliman B, Kjellberg RN. Tissue culture studies on human pituitary tumours; radioimmunoassayable anterior pituitary hormones in the culture medium. Acta Endocrinol (Copenh) *88*:239–249, 1978.

38. Kameya T, Tsumuraya M, Adachi I, Abe K, Ichikizaki K, Toya S, Demura R. Ultrastructure, immunohistochemistry and hormone release of pituitary adenomas in relation to prolactin production. Virchows Arch [Pathol Anat] *387*:31–46, 1980.

39. Kawakita S, Asa SL, Kovacs K. Effects of growth hormone-releasing hormone (GHRH) on densely granulated somatotroph adenomas and sparsely granulated somatotroph adenomas *in vitro*; a morphological and functional investigation. J Endocrinol Invest *12*:443–448, 1989.

40. Hofland LJ, van Koetsveld PM, van Vroonhoven CCJ, Stefanko SZ, Lamberts SWJ. Heterogeneity of growth hormone (GH) release by individual pituitary adenoma cells from acromegalic patients, as determined by the reverse hemolytic plaque assay; effects of SMS 201-995, GH-releasing hormone and thyrotropin-releasing hormone. J Clin Endocrinol Metab *68*:613–620, 1989.

41. Beck-Peccoz P, Bassetti M, Spada A, Medri G, Arosio M, Giannattasio G, Faglia G. Glycoprotein hormone α-subunit response to growth hormone (GH)-releasing hormone in patients with active acromegaly. Evidence for α-subunit and GH coexistence in the same tumoral cell. J Clin Endocrinol Metab *61*:541–546, 1985.

42. White MC, Newland P, Daniels M, Turner SJ, Mathias D, Teasdale G, Kendall-Taylor P. Growth hormone secreting pituitary adenomas are heterogeneous in cell culture and commonly secrete glycoprotein hormone α-subunit. Clin Endocrinol (Oxf) *25*:173–179, 1986.

43. Ishibashi M, Yamaji T, Takaku F, Teramoto A, Fukushima T. Secretion of glycoprotein hormone α-subunit by pituitary tumors. J Clin Endocrinol Metab *64*:1187–1193, 1987.

44. Adams EF, Winslow CLJ, Mashiter K. Pancreatic growth hormone releasing factor stimulates growth hormone secretion by pituitary cells. Lancet *1*:1100–1101, 1983.

45. Webb CB, Thominet L, Frohman LA. Ectopic growth hormone releasing factor stimulates growth hormone release from human somatotroph adenomas in vitro. J Clin Endocrinol Metab *56*:417–419, 1983.

46. Adams EF, Bhuttacharji SC, Halliwell CLJ, Loizou M, Birch G, Mashiter K. Effect of pancreatic growth hormone releasing factors on GH secretion by human somatotrophic pituitary tumours in cell culture. Clin Endocrinol (Oxf) *21*:709–718, 1984.

47. Lamberts SWJ, Verleun T, Oosterom R. The interrelationship between the effects of somatostatin and human pancreatic growth hormone-releasing factor on growth hormone release by cultured pituitary tumor cells from patients with acromegaly. J Clin Endocrinol Metab *58*:250–254, 1984.

48. Ishibashi M, Yamaji T. Effects of hypophysiotropic factors on growth hormone and prolactin secretion from somatotroph adenomas in culture. J Clin Endocrinol Metab *60*:985–993, 1985.

49. Loras B, Li JY, Durand A, Trouillas J, Sassolas G, Girod C. GRF et adénomes somatotropes humains. Corrélations *in vivo* et *in vitro* entre la libération de GH et les aspects morphologiques et immunocytochimiques. Ann Endocrinol (Paris) *46*:373–382, 1985.

50. Spada A, Elahi FR, Arosio M, Sartorio A, Guglielmo L, Vallar L, Faglia G. Lack of desensitization of adenomatous somatotrophs to growth hormone-releasing hormone in acromegaly. J Clin Endocrinol Metab *64*:585–591, 1987.

51. Davis JRE, Wilson EM, Vidal ME, Johnson AP, Lynch SS, Sheppard MC. Regulation of growth hormone secretion and messenger ribonucleic acid accumulation in human somatotropinoma cells *in vitro*. J Clin Endocrinol Metab *69*:704–708, 1989.

52. Herman V, Weiss M, Becker D, Melmed S. Hypothalamic hormonal regulation of human growth hormone gene expression in somatotroph adenoma cell cultures. Endocr Pathol *1*:236–244, 1990.

53. Shibasaki T, Hotta M, Yamauchi N, Masuda A, Imaki T, Demura H, Ling N, Shizume K. Desensitization of rat pituitary somatotrophs to growth hormone-releasing factor occurs *in vitro*. Endocrinol Jpn *34*:799–807, 1987.

54. Schulte HM, Benker G, Windeck R, Olbricht T, Reinwein D. Failure to respond to growth hormone

releasing hormone (GHRH) in acromegaly due to a GHRH secreting pancreatic tumor: Dynamics of multiple endocrine testing. J Clin Endocrinol Metab 61:585–587, 1985.

55. Billestrup N, Swanson LW, Vale W. Growth hormone-releasing factor stimulates proliferation of somatotrophs *in vitro*. Proc Natl Acad Sci USA 83:6854–6857, 1986.

56. Sano T, Asa SL, Kovacs K. Growth hormone-releasing hormone-producing tumors; clinical, biochemical, and morphological manifestations. Endocr Rev 9:357–373, 1988.

57. Stefaneanu L, Kovacs K, Horvath E, Asa SL, Losinski NE, Billestrup N, Price J, Vale W. Adenohypophysial changes in mice transgenic for human growth hormone-releasing factor: A histological, immunocytochemical, and electron microscopic investigation. Endocrinology 125:2710–2718, 1989.

58. Asa SL, Kovacs K, Stefaneanu L, Horvath E, Billestrup N, Gonzalez-Manchon C, Vale W. Pituitary mammosomatotroph adenomas develop in old mice transgenic for growth hormone-releasing hormone. Proc Soc Exp Biol Med 193:232–235, 1990.

59. Adams EF, Brajkovich IE, Mashiter K. Hormone secretion by dispersed cell cultures of human pituitary adenomas: Effects of theophylline, thyrotropin-releasing hormone, somatostatin, and 2-bromo-α-ergocriptine. J Clin Endocrinol Metab 49:120–126, 1979.

60. Marcovitz S, Goodyer CG, Guyda H, Gardiner RJ, Hardy J. Comparative study of human fetal, normal adult, and somatotropic adenoma pituitary function in tissue culture. J Clin Endocrinol Metab 54:6–16, 1982.

61. Le Dafniet M, Garnier P, Bression D, Brandi AM, Racadot J, Peillon F. Correlative studies between the presence of thyrotropin-releasing hormone (TRH) receptors and the in vitro stimulation of growth-hormone (GH) secretion in human GH-secreting adenomas. Horm Metab Res 17:476–479, 1985.

62. White MC, Daniels M, Kendall-Taylor P, Turner SJ, Mathias D, Teasdale G. Effects of growth hormone-releasing factor (1–44) on growth hormone release from human somatotrophinomas *in vitro*; interaction with somatostatin, dopamine, vasoactive intestinal peptide and cycloheximide. J Endocrinol 105:269–276, 1985.

63. Oosterom R, Verleun T, Lamberts SWJ. Human growth hormone-secreting pituitary adenoma cells in long-term culture; effects of dexamethasone and growth hormone releasing factor. J Endocrinol 100:353–360, 1984.

64. Daniels M, White MC, Kendall-Taylor P. Long-term in-vitro maintenance of growth hormone secretion from human somatotrophinomas with cortisol, and its effects on growth hormone-releasing factor. J Endocrinol 114:503–509, 1987.

65. Prysor-Jones RA, Kennedy SJ, O'Sullivan JP, Jenkins JS. Effect of bromocriptine, somatostatin, and oestradiol-17β on hormone secretion and ultrastructure of human pituitary tumours in vitro. Acta Endocrinol (Copenh) 98:14–23, 1981.

66. Lamberts SWJ, Verleun T, Hofland L, Del Pozo E. A comparison between the effects of SMS 201–995, bromocriptine and a combination of both drugs on hormone release by the cultured pituitary tumour cells of acromegalic patients. Clin Endocrinol (Oxf) 27:11–23, 1987.

67. Asa SL, Felix I, Kovacs K, Ramyar L. Effects of somatostatin on somatotroph adenomas of the human pituitary: An in vitro functional and morphological study. Endocr Pathol 1:228–235, 1990.

68. Peillon F, Cesselin F, Bression D, Zygelman N, Brandi AM, Nousbaum A, Mauborgne A. *In vitro* effect of dopamine and L-dopa on prolactin and growth hormone release from human pituitary adenomas. J Clin Endocrinol Metab 49:737–741, 1979.

69. Tallo D, Malarkey WB. Adrenergic and dopaminergic modulation of growth hormone and prolactin secretion in normal and tumor-bearing human pituitaries in monolayer culture. J Clin Endocrinol Metab 53:1278–1284, 1981.

70. Lawton NF, Evans AJ, Weller RO. Dopaminergic inhibition of growth hormone and prolactin release during continuous in vitro perifusion of normal and adenomatous human pituitary. J Neurol Sci 49:229–239, 1981.

71. Vallar L, Spada A, Giannattasio G. Altered G_S and adenylate cyclase activity in human GH-secreting pituitary adenomas. Nature 330:566–568, 1987.

72. Knazek RA, Skyler JS. Secretion of human prolactin *in vitro*. Proc Soc Exp Biol Med 151:561–564, 1976.

73. Bethea CL, Weiner RI. Human prolactin secreting adenoma cells maintained on extracellar matrix. Endocrinology 108:357–360, 1981.

74. Lamberts SWJ. Interactions of steroids with prolactin secretion in vitro. Horm Res 22:172–178, 1985.

75. Prysor-Jones RA, Silverlight JJ, Jenkins JS. Oestradiol, vasoactive intestinal peptide and fibroblast growth factor in the growth of human pituitary tumour cells *in vitro*. J Endocrinol 120:171–177, 1989.

76. Jaquet P, Gunz G, Grisoli F. Hormonal regulation of prolactin release by human prolactinoma cells cultured in serum-free conditions. Horm Res 22:153–163, 1985.

77. Chihara K, Iwasaki J, Minamitani N, Kaji H, Kodama H, Fujita T, Shirataki K, Tamaki N, Matsumoto S. Prolactin secretion from human prolactinomas perifused in vitro; effect of TRH, prostaglandin E, theophylline, dopamine and dopamine receptor blockers. Acta Endocrinol (Copenh) 105:6–13, 1984.

78. Spada A, Nicosia S, Cortelazzi L, Pezzo G, Bassetti M, Sartorio A, Giannattasio G. *In vitro* studies on prolactin release and adenylate cyclase activity in human prolactin-secreting pituitary adenomas. Different sensitivity of macro- and microadenomas to dopamine and vasoactive intestinal polypeptide. J Clin Endocrinol Metab 56:1–10, 1983.

79. Prysor-Jones RA, Silverlight JJ, Jenkins JS. Vasoactive intestinal peptide increases intracellular free calcium in rat and human pituitary tumour cells *in vitro*. J Endocrinol 114:119–123, 1987.

80. Hassoun J, Jaquet P, Devictor B, Andonian C, Grisoli F, Gunz G, Toga M. Bromocriptine effects on cultured human prolactin-producing pituitary adenomas: *In vitro* ultrastructural, morphometric, and immunoelectron microscopic studies. J Clin Endocrinol Metab 61:686–692, 1985.

81. Ishibashi M, Yamaji T. Mechanism of the inhibitory action of dopamine and somatostatin on prolactin secretion from human lactotrophs in culture. J Clin Endocrinol Metab 60:599–606, 1985.

82. Duffy AE, Asa SL, Kovacs K. Effect of bromocrip-

tine on secretion and morphology of human pro-lactin cell adenomas in vitro. Horm Res *30*:32–38, 1988.

83. Niwa J, Mori M, Minase T, Hashi K. Immunofluo-rescence demonstration of tubulin and actin in estrogen-induced rat prolactinoma cells in vitro. Exp Cell Res *161*:517–524, 1985.

84. Castanas E, Jaquet P, Gunz G, Cantau P, Giraud P. Direct action of opiates on bromocriptine-inhib-ited prolactin release by human prolactinoma cells in primary culture. J Clin Endocrinol Metab *61*:963–968, 1985.

85. Ishibashi M, Yamaji T, Takaku F, Teramoto A, Fukushima T, Toyama M, Kamoi K. Effect of GnRH-associated peptide on prolactin secretion from human lactotrope adenoma cells in culture. Acta Endocrinol (Copenh) *116*:81–84, 1987.

86. Lamberts SWJ, Uitterlinden P, Reubi JC, de Jong FH. Effects of gonadotropin-releasing hormone and its agonists on prolactin secretion from normal and tumorous pituitary cells. Neuroendocrinology *49*:157–163, 1989.

87. Goluboff LG, Ezrin C. Effect of pregnancy on the somatotroph and the prolactin cell of the human adenohypophysis. J Clin Endocrinol *29*:1533–1538, 1969.

88. Skyler JS, Rogol AD, Lovenberg W, Knazek RA. Characterization of growth hormone and prolactin produced by human pituitary in culture. Endocri-nology *100*:283–291, 1977.

89. Mashiter K, Van Noorden S, De Marco L, Adams E, Joplin GF. Hormone secretion by human so-matotrophic, lactotrophic, and mixed pituitary ad-enomas in culture. J Clin Endocrinol Metab *48*:108–113, 1979.

90. Loras B, Trouillas J, Li Y, Durand A, Girod C, Bertrand J. Inversely related evolution of growth hormone and prolactin secretions in long-term tissue cultures of human pituitary adenomas from acromegalic patients. In Vitro Cell Dev Biol *24*:1064–1070, 1988.

91. Hofland LJ, van Koetsveld PM, Verleun TM, Lam-berts SWJ. Glycoprotein hormone alpha-subunit and prolactin release by cultured pituitary ade-noma cells from acromegalic patients: Correlation with GH release. Clin Endocrinol (Oxf) *30*:601–611, 1989.

92. Kashio Y, Chomczynski P. Downs TR, Frohman LA. Growth hormone and prolactin secretion in cultured somatomammotroph cells. Endocrinology *127*:1129–1135, 1990.

93. Kovacs K, Horvath E. Tumors of the pituitary gland. In: Atlas of Tumor Pathology. 2nd Series. Fascicle 21. Washington, DC, Armed Forces Insti-tute of Pathology, 1986.

94. Asa SL, Kovacs K, Singer W, Smyth HS. Hormone secretion *in vitro* by plurihormonal pituitary tumors of the acidophil cell line. Abstract. J Endocrinol Invest 14(suppl 1):69, 1991.

95. Leong DA, Lau SK, Sinha YN, Kaiser DL, Thorner MO. Enumeration of lactotropes and somatotropes among male and female pituitary cells in culture; evidence in favor of a mammosomatotrope sub-population in the rat. Endocrinology *116*:1371–1378, 1985.

96. Mulchahey JJ, Jaffe RB. Detection of a potential progenitor cell in the human fetal pituitary that secretes both growth hormone and prolactin. J Clin Endocrinol Metab *66*:24–32, 1987.

97. Asa SL, Kovacs K, Horvath E, Losinski NE, Laszlo FA, Domokos I, Halliday WC. Human fetal ade-nohypophysis. Electron microscopic and ultra-structural immunocytochemical analysis. Neuroen-docrinology *48*:423–431, 1988.

98. Asa SL, Kovacs K, Singer W. Human fetal adeno-hypophysis: Morphologic and functional analysis in vitro. Neuroendocrinology *53*:562–572, 1991.

99. Moran A, Asa SL, Kovacs K, Horvath E, Singer W, Sagman U, Reubi JC, Wilson CB, Larson R, Pescovitz OH. Gigantism due to pituitary mam-mosomatotroph hyperplasia. N Engl J Med *323*:322–327, 1990.

100. Serri O. Growth hormone releasing factor stimu-lates and somatostatin inhibits prolactin release from human mixed somatotroph-lactotroph ade-nomas in perifusion. Clin Endocrinol (Oxf) *27*:675–682, 1987.

101. Ishibashi M, Yamaji T. Direct effects of catechol-amines, thyrotropin-releasing hormone, and so-matostatin on growth hormone and prolactin se-cretion from adenomatous and nonadenomatous human pituitary cells in culture. J Clin Invest *73*:66–78, 1984.

102. Boudouresque F, Lissitzky JC, Jaquet P, Guibout M, Goldstein E, Grisoli F, Oliver C. Peptides lipo-corticotropes dans la maladie de Cushing: Etudes in vitro. Horm Res *13*:242–258, 1980.

103. Gillies G, Ratter S, Grossman A, Gaillard R, Lowry PJ, Besser GM, Rees LH. ACTH, LPH and β-endorphin secretion from perfused isolated human pituitary tumour cells in vitro. Horm Res *13*:280–290, 1980.

104. Fuller PJ, Lim ATW, Barlow JW, White EL, Khalid BAK, Copolov DL, Lolait S, Funder JW, Stockigt JR. A pituitary tumor producing high molecular weight adrenocorticotropin-related peptides: Clin-ical and cell culture studies. J Clin Endocrinol Metab *58*:134–142, 1984.

105. Krieger DT. Physiopathology of Cushing's disease. Endocr Rev *4*:22–43, 1983.

106. Shibasaki T, Nakahara M, Shizume K, Kiyosawa Y, Suda T, Demura H, Kuwayama A, Kageyama N, Benoit R, Ling N. Pituitary adenomas that caused Cushing's disease or Nelson's syndrome are not responsive to ovine corticotropin-releasing fac-tor *in vitro*. J Clin Endocrinol Metab *56*:414–416, 1983.

107. White MC, Adams EF, Loizou M, Mashiter K, Fahlbusch R. Corticotropin releasing factor stim-ulates ACTH release from human pituitary corti-cotropic tumour cell in culture. Lancet *1*:1251–1252, 1982.

108. Suda T, Tozawa F, Mouri T, Sasaki A, Shibasaki T, Demura H, Shizume K. Effects of cyprohepta-dine, reserpine, and synthetic corticotropin-releas-ing factor on pituitary glands from patients with Cushing's disease. J Clin Endocrinol Metab *56*:1094–1099, 1983.

109. Lamberts SWJ, Verleun T, Oosterom R, De Jong F, Hackeng WHL. Corticotropin-releasing factor (ovine) and vasopressin exert synergistic effect on adrenocorticotropin release in man. J Clin Endo-crinol Metab *58*:298–303, 1984.

110. Suda T, Tomori N, Tozawa F, Demura H, Shizume K. Effects of corticotropin-releasing factor and other materials on adrenocorticotropin secretion from pituitary glands of patients with Cushing's disease *in vitro*. J Clin Endocrinol Metab *59*:840–845, 1984.

111. Oosterom R, Verleun T, Uitterlinden P, Hackeng

WHL, Burbach JPH, Wiegant VM, Lamberts SWJ. ACTH and β-endorphin secretion by three corticotrophic adenomas in culture. Effects of culture time, dexamethasone, vasopressin and synthetic corticotrophin releasing factor. Acta Endocrinol (Copenh) *106*:21–29, 1984.

112. White MC, Adams EF, Loizou M, Mashiter K, Fahlbusch R. Ovine corticotrophin releasing factor stimulates ACTH release from human corticotrophinoma cells in culture; interaction with hydrocortisone and arginine vasopressin. Clin Endocrinol (Oxf) *23*:295–302, 1985.

113. Westphal M, Jaquet P, Wilson CB. Long-term culture of human corticotropin-secreting adenomas on extracellular matrix and evaluation of serum-free conditions. Secretory aspects. Acta Neuropathol (Berl) *71*:111–118, 1986.

114. Westphal M, Jaquet P, Wilson CB. Long-term culture of human corticotropin-secreting adenomas on extracellular matrix and evaluation of serum-free conditions. Morphological aspects. Acta Neuropathol (Berl) *71*:142–149, 1986.

115. Grino M, Boudouresque F, Conte-Devolx B, Gunz G, Grisoli F, Oliver C, Jaquet P. *In vitro* corticotropin-releasing hormone (CRH) stimulation of adrenocorticotropin release from corticotroph adenoma cells: Effect of prolonged exposure to CRH and its interaction with cortisol. J Clin Endocrinol Metab *66*:770–775, 1988.

116. Horvath SE, Asa SL, Kovacs K, Adams LA, Singer W, Smyth HS. Human pituitary corticotroph adenomas in vitro: Morphologic and functional responses to corticotropin-releasing hormone and cortisol. Neuroendocrinology *51*:241–248, 1990.

117. Suda T, Tozawa F, Yamada M, Ushiyama T, Tomori N, Sumitomo T, Nakagami Y, Demura H, Shizume K. Effects of corticotropin-releasing hormone and dexamethasone on proopiomelanocortin messenger RNA level in human corticotroph adenoma cells in vitro. J Clin Invest *82*:110–114, 1988.

118. Mashiter K, Adams EF, Gillies G, Van Noorden S, Ratter S. Adrenocorticotropin and lipotropin secretion by dispersed cell cultures of a human corticotropic adenoma: Effect of hypothalamic extract, arginine vasopressin, hydrocortisone, and serotonin. J Clin Endocrinol Metab *51*:566–572, 1980.

119. White MC, Adams EF, Loizou M, Mashiter K. Vasoactive intestinal peptide stimulates adrenocorticotropin release from human corticotropinoma cells in culture: Interaction with arginine vasopressin and hydrocortisone. J Clin Endocrinol Metab *55*:967–972, 1982.

120. Shibasaki T, Masui H. Effects of various neuropeptides on the secretion of proopiomelanocortin-derived peptides by a cultured pituitary adenoma causing Nelson's syndrome. J Clin Endocrinol Metab *55*:872–876, 1982.

121. Mollard P, Vacher P, Rogawski MA, Dufy B. Vasopressin enhances a calcium current in human ACTH-secreting pituitary adenoma cells. FASEB J *2*:2907–2912, 1988.

122. Ishibashi M, Yamaji T. Direct effects of thyrotropin-releasing hormone, cyproheptadine, and dopamine on adrenocorticotropin secretion from human corticotroph adenoma cells in vitro. J Clin Invest *68*:1018–1027, 1981.

123. Lüdecke DK, Westphal M, Schabet M, Höllt V. In vitro secretion of ACTH, β-endorphin and β-lipotropin in Cushing's disease and Nelson's syndrome. Horm Res *13*:259–279, 1980.

124. Thorén M, Anniko M. Glucocorticoid incubation of human ACTH-producing pituitary tumours in vitro. A study on ACTH secretion and cell morphology. Arch Otorhinolaryngol *243*:96–101, 1986.

125. Hale AC, Coates PJ, Doniach I, Howlett TA, Grossman A, Rees LH, Besser GM. A bromocriptine-responsive corticotroph adenoma secreting alpha-MSH in a patient with Cushing's disease. Clin Endocrinol (Oxf) *28*:215–223, 1988.

126. Jimenez Reina L, Leal-Cerro A, Garcia J, Garcia-Luna PP, Astorga R, Bernal G. In vitro effects of ketoconazole on corticotrope cell morphology and ACTH secretion of two pituitary adenomas removed from patients with Nelson's syndrome. Acta Endocrinol (Copenh) *121*:185–190, 1989.

127. Bateman A, Singh A, Kral T, Solomon S. The immune-hypothalamic-pituitary-adrenal axis. Endocr Rev *10*:92–112, 1989.

128. Berczi I. Neurohormonal immunoregulation. Endocr Pathol 1:197–219, 1990.

129. Malarkey WB, Zvara BJ. Interleukin-1β and other cytokines stimulate adrenocorticotropin release from cultured pituitary cells of patients with Cushing's disease. J Clin Endocrinol Metab 69:196–199, 1989.

130. Yovos JG, Falko JM, O'Dorisio TM, Malarkey WB, Cataland S, Capen CC. Thyrotoxicosis and a thyrotropin-secreting pituitary tumor causing unilateral exophthalmos. J Clin Endocrinol Metab *53*:338–343, 1981.

131. Filetti S, Rapoport B, Aron DC, Greenspan FC, Wilson CB, Fraser W. TSH and TSH-subunit production by human thyrotrophic tumour cells in monolayer culture. Acta Endocrinol (Copenh) *99*:224–231, 1982.

132. Mashiter K, Van Noorden S, Fahlbusch R, Fill H, Skrabal K. Hyperthyroidism due to a TSH secreting pituitary adenoma: Case report, treatment and evidence for adenoma TSH by morphological and cell culture studies. Clin Endocrinol (Oxf) *18*:473–483, 1983.

133. Spada A, Bassetti M, Martino E, Giannattasio G, Beck-Peccoz P, Sartorio A, Vallar L, Baschieri L, Pinchera A, Faglia G. *In vitro* studies on TSH secretion and adenylate cyclase activity in a human TSH-secreting pituitary adenoma. Effects of somatostatin and dopamine. J Endocrinol Invest *8*:193–198, 1985.

134. Trouillas J, Girod C, Loras B, Claustrat B, Sassolas G, Perrin G, Buonaguidi R. The TSH secretion in the human pituitary adenomas. Pathol Res Pract *183*:596–600, 1988.

135. Bevan JS, Burke CW, Esiri MM, Adams CBT, Ballabio M, Nissim M, Faglia G. Studies of two thyrotrophin-secreting pituitary adenomas: Evidence for dopamine receptor deficiency. Clin Endocrinol (Oxf) *31*:59–70, 1989.

136. Demura R, Kubo O, Demura H, Shizume K. FSH and LH secreting pituitary adenoma. J Clin Endocrinol Metab *45*:653–657, 1977.

137. Takeuchi J, Handa H, Suda K, Aso T. In vitro secretion of follicle-stimulating hormone by pituitary chromophobe adenomas. Surg Neurol *14*:303–309, 1980.

138. Snyder PJ, Bashey HM, Kim SU, Chappel SC. Secretion of uncombined subunits of luteinizing

hormone by gonadotroph cell adenomas. J Clin
Endocrinol Metab 59:1169–1175, 1984.

139. Asa SL, Gerrie BM, Kovacs K, Horvath E, Singer
W, Killinger DW, Smyth HS. Structure-function
correlations of human pituitary gonadotroph adenomas *in vitro*. Lab Invest 58:403–410, 1988.

140. Asa SL, Gerrie BM, Singer W, Horvath E, Kovacs
K, Smyth HS. Gonadotropin secretion *in vitro* by
human pituitary null cell adenomas and oncocytomas. J Clin Endocrinol Metab 62:1011–1019,
1986.

141. Snyder PJ. Gonadotroph cell adenomas of the
pituitary. Endocr Rev 6:552–563, 1985.

142. Lamberts SWJ, Verleun T, Oosterom R, Hofland
L, van Ginkel LA, Loeber JG, van Vroonhoven
CCJ, Stefanko SZ, de Jong FH. The effects of
bromocriptine, thyrotropin-releasing hormone,
and gonadotropin-releasing hormone on hormone
secretion by gonadotropin-secreting pituitary adenomas *in vivo* and *in vitro*. J Clin Endocrinol Metab
64:524–530, 1987.

143. Daniels M, Newland P, Dunn J, Kendall-Taylor P,
White MC. Long-term effects of a gonadotro-
phin-releasing hormone agonist ([D-Ser([Buᵗ)⁶]-
GnRH(1–9) nonapeptide-ethylamide) on gonadotrophin secretion from human pituitary gonadotroph cell adenomas *in vitro*. J Endocrinol 118:491–
496, 1988.

144. Kwekkeboom DJ, de Jong FH, Lamberts SWJ.
Gonadotropin release by clinically nonfunctioning
and gonadotroph pituitary adenomas *in vivo* and
in vitro; relation to sex and effects of thyrotropin-
releasing hormone, gonadotropin-releasing hormone, and bromocriptine. J Clin Endocrinol Metab
68:1128–1135, 1989.

145. Song JY, Jin L, Chandler WF, England BG, Smart
JB, Landefeld TD, Lloyd RV. Gonadotropin-releasing hormone regulates gonadotropin β-subunit
and chromogranin-B messenger ribonucleic acids
in cultured chromogranin-A–positive pituitary adenomas. J Clin Endocrinol Metab 71:622–630,
1990.

146. Mashiter K, Adams E, Van Noorden S. Secretion
of LH, FSH and PRL shown by cell culture and
immunocytochemistry of human functionless pituitary adenomas. Clin Endocrinol 15:103–112,
1981.

147. Surmont DWA, Winslow CLJ, Loizou M, White
MC, Adams EF, Mashiter K. Gonadotrophin and
alpha subunit secretion by human 'functionless'
pituitary adenomas in cell culture: Long term effects of luteinizing hormone releasing hormone
and thyrotrophin releasing hormone. Clin Endocrinol (Oxf) 19:325–336, 1983.

148. Kovacs K, Lloyd R, Horvath E, Asa SL, Stefaneanu
L, Killinger DW, Smyth HS. Silent somatotroph
adenomas of the human pituitary. A morphologic
study of three cases including immunocytochemistry, electron microscopy, *in vitro* examination, and
in situ hybridization. Am J Pathol 134:345–353,
1989.

149. Lloyd RV, Fields K, Jin L, Horvath E, Kovacs K.
Analysis of endocrine active and clinically silent
corticotropic adenomas by *in situ* hybridization. Am
J Pathol 137:479–488, 1990.

150. Reincke M, Allolio B, Saeger W, Kaulen D, Winkelmann W. A pituitary adenoma secreting high
molecular weight adrenocorticotropin without evidence of Cushing's disease. J Clin Endocrinol
Metab 65:1296–1300, 1987.

151. Chabre O, Martinie M, Vivier J, Eimin-Richard E,
Bertagna X, Bachelot I. A clinically silent corticotrophic pituitary adenoma (CSCPA) secreting a
biologically inactive but immunoreactive assayable
ACTH. Abstract. J Endocrinol Invest 14(Suppl
1):87, 1991.

152. Yamada S, Asa SL, Kovacs K. Oncocytomas and
null cell adenomas of the human pituitary; morphometric and in vitro functional comparison. Virchows Arch [A] 413:333–339, 1988.

153. Kovacs K, Asa SL, Horvath E, Ryan N, Singer W,
Killinger DW, Smyth HS, Scheithauer BW, Eber-
sold MJ. Null cell adenomas of the pituitary: At-
tempts to resolve their cytogenesis. In: Lechago J,
Kameya T (eds). Endocrine Pathology Update.
New York, Field and Wood, 1990, pp 17–31.

154. Asa SL, Cheng Z, Ranyar L, Singer W, Kovacs K,
Smyth HS, Muller P. Human pituitary null cell
adenomas and oncocytomas *in vitro*: Effects of
adenohypophysiotropic hormones and gonadal
steroids on hormone secretion and tumor cell morphology. J Clin Endocrinol Metab 74:1128–1134,
1992.

155. Levy A, Lightman SL. Effects of thyrotropin-releasing hormone and gonadotropin-releasing hormone on inositol phospholipid turnover in endocrinologically inactive pituitary adenomas and
prolactinomas. J Clin Endocrinol Metab 69:122–
126, 1989.

156. Kwekkeboom DJ, Hofland LJ, van Koetsveld PM,
Singh R, van den Berge JH, Lamberts SWJ. Bromocriptine increasingly suppresses the *in vitro* gonadotropin and α-subunit release from pituitary
adenomas during long term culture. J Clin Endocrinol Metab 71:718–724, 1990.

157. Klibanski A, Shupnik MA, Bikkal HA, Black PM,
Kliman B, Zervas NT. Dopaminergic regulation of
α-subunit secretion and messenger ribonucleic acid
levels in α-secreting pituitary tumors. J Clin Endocrinol Metab 66:96–102, 1988.

158. Kovacs K, Horvath E, Asa SL, Stefaneanu L, Sano
T. Pituitary cells producing more than one hormone. Human pituitary adenomas. Trends Endocrinol Metab 1:104–107, 1989.

159. Jaquet P, Hassoun J, Delori P, Gunz G, Grisoli F,
Weintraub BD. A human pituitary adenoma secreting thyrotropin and prolactin; immunohistochemical, biochemical, and cell culture studies. J
Clin Endocrinol Metab 59:817–824, 1984.

160. Lamberts SWJ, Oosterom R, Verleun T, Krenning
EP, Assies H. Regulation of hormone release by
cultured cells from a thyrotropin-growth hormone-
secreting pituitary tumor. Direct inhibiting effects
of 3,5,3′-triiodothyronine and dexamethasone on
thyrotropin secretion. J Endocrinol Invest 7:313–
317, 1984.

161. Beck-Peccoz P, Piscitelli G, Amr S, Ballabio M,
Bassetti M, Giannattasio G, Spada A, Nissim M,
Weintraub BD, Faglia G. Endocrine, biochemical,
and morphological studies of a pituitary adenoma
secreting growth hormone, thyrotropin (TSH), and
α-subunit: Evidence for secretion of TSH with
increased bioactivity. J Clin Endocrinol Metab
62:704–711, 1986.

162. Simard M, Mirell CJ, Pekary AE, Drexler J, Kovacs
K, Hershman JM. Hormonal control of thyrotropin and growth hormone secretion in a human
thyrotrope pituitary adenoma studied in vitro. Acta
Endocrinol (Copenh) 119:283–290, 1988.

163. Malarkey WB, Kovacs K, O'Dorisio TM. Response

of a GH- and TSH-secreting pituitary adenoma to a somatostatin analogue (SMS 201–995); evidence that GH and TSH coexist in the same cell and secretory granules. Neuroendocrinology 49:267–274, 1989.

164. Kuzuya N, Inoue K, Ishibashi M, Murayama Y, Koide Y, Ito K, Yamaji T, Yamashita K. Endocrine and immunohistochemical studies on thyrotropin (TSH)-secreting pituitary adenomas; responses of TSH, α-subunit, and growth hormone to hypothalamic releasing hormones and their distribution in adenoma cells. J Clin Endocrinol Metab 71:1103–1111, 1990.

165. Sano T, Kovacs K, Asa SL, Smyth HS. Immunoreactive luteinizing hormone in functioning corticotroph adenomas of the pituitary. Immunohistochemical and tissue culture studies of two cases. Virchows Arch [A] 417:361–367, 1990.

166. Felix I, Asa SL, Kovacs K, Horvath E. Changes in hormone production of a recurrent silent corticotroph adenoma of the pituitary: A histologic, immunohistochemical, ultrastructural, and tissue culture study. Hum Pathol 22:719–721, 1991.

167. Lloyd RV, Jin L, Song J. Ultrastructural localization of prolactin and chromogranin B messenger ribonucleic acids with biotinylated oligonucleotide probes in cultured pituitary cells. Lab Invest 63:413–419, 1990.

168. Joubert (Bression) D, Benlot C, Lagoguey A, Garnier P, Brandi AM, Gautron JP, LeGrand JC, Peillon F. Normal and growth hormone (GH)-secreting adenomatous human pituitaries release somatostatin and GH-releasing hormone. J Clin Endocrinol Metab 68:572–577, 1989.

169. May V, Wilber JF, U'Prichard DC, Childs GV. Persistence of immunoreactive TRH and GnRH in long-term primary anterior pituitary cultures. Peptides 8:543–558, 1987.

170. Le Dafniet M, Lefebvre P, Barret A, Mechain C, Feinstein MC, Brandi AM, Peillon F. Normal and adenomatous human pituitaries secrete thyrotropin-releasing hormone in vitro; modulation by dopamine, haloperidol, and somatostatin. J Clin Endocrinol Metab 71:480–486, 1990.

171. Lam KSL, Reichlin S. Pituitary vasoactive intestinal peptide regulates prolactin secretion in the hypothyroid rat. Neuroendocrinology 50:524–528, 1989.

172. Vankelecom H, Carmeliet P, van Damme J, Billiau A, Denef C. Production of interleukin-6 by folliculo-stellate cells of the anterior pituitary gland in a histiotypic cell aggregate culture system. Neuroendocrinology 49:102–106, 1989.

173. Spangelo BL, Judd AM, Isakson PC, MacLeod RM. Interleukin-6 stimulates anterior pituitary hormone release in vitro. Endocrinology 125:575–577, 1989.

174. Walton PE, Cronin MJ. Tumor necrosis factor-α and interferon-gamma reduce prolactin release in vitro. Am J Physiol 259:E672–E676, 1990.

175. Yamaguchi M, Sakata M, Matsuzaki N, Koike K, Miyake A, Tanizawa O. Induction by tumor necrosis factor-alpha of rapid release of immunoreactive and bioactive luteinizing hormone from rat pituitary cells in vitro. Neuroendocrinology 52:468–472, 1990.

176. Webster J, Ham J, Bevan JS, Scanlon MF. Growth factors and pituitary tumors. Trends Endocrinol Metab 1:95–98, 1989.

177. Ezzat S, Melmed S. The role of growth factors in

the pituitary. J Endocrinol Invest 13:691–698, 1990.

178. Kobrin MS, Asa SL, Samsoondar J, Kudlow JE. α-Transforming growth factor in the bovine anterior pituitary gland; secretion by dispersed cells and immunohistochemical localization. Endocrinology 121:1412–1416, 1987.

179. Gertz BJ, Contreras LN, McComb DJ, Kovacs K, Tyrrell JB, Dallman MF. Chronic administration of corticotropin-releasing factor increases pituitary corticotroph number. Endocrinology 120:381–388, 1987.

180. Fagin JA, Pixley S, Slanina S, Ong J, Melmed S. Insulin-like growth factor I gene expression in GH₃ rat pituitary cells; messenger ribonucleic acid content, immunocytochemistry, and secretion. Endocrinology 120:2037–2043, 1987.

181. Ceda GP, Hoffman AR, Silverberg GD, Wilson DM, Rosenfeld RG. Regulation of growth hormone release from cultured human pituitary adenomas by somatomedins and insulin. J Clin Endocrinol Metab 60:1204–1209, 1985.

182. Yamashita S, Weiss M, Melmed S. Insulin-like growth factor I regulates growth hormone secretion and messenger ribonucleic acid levels in human pituitary tumor cells. J Clin Endocrinol Metab 63:730–735, 1986.

183. Kasselberg AG, Orth DN, Gray ME, Stahlman MT. Immunocytochemical localization of human epidermal growth factor/urogastrone in several human tissues. J Histochem Cytochem 33:315–322, 1985.

184. Ikeda H, Mitsuhashi T, Kubota K, Kuzuya N, Uchimura H. Epidermal growth factor stimulates growth hormone secretion from superfused rat adenohypophyseal fragments. Endocrinology 115:556–558, 1984.

185. Birman P, Michard M, Li JY, Peillon F, Bression D. Epidermal growth factor-binding sites, present in normal human and rat pituitaries, are absent in human pituitary adenomas. J Clin Endocrinol Metab 65:275–281, 1987.

186. Ying S-Y. Inhibins, activins, and follistatins: Gonadal proteins modulating the secretion of follicle-stimulating hormone. Endocr Rev 9:267–293, 1988.

187. Roberts V, Meunier H, Vaughan J, Rivier J, Rivier C, Vale W, Sawchenko P. Production and regulation of inhibin subunits in pituitary gonadotropes. Endocrinology 124:552–554, 1989.

188. Baird A, Mormède P, Ying S-Y, Wehrenberg WB, Ueno N, Ling N, Guillemin R. A nonmitogenic pituitary function of fibroblast growth factor; regulation of thyrotropin and prolactin secretion. Proc Natl Acad Sci USA 82:5545–5549, 1985.

189. Gospodarowicz D, Ferrara N, Schweigerer L, Neufeld G. Structural characterization and biological functions of fibroblast growth factor. Endocr Rev 8:95–114, 1987.

190. Larson GH, Koos RD, Sortino MA, Wise PM. Acute effect of basic fibroblast growth factor on secretion of prolactin as assessed by the reverse hemolytic plaque assay. Endocrinology 126:927–932, 1990.

191. Jones KL, Villela JF, Lewis UJ. The growth of cultured rabbit articular chondrocytes is stimulated by pituitary growth factors but not by purified human growth hormone or ovine prolactin. Endocrinology 118:2588–2593, 1986.

192. Kasper S, Friesen HG. Human pituitary tissue secretes a potent growth factor for chondrocyte

proliferation. J Clin Endocrinol Metab 62:70–76, 1986.

193. Webster J, Ham J, Bevan JS, ten Horn CD, Scanlon MF. Preliminary characterization of growth factors secreted by human pituitary tumors. J Clin Endocrinol Metab 72:687–692, 1991.

194. Denef C, Andries M. Evidence for paracrine interaction between gonadotrophs and lactotrophs in pituitary cell aggregates. Endocrinology 112:813–822, 1983.

195. Lloyd RV, Mailloux J. Analysis of S-100 protein positive folliculo-stellate cells in rat pituitary tissues. Am J Pathol 133:338–346, 1988.

196. Lapp CA, Tyler JM, Lee YS, Stachura ME. Autocrine-paracrine inhibition of growth hormone and prolactin production by GH$_3$ cell-conditioned medium. In Vitro Cell Dev Biol 25:528–534, 1989.

197. Miller MJ, Fels EC, Shapiro LE, Surks MI. L-triiodothyronine stimulates growth by means of an autocrine factor in a cultured growth-hormone–producing cell line. J Clin Invest 79:1773–1781, 1987.

10

ECTOPIC PITUITARY ADENOMAS

Ricardo V. Lloyd

A portion of the stalk of Rathke's pouch persists throughout life as a structure with the distinct histological features of the pars distalis and is referred to as the "pharyngeal pituitary gland" (Fig. 10–1) (1–4). With elaborate dissection of a block that included the body of the sphenoid bone, the body of the nasal septum and the posterior nasopharynx and subsequent examination of 8800 mounted sections, the pharyngeal pituitary gland was found in 51 (93.4%) of the 54 autopsy cases studied by Melchionna and Moore (1). It was most frequently located in the midline deep in the mucosa or in the periosteum beneath or near the vomerosphenoidal articulation. It was most frequently seen as a single well-circumscribed and encapsulated structure. These studies confirmed earlier observations that the pharyngeal pituitary grows during fetal life and in the first few months of life after birth, with little growth during childhood or adulthood. The glands ranged from 0.22 mm to 6.6 mm in length. Histological features included epithelial cells similar to those of the par distalis. Colloid material was present in some cases, and the interstitial tissue and vascular supply of the pharyngeal pituitary were similar to those in the pituitary. Early studies suggested that the pharyngeal pituitary cells did not respond to altered hormonal conditions of pregnancy. The studies of McGrath (4) revealed that a direct vascular communication between the hypothalamus

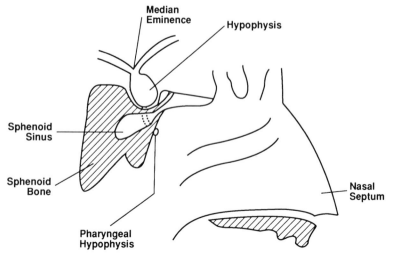

Figure 10–1. Diagram illustrating the pharyngeal hypophysis. The dashed lines show the most common location of ectopic pituitary adenomas within the sphenoid sinus or in adjacent areas.

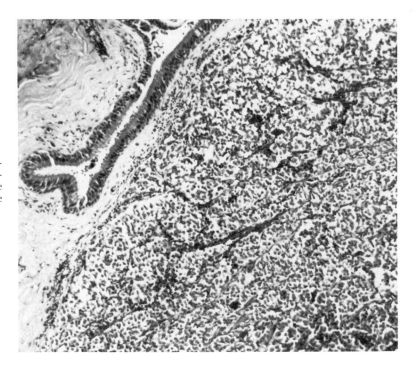

Figure 10–2. Ectopic ACTH-producing adenoma from a patient with Cushing's disease. The adenoma was present in the sphenoid sinus (×150).

and human pharyngeal hypophysis was unlikely and that the gland functioned as an isolated graft of pars distalis tissue responding to factors circulating in the systemic blood. (3) She also observed that there was usually a marked increase in the vascularity around the pharyngeal pituitary after age 50 (4).

In one immunohistochemical study of eight adult pharyngeal pituitary glands, Ciocca *et al.* detected immunoreactivity for adrenocorticotropic hormone (ACTH), folli-

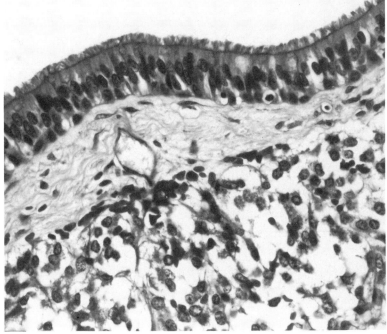

Figure 10–3. Higher magnification of an ectopic ACTH adenoma. The tumor is present beneath the ciliated epithelial lining of the sphenoid sinus (×350).

Table 10–1. Clinicopathological Data on Patients With Ectopic Pituitary Adenomas and Normal Intrasellar Pituitaries

Author (Ref.)	Age/Sex	Presenting Signs/Symptoms	Location/Size	H & E	IP	Follow-up
Erdheim (7)	53/M	Acromegaly	Sphenoid	Eosinophilic adenoma	—	Autopsy finding
Kepes and Fritzlen (8)	40/M	Pain, right eye	Sphenoid (7.5 × 7.5 × 5 cm)	Chromophobe (invasive adenoma)	—	Died in status epilepticus; autopsy results: normal pituitary
Rothman et al (9)	15/M	Seizures	Inferior third ventricle (1.5 cm)	Chromophobe adenoma	—	Hypothyroid, hypothalamic pituitary insufficiency
Chessin et al (10)	64/F	Nasal congestion	Nasopharynx	Chromophobe adenoma	—	NED, 17 mo
Borit and Blanshard (11)	62/F	Diplopia	Sphenoid	Chromophobe adenoma	—	Recurrent tumor; died 1 yr after surgery
Kammer and George (12)	51/F	Cushing's disease	Sphenoid	Chromophobe adenoma	—	NED, 3 yr
Warner et al (13)	40/F	Acromegaly	Sphenoid	Chromophobe adenoma	GH/PRL	NED, 1 yr
Matsushita et al (14)	40/F	Headache	Sphenoid (4.5 cm)	Chromophobe adenoma	PRL	Died 1 mo after surgery; autopsy results: normal pituitary
Burch et al (15)	43/F	Cushing's disease	Sphenoid (1.0 cm)	Chromophobe adenoma	ACTH, TSH	NED, 2 yr
Lloyd et al (16)	54/F	Cushing's disease	Sphenoid (0.7 cm)	Chromophobe adenoma	—	
Lloyd et al (16)	49/M	Hyperparathyroidism	Sphenoid	Chromophobe adenoma	PRL	Treated with medical therapy after surgery
Tovi et al (17)	68/F	Headaches, epistaxis	Sphenoid	Acidophilic adenoma	PRL	Invasive adenoma—radiotherapy, bromocriptine; persistent disease after 1 yr

cle-stimulating hormone (FSH), luteinizing hormone (LH), thyroid-stimulating hormone (TSH), prolactin (PRL) and growth hormone (GH) in patients with no evidence of endocrine disorders. The percentage of the various hormones ranged from 1% to 30%. The glands were 2 to 3 mm in length and 0.5 mm in diameter. Glands with squamous nests and mucinous acini were noted in some cases.

The ability of the pharyngeal pituitary to respond to feedback mechanisms has been suggested by several observations, including the presence of increased PRL cells in a patient on metoclopramide, a dopamine receptor blocking drug. There was also a reported increase in TSH cells in a patient with primary hypothyroidism (6). Although these two cases of hyperplasia were documented by quantitation of cell type after immunostaining, the ability of the pharyngeal pituitary to respond to negative feedback stimuli remains controversial, since other studies have not found changes in this gland with pregnancy (4).

The development of adenomas in ectopic pituitary tissue has been well documented in various reports (Figs. 10–2 and 10–3; Table 10–1). In a few cases, patients have had normal intrasellar pituitaries with ectopic adenomas (7–17), while in other cases there has been neoplastic involvement of the pituitary as well as ectopic sites (18–23).

The sphenoid sinus has usually been the most common site of ectopic pituitary adenomas. Aggressive tumors have been reported in some cases (8, 17, 22); immunohistochemical stains have been done to characterize these tumors. PRL- and GH-producing tumors have been the most common adenomas revealed by immunostaining, which is similar to the general incidence of surgically resected adenomas (24). In 12 patients with ectopic pituitary tissue and normal pituitaries, the sphenoid sinus was the most common location of these neoplasms. Although a few patients were cured by surgery alone, many patients had persistent disease requiring medical therapy such as bromocriptine and radiation therapy.

Another subtype of ectopic pituitary adenomas includes the suprasellar or subdiaphragmatic tumors, which may arise from anterior lobe cells attached to the supradiaphragmatic portion of the pituitary stalk (25, 26). Suprasellar tumors may compress the optic chiasm and expand against the base of the brain without destroying the sella. Cushing postulated that these tumors originated in the stalk or possibly developed in a superficial portion of the pituitary and escaped through the diaphragm without having previously expanded the sella (25). Kepes and Fritzlen (8) reported on a pituitary adenoma that involved both the sphenoid bone and the suprasellar area. This tumor may have originated from the suprasellar region, but definite evidence is not available. In rare cases, craniopharyngiomas have also been reported to arise from the pharyngeal hypophysis (27).

Although most ectopic pituitary adenomas are solitary, the report of Borit and Blanshard included two separate ectopic adenomas that originated in the sphenoid and suprasellar areas (11). Patients with ectopic adenomas commonly present with evidence of an expanding mass and compression of adjacent structures. Although some ectopic adenomas have been designated as invasive adenomas, suggesting malignancy, they are usually low-grade neoplasms. The use of computed tomographic scans can be helpful in the diagnosis of ectopic adenomas, although ectopic tumors in the sphenoid region may not be readily diagnosed by magnetic resonance imaging (17).

The definitive diagnosis of ectopic pituitary tumors depends on a tissue biopsy of the lesion. Because the sphenoid sinus is the most common location of these rare adenomas, patients with normal intrasellar pituitaries who have markedly elevated hormone levels should be evaluated for a possible ectopic adenoma in the sphenoid sinus or in contiguous areas that may harbor an ectopic pituitary adenoma.

REFERENCES

1. Melchionna RH, Moore RA. The pharyngeal pituitary gland. Am J Pathol *14*:763–771, 1938.
2. Boyd JD. Observations on the human pharyngeal hypophysis. J Endocrinol *14*:66–77, 1956.
3. McPhie JL, Beck JS. The histological features and human growth hormone content of the pharyngeal pituitary gland in normal and endocrinologically-disturbed patients. Clin Endocrinol *2*:157–173, 1973.
4. McGrath P. Vascularity of the environs of the human pharyngeal hypophysis as a possible indication of the mechanism of its control. J Anat *112*:185–193, 1972.
5. Ciocca DR, Puy LA, Stati AO. Identification of seven hormone-producing cell types in the human pha-

ryngeal hypophysis. J Clin Endocrinol Metab *60*:212–216, 1985.

6. Ciocca DR, Puy LA, Stati AO. Immunocytochemical evidence for the ability of the human pharyngeal hypophysis to respond to change in endocrine feedback. Virchows Arch (Pathol Anat) *405*:497–502, 1985.

7. Erdheim J. Uber Einen Hypophysentumor von ungewohnlichem Sitz. Beitr Pathol *46*:233–240, 1909.

8. Kepes JJ, Fritzlen TJ. Large invasive chromophobe adenoma with well-preserved pituitary gland: Report of a case. Neurology *14*:537–541, 1964.

9. Rothman LM, Sher J, Quencer RM, Tenner MS. Intracranial ectopic pituitary adenoma: Case report. J Neurosurg *44*:96–99, 1976.

10. Chessin H, Urdaneta N, Smith H, Van Gilder J. Chromophobe adenoma manifesting as a nasopharyngeal mass. Arch Otolaryngol *102*:631–633, 1976.

11. Borit A, Blanshard TP. Sphenoidal pituitary adenoma. Hum Pathol *10*:93–96, 1979.

12. Kammer H, George R. Cushing's disease in a patient with an ectopic pituitary adenoma. JAMA *246*:2722–2724, 1981.

13. Warner BA, Santen RJ, Page RB. Growth of hormone and prolactin secretion by a tumor of the pharyngeal pituitary. Ann Intern Med *96*:65–66, 1982.

14. Matsushita H, Matsuya S, Endo Y, Hara M, Shishiba Y, Yamaguchi H, Kameya T. A prolactin producing tumor originated in the sphenoid sinus. Acta Pathol Jpn *34*:103–109, 1984.

15. Burch WM, Kramer RS, Kenan PA, Hammond CB. Cushing's disease caused by an ectopic pituitary adenoma within the sphenoid sinus. N Engl J Med *312*:587–588, 1985.

16. Lloyd RV, Chandler WF, Kovacs K, Ryan N. Ectopic pituitary adenomas with normal anterior pituitary glands. Am J Surg Pathol *10*:546–552, 1986.

17. Tovi F, Hirsch M, Sacks M, Leiberman A. Ectopic pituitary adenoma of the sphenoid sinus: Report of a case and review of the literature. Head Neck *12*:264–268, 1990.

18. Corenblum B, LeBlanc FE, Watanabe M. Acromegaly with an adenomatous pharyngeal pituitary. JAMA *243*:1456–1457, 1980.

19. Garschin W. Ein Fall der intrasphenoidalen Hypophysenganggeschwulst. Z Krebsforsch *31*:432–436, 1930.

20. Kay S, Lees JK, Stout AP. Pituitary chromophobe tumors of the nasal cavity. Cancer *3*:695–704, 1950.

21. Lindholm J, Korsgaard O, Rasmussen P. Ectopic pituitary function. Acta Med Scand *198*:299–302, 1975.

22. Oglivy KM, Jakubowski J. Intracranial dissemination of pituitary adenomas. J Neurol Neurosurg Psychiatry *36*:199–205, 1973.

23. Solitaire GR, Jatlow P. Adenohypophyseal carcinoma. J Neurosurg *26*:624–632, 1959.

24. Kovacs K, Horvath E. Tumors of the pituitary gland. In: Hartmann WH, Sobin LH (eds). Atlas of Tumor Pathology. 2nd Series. Fascicle 21. Washington, DC, Armed Forces Institute of Pathology, 1986, pp 51–56.

25. Cushing H, Davidhoff LM. The pathological findings in four autopsied cases of acromegaly with a discussion of their significance. Monogr Rockefeller Inst Med Res, No. 22, April 23, 1927.

26. Henderson WR. Sexual dysfunction in adenomas of the pituitary body. Endocrinology *15*:111–127, 1931.

27. Levin R, Ruffolo E, Saracero C. Craniopharyngioma arising in the pharyngeal hypophysis. South Med J *77*:1519–1523, 1984.

11

INVASIVE PITUITARY ADENOMAS AND PITUITARY CARCINOMAS

PETER J. PERNICONE **and** BERND W. SCHEITHAUER

Pituitary tumors are relatively common, comprising nearly 10% of all intracranial neoplasms. The vast majority originate in the adenohypophysis. Classically, tumors of anterior pituitary cells have been categorized as adenomas, invasive adenomas, and carcinomas. This chapter will discuss the clinicopathologic features of invasive adenomas and primary pituitary carcinomas.

Adenomas, the most frequently occurring tumors of the sellar region, consist of a proliferation of adenohypophyseal endocrine cells of varying type. Most are cytologically benign. Their natural history is often one of slow expansile growth with compression of surrounding structures. Despite gradual enlargement, some may become remarkably large without appreciable clinical abnormalities. When evident, such abnormalities include headache; subtle, often temporal visual field deficits; hyperprolactinemia due to compression of the pituitary stalk; and a number of endocrine abnormalities due to tumoral hormone production. Although tumors are often small and confined to the sella, others may be large, exhibit invasiveness, and, rarely, behave in a frankly malignant manner, exhibiting cerebrospinal or distant metastases.

INVASIVE ADENOMAS

A number of excellent descriptions of invasive adenomas have appeared in the liter-

ature (1–6). Unlike typical expansile adenomas, invasive tumors infiltrate surrounding tissues by either ragged single-cell extensions or by blunt projection of tumor dissecting along connective tissue planes. Though invasive adenomas often display minor degrees of pleomorphism, increased cellularity and accelerated mitotic activity, these findings are neither universal in invasive lesions nor sufficiently expressed in rare metastasizing tumors to permit a diagnosis of pituitary carcinoma.

Adenomas may invade in any of a number of directions (Figs. 11–1 to 11–3). Superiorly, they infiltrate and permeate the sellar diaphragm, extend into the suprasellar cistern and cause compression of the optic apparatus, hypothalamus and third ventricle (Figs. 11–1 and 11–2). Upward extension may be either pre- or retrochiasmal. Inferiorly, invasive adenomas penetrate the sellar floor and may ultimately gain access not only to the sphenoid sinus, but also to the nasal cavity (Fig. 11–4). Tumors showing lateral invasion permeate the interstices of the cavernous sinus wherein they compress, but rarely invade, cranial nerves and vessels (Figs. 11–1 to 11–3 and 11–5). Specifically, cavernous sinus involvement may be clinically manifest as neuropathies of cranial nerves III (oculomotor), IV (trochlear), V (trigeminal), and VI (abducens). Further lateral invasion or extension may result in temporal and parietal lobe compression (Figs. 11–6 and 11–7). Tumors that invade anteriorly may result in

Text continued on page 127

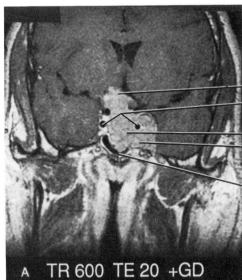

Optic chiasm
Internal carotid arteries

Invasive adenoma
Region of
 left cavernous sinus

Sphenoid sinus

A TR 600 TE 20 +GD

Figure 11–1. *A,* Coronal MRI scan of the head showing an invasive adenoma extensively involving the right and left cavernous sinuses and the sphenoid sinus. There is marked suprasellar extension with compression of the optic chiasm. *B,* Sagittal MRI scan of the head showing an invasive adenoma extending deeply into the sphenoid sinus. The optic chiasm is stretched and displaced superiorly.

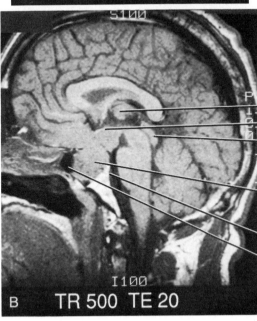

Thalamus
Optic chiasm
Pineal gland

Invasive adenoma

Clivus

Sphenoid sinus

B TR 500 TE 20

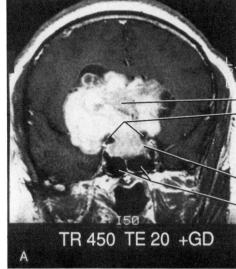

Invasive adenoma
Internal carotid arteries

Cavernous sinus invasion

Sphenoid sinus

Figure 11–2. *A,* Coronal MRI scan of the head showing a massive invasive adenoma extensively replacing both cavernous sinuses and extending into the sphenoid sinus. There is remarkable suprasellar extension with involvement of the third ventricle and effacement of the hypothalamus. *B,* Sagittal MRI scan of the head showing invasion of the sella and sphenoid sinus, as well as marked suprasellar extension. The optic tracts are displaced superiorly.

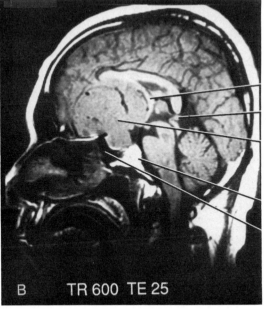

Fornix

Pineal gland

Invasive adenoma

Clivus

Sphenoid sinus

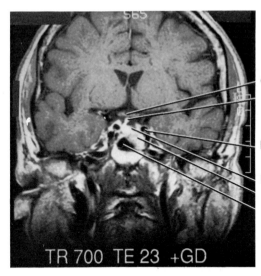

Optic chiasm
Pituitary stalk

Internal carotid artery

Microadenoma
Left cavernous sinus
Sphenoid sinus

Figure 11–3. Coronal MRI scan of the head showing an invasive microadenoma involving the left cavernous sinus and extending into the sphenoid sinus.

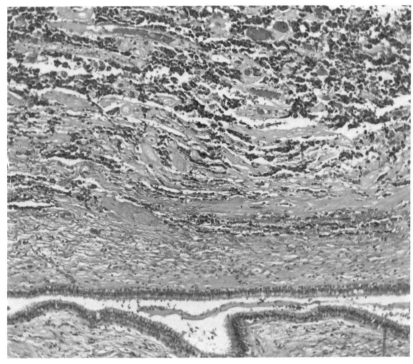

Figure 11–4. Invasive adenoma involving the submucosa of the sphenoid sinus. Note the permeative pattern of tumor spread (H & E; × 40).

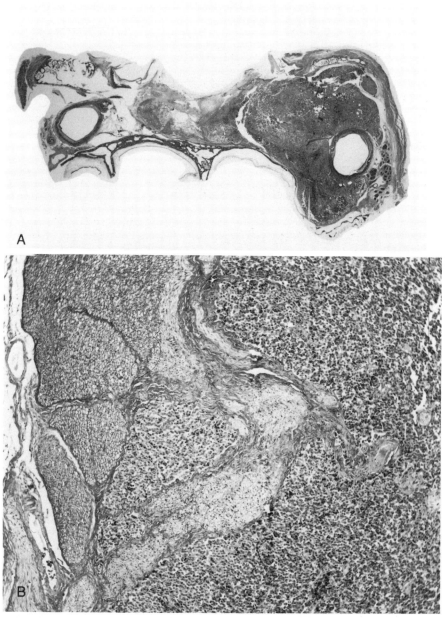

Figure 11–5. *A*, The pituitary and sellar region in a coronal section showing invasive adenoma replacing the left cavernous sinus. Note ensheathement of cranial nerves and the internal carotid artery by tumor (H & E; × 6). *B*, Prominent perineural involvement by invasive adenoma within the cavernous sinus (H & E; × 100).

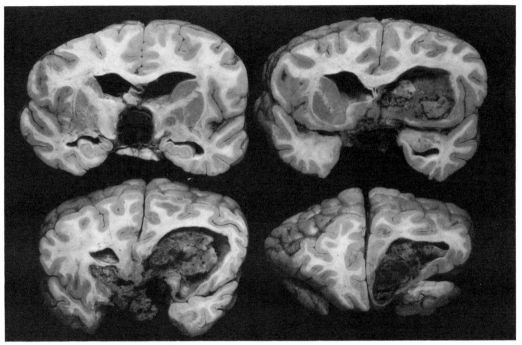

Figure 11–6. Coronal sections of the brain showing a large invasive adenoma that has extended into the third ventricle and displaced the parietal and frontal lobes.

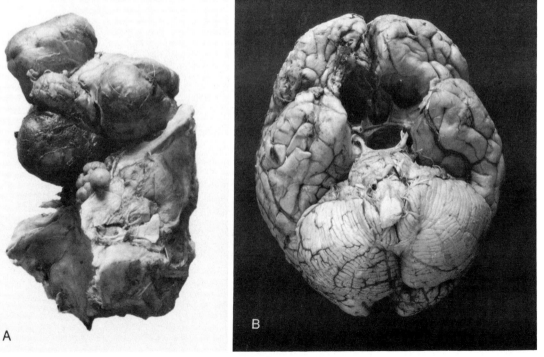

Figure 11–7. Ventral view of the tumor (A) and brain (B) showing the marked compressive effect produced by prominent extension of pituitary adenoma.

compression of the optic or olfactory nerves. Finally, posterior invasion causes clival destruction and, with further extension, may result in compression of vital midbrain or brain stem structures. Extensive sellar remodeling due to an invasive adenoma may permit direct compression of the trigeminal ganglion, a structure normally somewhat protected medially by the internal carotid artery (5).

It is important to distinguish tumor extension from invasion. "Invasion" implies destructive permeation of underlying tissue, while "extension" suggests directional tumor growth with compression of underlying tissue (Fig. 11–7). Often, invasive adenomas exhibit both qualities (see Figs. 11–6 and 11–7).

The clinical presentation of invasive adenomas is sometimes quite spectacular. Jefferson (5) described a case of a female acromegalic patient who worked until 1 week prior to admission and then died the next day. Autopsy revealed a tumor that completely filled the cavernous sinuses, along with massive posterior extension.

Pituitary adenomas have been arbitrarily classified as either micro- or macroadenomas. Histologically, the two types are indistinguishable. The former are defined as those tumors measuring less than 10 mm in greatest dimension, while the latter measure 10 mm or more. The somewhat less specific term "diffuse adenoma" implies filling of the sellar volume by tumor; most of these are small macroadenomas. Using computerized tomography (CT) or magnetic resonance imaging (MRI), neuroradiologists categorize tumors by size, invasiveness and degree of suprasellar extension. From a clinical point of view the distinction is important, as macroadenomas are more likely to show dural invasion than microadenomas (3). Therefore, microadenomas are more likely to be cured by surgical resection than macroadenomas. Microscopic dural invasion has been identified in 66% of microadenomas, 87% of intrasellar macroadenomas, and 94% of macroadenomas with suprasellar extension (4). Although microadenomas are less likely than macroadenomas to be invasive, such tumors do occur, and despite their small size, they may be unresectable when they involve the cavernous sinuses (see Fig. 11–3).

The frequency of invasion ranges considerably, with 10% being noted on routine radiographs, 35% to 40% on intraoperative gross inspection (3, 4), and nearly 90% in instances where the dura is systematically inspected on histological sections (4). It appears, therefore, that tissue invasion as judged by intraoperative findings is clinically more meaningful than ubiquitous microscopic dural invasion. Indeed, if diligently sought, small foci of microscopic invasion can be found in even the most clinically indolent adenomas.

Not all adenomas exhibit the same frequency of invasiveness. In fact, tumors of varying hormonal type, regardless of whether they are clinically functional, show differing frequencies of invasion (3).

Growth Hormone Cell Adenoma

Growth hormone (GH)-producing adenomas comprise about 10% of pituitary adenomas and typically cause acromegaly in adults and gigantism in children. In addition, GH hypersecretion may be complicated by diabetes mellitus; visceromegaly, including cardiomegaly; congestive heart failure; and peripheral neuropathy. Biochemical testing reveals elevations in plasma GH levels, which may show wide fluctuations. The normally occurring GH rise during sleep is typically absent. Somatomedin C, or insulin-like growth factor I, a GH-dependent growth factor that is insufficiently produced in Laron dwarfism, is elevated in acromegalic and giant patients.

GH-producing pituitary adenomas have been divided into densely granulated and sparsely granulated types based on their light microscopic and ultrastructural features. They occur with approximately equal frequency. Densely granulated adenomas present most often in middle-aged adults and are composed of cells having deeply acidophilic cytoplasm, whereas sparsely granulated tumors are composed of chromophobic cells. Although some tumors do show intermediate granulation, the distinction between the two is significant, as sparsely granulated GH adenomas are more likely to recur and to exhibit invasive growth. In one study, sparsely granulated GH adenomas were as likely as densely granulated adenomas to be macroadenomas and were more likely to be invasive (7).

Mixed Growth Hormone–Prolactin Cell Adenoma

The GH- and prolactin-producing adenoma is bicellular, being composed of both lactotrophs and somatotrophs. Not unexpectedly, these tumors are associated with acromegaly or gigantism, as well as amenorrhea-galactorrhea, decreased libido and impotence. They grow slowly and show invasiveness in only 30% of cases (3).

Acidophil–Stem Cell Adenoma

A rare tumor, the acidophil–stem cell adenoma comprises at best, 1% of pituitary adenomas and is composed of cells thought to represent precursors of both lactotrophs and somatotrophs (8). Patients with this lesion usually exhibit hyperprolactinemia but have normal GH levels. The clinical manifestations include amenorrhea-galactorrhea in women and impotence and loss of libido in men. Acromegalic features are unusual. Its tendency to exhibit rapid growth and invasiveness makes complete surgical removal difficult, if not impossible, and underlies the importance of recognizing this rare tumor early. Invasion of the sphenoid sinus is present in up to 50% of cases. Acidophil–stem cell adenomas consistently exhibit immunoreactivity for prolactin, but GH staining is often spotty. Ultrastructurally, they are composed of a single cell type characterized by sparse granulation, atypical mitochondria containing tubular structures and occasional misplaced exocytoses as well as fibrous bodies. Mitochondria may assume giant proportions and be visible at the light microscopic level as cytoplasmic vacuolation.

Prolactin Cell Adenoma

Prolactin-producing adenomas, which compose about 30% of pituitary adenomas, become clinically apparent by producing galactorrhea-amenorrhea in women and impotence and decreased libido in men. Amenorrhea-galactorrhea, a prominent symptom, prompts early evaluation of female patients, whose tumors are often microadenomas, whereas late presentation with mass effect typifies male prolactinomas, nearly all of which are macroadenomas.

The biological behavior of prolactinomas is quite variable. Some show indolent growth and are confined to the sella, while others demonstrate early invasive growth. Overall, surgically observed gross invasion has been detected in up to 52% of prolactinomas (3). Like other pituitary adenomas, there is no definite correlation between histomorphology and the propensity for invasiveness.

ACTH-Cell Adenoma

Adrenocorticotropic hormone (ACTH)–producing adenomas associated with Cushing's disease are typically intrasellar microadenomas with little tendency to invade surrounding structures. Surgically observed invasiveness occurs in less than 10% of such tumors (3). Macroadenomas, on the other hand, represent about 13% of Cushing's adenomas; 62% are grossly invasive (3). Basophilic corticotrophic adenomas are more likely to remain intrasellar, while chromophobic examples often exhibit local invasiveness.

Nelson's syndrome, a far less common condition than Cushing's disease, is characterized by an ACTH-producing adenoma that is undetectable at the onset of disease, thus prompting bilateral adrenalectomy for cure of hypercortisolism. The disorder is becoming rare with the advent of sophisticated and more sensitive imaging techniques capable of detecting minute adenomas. Patients with Nelson's syndrome present with elevated ACTH, pituitary tumor and mass effect an average of 10 years following adrenalectomy. More often than not, they have macroadenomas, with approximately 64% being grossly invasive (3). Large tumor size and aggressiveness is not unexpected considering that neoplastic corticotrophs lose their negative feedback following adrenalectomy. Thus normal, and presumably adenomatous, corticotrophs are driven to produce ACTH. Though Nelson's syndrome is becoming rare, prompt diagnosis is important in order to provide this subset of patients a reasonable chance for successful treatment.

Silent ACTH Cell Adenoma

Silent corticotroph adenomas, once thought rare, are now known to represent up to 30% of corticotropic adenomas (9). By strict definition, these tumors are not associated with clinical or biochemical evidence of hypercortisolism. Unfortunately, however, the term has been loosely applied to clinically nonfunctioning tumors with minimal ACTH elevation. Given their lack of function, these tumors present with mass symptoms (e.g., headache, ophthalmoplegia, and even blindness) (9). Tumor cells appear basophilic by light microscopy and show variable immunoreactivity for ACTH, β-lipotropin and α-endorphin. Ultrastructurally, most are composed of densely granulated corticotrophs, though sparsely granulated, and hence chromophobic, examples also occur. The silent nature of these adenomas has been attributed to defective packaging of hormone, intracellular lysosomal disposal of hormone and production of an immunoreactive but biochemically nonfunctioning hormone (9). Characteristics of silent corticotroph adenomas include a striking tendency to undergo infarction, rapid growth and recurrence (9). Overall, invasiveness has been found in 82% of cases; not surprisingly, all symptomatic lesions are macroadenomas (3).

TSH Cell Adenoma

One of the rarest of pituitary tumors, the thyroid-stimulating hormone (TSH)–producing adenoma is characterized by elongate cells with chromophobic, delicate periodic acid—Schiff (PAS)–positive cytoplasm. Small, peripherally disposed neurosecretory granules are the rule, as are occasional prominent lysosomes.

TSH adenomas may present as hypo- or hyperthyroidism, or patients may be euthyroid. Hyperthyroid patients have elevated levels of total thyroxine (T_4), unbound thyroxine (free T_4) and serum TSH. Interestingly, in one study, no correlation was noted between serum TSH levels and tumor size or invasiveness (10). Some examples of TSH-producing adenomas that are classified as "plurihormonal adenomas" also produce significant quantities of GH and may be associated with acromegaly (see later discussion). If patients with TSH adenomas are misdiagnosed and treated for primary hyperthyroidism, the resulting hypothyroid state may actually hasten tumor growth, a situation analogous to the Nelson-Salassa syndrome. In one study, serum α subunit was found to be the most specific marker for the presence of pituitary adenoma in patients with inappropriately elevated serum TSH (10). An important attribute of TSH-producing adenomas is their relentless and aggressive growth. Most are characterized by invasion of surrounding structures, including the cavernous sinuses, sphenoid sinus, clivus, orbit and brain (11). Suprasellar growth may compress the pituitary stalk, causing hyperprolactinemia, and, by further extension, may lead to hypothalamic insufficiency. A substantial proportion of patients present with marked visual field deficits.

Null Cell Adenoma

Comprising approximately 25% of pituitary adenomas, null cell adenomas are defined as those tumors showing no significant morphological or immunohistochemical evidence of functional differentiation. They are not associated with either clinical or biochemical evidence of hormone production. Clinically, null cell tumors are not particularly aggressive. Nonetheless, such tumors may extend beyond the confines of the sella and exhibit chiasmal compression, hypothalamic compromise and even cavernous sinus invasion at the time of diagnosis (12). In one study (3), 42% of null cell adenomas were grossly invasive, with 98% of tumors being macroadenomas. Their large size at the time of diagnosis is primarily attributed to their endocrinologic and biochemical silence. Careful immunohistochemical study often shows focal or minimal evidence of glycoprotein differentiation. Ultrastructurally, null cell adenomas possess poorly differentiated, occasionally oncocytic cytoplasm and sparse, small secretory granules (12).

Plurihormonal Adenomas

Plurihormonal adenomas, which comprise approximately 10% to 15% of all pituitary adenomas, are defined as tumors that produce unusual combinations of hormones, including GH, prolactin, and one or more glycoprotein hormone, (e.g., TSH, ACTH, or follicle-stimulating hormone [FSH]/luteinizing hormone [LH]). In one study (13), 83% of plurihormonal adenomas contained a component of GH-producing cells, and 67% of all evaluated patients exhibited evidence of GH excess. The majority of plurihormonal adenomas are macroadenomas, with approximately 50% of these being invasive (13).

LABORATORY EVALUATION OF TUMOR AGGRESSIVENESS

A variety of laboratory techniques have been applied in an effort to assess the growth potential of pituitary adenomas. Light microscopy supplemented with immunohistochemical staining of hormonal products provides little insight into the growth potential of these tumors. Adenomas showing rank invasion either appear cytologically bland or show varying degrees of nuclear pleomorphism and mitotic activity. The crude correlation between these features and tumor aggressiveness severely limits their diagnostic and prognostic value. Adenomas with monotonous cytology and little or no mitotic activity are particularly vexing and must be evaluated by other means.

Immunoperoxidase staining of the cell cycle–associated antigen Ki-67 has shed some light on this important problem. Invasive adenomas show a significantly increased expression of Ki-67 antigen (14,15). In one study, however, no significant correlation was demonstrated between hormonal content of adenomas and expression of Ki-67 antigen (14).

Flow cytometry has been used to evaluate DNA-ploidy. Generally, most such studies show that the majority of pituitary adenomas are diploid, although estimates of aneuploidy range from 0% to 49% in the literature (16–18). In one study, no statistically significant correlation was found between aneuploidy and tumor aggressiveness (17).

The fraction of cells in the S phase of the cell cycle has been accurately determined using preoperative infusions of 5-bromodeoxyuridine (BUDU), followed by postoperative staining of the adenoma using a monoclonal antibody to BUDU (19). Not surprisingly, the S-phase fraction of most pituitary adenomas is quite low, in most cases less than 0.5%. Interestingly, however, adenomas occurring in Nelson's syndrome, tumors typified by invasiveness, show a significantly increased S-phase fraction, usually greater than 1% (19).

Finally, a study that evaluated the expression of the proliferation-associated antigen P105 and the DNA content of adenomas found a significantly increased G2M/G0G1 fluorescence ratio for P105 in recurrent diploid tumors (18).

In summary, expression of the antigens Ki-67 and P105, as well as measurement of the S-phase fraction may provide clinically and prognostically useful data. The degree to which it correlates with the functional status or immunotype of adenomas remains to be seen.

PITUITARY GLAND CARCINOMA

While grossly invasive adenomas are fairly common, constituting at least one third of pituitary adenomas, pituitary carcinomas are extremely rare. Strictly defined, pituitary carcinoma is a primary neoplasm of adenohypophysial endocrine cells that exhibits craniospinal and/or extracranial metastases. Metastatic potential distinguishes pituitary carcinoma as unique from the invasive adenomas discussed earlier (Figs. 11–8 to 11–12). Approximately 36 such cases have been reported in the literature since 1900 (20–55). The patients have ranged in age from 1.5 to 75 years, with a slight female predominance. Presenting signs and symptoms have covered a broad spectrum and include headache, visual loss, diplopia, loss of libido, amenorrhea, loss of consciousness and even coma. Specific endocrine syndromes, including Cushing's disease, Nelson-Salassa syndrome, acromegaly and hyperprolactinemia, have been reported, but many tumors have been described as clinically inactive. In the majority of cases, an adenoma was suspected on the basis of clinical and radiographical findings, and treatment consisted of surgery, often transsphenoidal resection.

While pituitary carcinoma is, by definition, capable of metastasizing, to date no patient has died directly from the effects of extracranial metastatic disease. On the contrary, the most common cause of death appears to be intracranial tumor expansion and invasion accompanied by brain herniation.

On the basis of histology alone, it is not possible to make an unequivocal diagnosis of pituitary carcinoma when examining an adenohypophyseal tumor limited to the sellar region. Some tumors are composed of cells with rare bland cytological features, little pleomorphism and no appreciable mitotic activity in the primary tumor, but marked nuclear atypia and mitotic activity in metastatic deposits (see Fig. 11–9B, C). In such cases, a transformation occurred from a locally aggressive tumor to a malignant neoplasm with

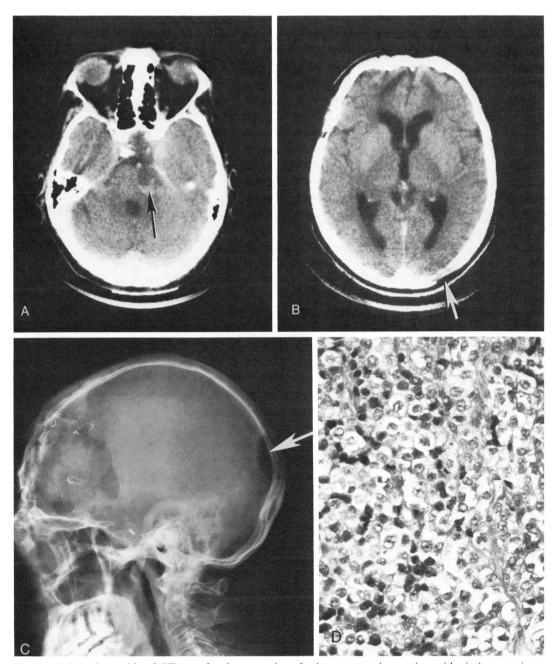

Figure 11–8. *A*, Coronal head CT scan showing extension of primary tumor in a patient with pituitary carcinoma. Note the peripherally enhancing tumor mass in the region of the cerebellopontine angle (*arrows*), representing tumor extension. *B*, Coronal head CT scan of the same patient showing a lytic metastatic lesion in the occipital bone (*arrow*), *C*, Lateral skull radiograph showing lytic metastasis of pituitary carcinoma in occipital bone (*arrow*). *D*, Tissue curetted from lytic bone lesion showing pituitary carcinoma. Immunostaining of the primary and metastatic tumor showed reactivity for prolactin (H & E; × 400). (*A* from Scheithauer BW, *et al.* Prolactin cell carcinoma of the pituitary. Cancer 55:598–604, 1985, with permission of the Mayo Foundation.)

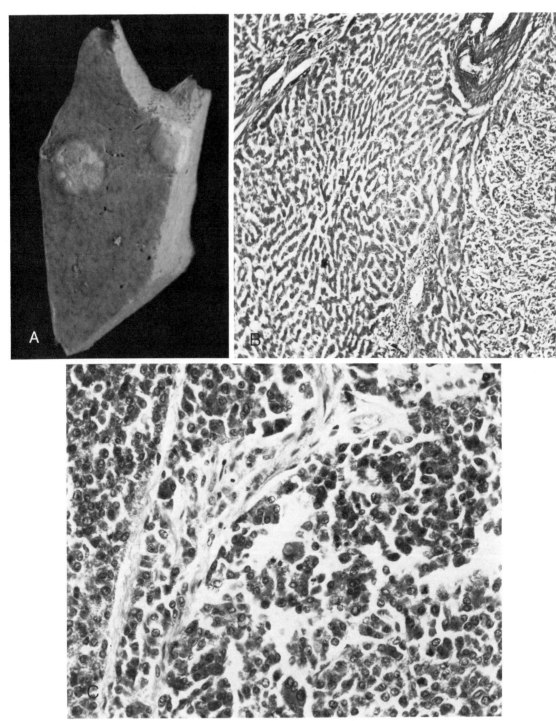

Figure 11–9. *A* Multiple liver metastases in a case of an ACTH-producing pituitary carcinoma in the setting of Nelson-Salassa syndrome. *B*, Focus of metastatic carcinoma in the liver, showing pleomorphism and mitotic activity (H & E; × 100). *C*, Prominent mitotic activity with atypical mitoses, multinucleated cells, and nuclear pleomorphism in pituitary carcinoma. (H & E; × 400). (*A* from Salassa RM, *et al.* Pituitary tumors in patients with Cushing's syndrome. J Clin Endocrinol Metab *19*:1523–1538, 1959, © by the Endocrine Society.)

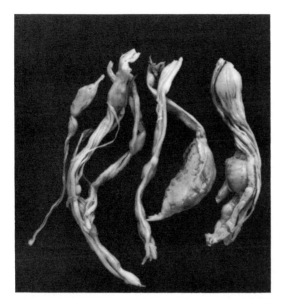

Figure 11–10. Tumor implants of metastatic ACTH-producing carcinoma involving the cauda equina. (From Scheithauer BW. Surgical pathology of the pituitary and sellar regions. In: Laws ER Jr. *et al* (eds). Management of Pituitary Adenomas and Related Lesions: With Emphasis on Transsphenoidal Microsurgery. New York, Appleton-Century-Crofts, 1982, pp 129–218, with permission of the Mayo Foundation.)

metastatic potential. Exceptionally, primary tumors have exhibited nuclear pleomorphism, hyperchromasia and brisk mitotic activity at initial presentation (43, 46, 50, 53, 54). The vast majority of pituitary carcinomas are described as chromophobic, whereas a small number are basophilic or acidophilic in appearance.

The diagnosis of pituitary carcinoma must be considered in a patient with a known pituitary adenoma, particularly one recently diagnosed, who presents with intracranial or extracranial metastases. If the microscopic features of such a metastasis resemble those of the primary, further studies, including electron microscopy, immunohistochemistry and review of the previous primary tumor are absolutely essential to confirm a diagnosis of pituitary gland carcinoma. The following criteria should be considered in making the diagnosis of pituitary gland adenocarcinoma:

1. The patient must have a history, usually recent, of an adenohypophyseal tumor, either an intrasellar or invasive adenoma.

2. The metastatic deposit(s) must be carcinoma. Its epithelial nature may be established by light microscopy, immunohistochemistry or electron microscopy.

3. The metastatic deposit(s) should exhibit a similar hormonal immunophenotype to that of the primary tumor, the exception being null cell tumors, in which no hormonal product may be demonstrable.

4. The tumor should demonstrate features of endocrine differentiation, both immunohistochemical and ultrastructural.

It is important in such situations to distinguish intracranial tumor extension from metastasis. Metastasis is defined as discontinuous or remote tumor growth (see Fig. 11–8). A thorough preoperative neuroradiologic evaluation is essential in establishing the discrete, isolated nature of intracranial metastases, either parenchymal or meningeal.

Although the mechanisms of spread are not fully understood, pituitary gland carcinomas may exhibit cerebrospinal dissemination as well as intracranial (parenchymal) and extracranial metastasis. Cerebrospinal dissemination presumably occurs by direct invasion of the subarachnoid space and subsequent transport of tumor cells via the cerebrospinal fluid to various locations along the craniospinal axis (see Figs. 11–10 and 11–11).

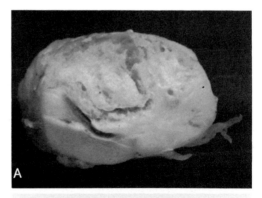

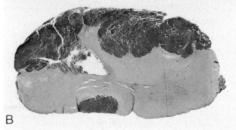

Figure 11–11. ACTH-producing pituitary carcinoma in the subarachnoid space with invasion of underlying spinal cord. (From Salassa RM, *et al.* Pituitary tumors in patients with Cushing's syndrome. J Clin Endocrinol Metab 19:1523–1538, 1959, © by the Endocrine Society.)

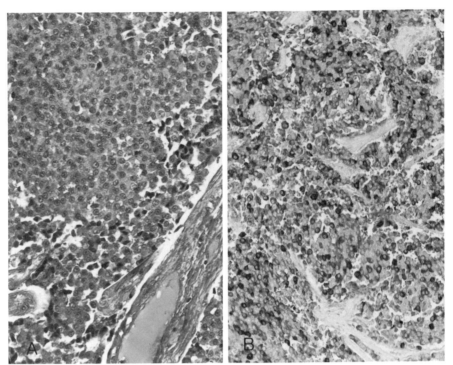

Figure 11–12. *A*, Lymph node metastasis in a patient with ACTH-producing pituitary carcinoma (H & E; × 400). *B*, Note positive staining for ACTH (immunostain; ×400).

A number of cases of parenchymal metastasis have been reported (20–35). They may be facilitated by either cerebrospinal dissemination, in which case access to the brain occurs by way of perivascular Virchow-Robin spaces or by venous sinus invasion. Specifically, cerebellar and cerebellopontine angle metastases may occur by way of cavernous sinus invasion with subsequent spread to the superior petrosal sinus. The latter provides a route by which cavernous sinus blood may gain access to the posterior fossa.

Extracranial metastasis of any primary intracranial neoplasm is a rare event. Basically, there are three potential routes of extracranial tumor spread: diversionary shunts, blood and lymphatic vessels. Conduits like ventriculo-peritoneal shunts provide a channel through which tumor cells may travel to an extracranial location (56). In the setting of a pituitary neoplasm that has extensively invaded the cavernous sinuses, one can easily imagine tumor gaining access to the internal jugular vein via the petrosal sinuses. From the jugular system, tumor cells could then travel by way of the right ventricle to the lung. Further systemic spread might occur following pulmonary metastases (see Fig. 11–

9). Cervical lymph node metastases may arise when aggressive pituitary neoplasms invade the submucosal lymphatics draining the sphenoid sinus and nasopharynx (see Figs. 11–4 and 11–12).

Craniotomy has been cited as a predisposing factor in the extracranial dissemination of central nervous system gliomas (56–58). Perhaps in a similar fashion, resection of pituitary carcinomas, regardless of method, increases the likelihood of lymphatic or vascular spread.

As with other forms of adenocarcinoma, treatment options for pituitary adenocarcinomas are limited. In the majority of reported cases, therapy has included surgery and radiotherapy. A few patients with prolactin or GH-producing neoplasms have been treated with the dopamine agonist bromocriptine, usually in combination with surgery and/or radiation therapy (23, 25, 34, 35, 55). The results have been disappointing, as bromocriptine has shown little efficacy in slowing tumor growth or lowering serum prolactin levels. In one unique case, pergolide mesylate, a dopamine agonist nearly 30 times more potent than bromocriptine, was administered (34). Surprisingly, the serum prolactin level, rather than falling, actually increased to nearly 10,000 ng/ml. Thus, unlike prolactin cell adenomas, which usually exhibit striking tumor shrinkage and decreased prolactin synthesis in the face of dopamine agonist therapy, pituitary carcinomas may be stubbornly unresponsive. Perhaps with transformation from adenoma to carcinoma dopamine receptors are lost, placing these neoplasms beyond pharmacological control.

Despite the rarity of primary carcinomas of the pituitary gland, pathologists should be aware of their existence. Early diagnosis, combined with radiotherapy and perhaps innovative pharmacological modalities, may bring this rare group of neoplasms under clinical control.

REFERENCES

1. Martins AN, Hayes GJ, Kempe LG. Invasive pituitary adenomas. J Neurosurg 22:268–276, 1965.
2. Trumble HC. Pituitary tumors: Observations on large tumours which have spread widely beyond the confines of the sella turcica. Br J Surg 39:7–24, 1951.
3. Scheithauer BW, Kovacs KT, Laws ER, Randall RV. Pathology of invasive pituitary tumors with special reference to functional classification. J Neurosurg 65:733–744, 1986.
4. Selman WR, Laws ER, Scheithauer BW, Carpenter SM. The occurrence of dural invasion in pituitary adenomas. J Neurosurg 64:402–407, 1986.
5. Jefferson G. The invasive adenomas of the anterior pituitary. Springfield, IL, Charles C Thomas, 1972.
6. Scheithauer BW. Pathol Annu 19 (part 2):269–329, 1984.
7. Robert F. Electron microscopy of human pituitary tumors. In: Tindall GT, Collins WF (eds). Clinical Management of Pituitary Disorders. New York, Raven, 1979, pp 113–131.
8. Horvath E, Kovacs K, Singer W, Smyth HS, Killinger DW, Erzin C, Weiss MH. Acidophil stem cell adenoma of the human pituitary: Clinicopathologic analysis of 15 cases. Cancer 47:761–771, 1981.
9. Horvath E, Kovacs K, Killinger DW, Smyth HS, Platts ME, Singer W. Silent corticotropic adenomas of the human pituitary gland. Am J Pathol 98:617–638, 1980.
10. Gesundheit N, Petrick PA, Nissim M, Dahlberg A, Doppman JL, Emerson CH, Breverman LE, Oldfield EH, Weintraub BD. Thyrotropin-secreting pituitary adenomas: clinical and biochemical heterogeneity. Case reports and follow-up of nine patients. Ann Intern Med 111: 827–835, 1989.
11. Hill SA, Falko JM, Wilson CB, Hunt WE. Thyrotropin-producing pituitary adenomas. J Neurosurg 57:515–519, 1982.
12. Martinez AJ. The pathology of nonfunctional pituitary adenomas. Semin Diagn Pathol 3:83–94, 1986.
13. Scheithauer BW, Horvath E, Kovacs K, Laws ER, Randall RV, Ryan N. Plurihormonal pituitary adenomas. Semin Diagn Pathol 3:69–82, 1986.
14. Knosp E, Kitz K, Perneczky A. Proliferation activity in pituitary adenomas: Measurement by monoclonal antibody Ki-67. Neurosurgery 25:927–930, 1989.
15. Landolt AM, Shibata T, Kleihues P. Growth rate of human pituitary adenomas. J Neurosurg 67:803–806, 1987.
16. Mork SJ, Laerum OD. Modal DNA content of human intracranial neoplasms studied by flow cytometry. J Neurosurg 53:198–204, 1980.
17. Fitzgibbons PL, Appley AJ, Turner RR, Bishop PC, Parker JW, Breeze RE, Weiss MH, Apuzzo MLJ. Flow cytometric analysis of pituitary tumors. Cancer 62:1556–1560, 1988.
18. Anniko M, Tribukait B, Wersall J. DNA ploidy and cell phase in human pituitary tumors. Cancer 53:1708–1713, 1984.
19. Nagashima T, Murovic JA, Hoshino T, Wilson CB, DeArmond SJ. The proliferative potential of human pituitary tumors in situ. J Neurosurg 64:588–593, 1986.
20. Newton TH, Burhenne HJ, Palubinskas AJ. Primary carcinoma of the pituitary. Am J Roentgenol Rad Ther Nucl Med 87:110–120, 1962.
21. Feiring EH, Davidoff LM, Zimmerman HM. Primary carcinoma of the pituitary. J Neuropath Exp Neurol 12:205–223, 1953.
22. Papotti M, Limone P, Riva C, Gatti G, Bussolati G. Malignant evolution of an ACTH-producing pituitary tumor treated with intrasellar implantation of 90Y. Appl Pathol 2:10–21, 1984.
23. Martin NA, Hales M, Wilson CB. Cerebellar metastasis from a prolactinoma during treatment with bromocriptine. J Neurosurg 55:615–619, 1981.
24. Cohen DL, Diengdoh JV, Thomas DGT, Himsworth RL. An intracranial metastasis from a PRL secreting pituitary tumor. Clin Endocrinol 18:259–264, 1983.
25. Hoi Sang U, Johnson C. Metastatic prolactin-secreting pituitary adenoma. Hum Pathol 15:94–96, 1984.
26. Fasske E. Uber einen primar maligner hypophysentumor bei einem saugling. Zentralbl Allg Pathol 98:281–286, 1958.
27. Madonick MJ, Rubinstein LJ, Rona Dacso M, Ribner H. Chromophobe adenoma of pituitary gland with subarachnoid metastases. Neurology 13:836–840, 1963.
28. Braun W, Tzonos T. Uber ein ungewohnlich rasch wachsendes hypophysencarcinom mit intracerebralen metastasen. Acta Neurochir 12:615–624, 1965.
29. Solitare GB, Jatlow P. Adenohypophysial carcinoma. J Neurosurg 26:624–632, 1967.
30. Fleischer AS, Reagan T, Ransohoff J. Primary carcinoma of the pituitary with metastasis to the brain stem. J Neurosurg 36:781–784, 1972.
31. Smoler F. Zur operation der hypophysentumoren auf nasalem wege. Wien Klin Wochenschr 22:1488–1489, 1909.
32. Gullotta F, Klein H. La microscopia elettronica nella diagnostica tumorale. neoplasia atipica della regione ipofisaria identificata con l'ultramicroscopio ("carcinoma" dell'ipofisi). Pathologica 65:353–355, 1973.
33. Ricoy J, Carrillo R, Garcia J, Bravo G. Dissemination of pituitary adenomas. Acta Neurochirurgica 31:123–130, 1974.
34. Scheithauer BW, Randall RV, Laws ER, Kovacs KT, Horvath E, Whitaker MD. Prolactin cell carcinoma of the pituitary. Cancer 55:598–604, 1985.
35. Ogilvy KM, Jakubowski J. Intracranial dissemination of pituitary adenomas. J Neurol Neurosurg Psychiatry 36:199–205, 1973.

36. Hashimoto N, Handa H, Nishi S. Intracranial and intraspinal dissemination from a growth hormone-secreting pituitary tumor. J Neurosurg 64:140–144, 1986.

37. Cagnetto G. Zur frage der anatomischen beziehung zwischen akromegalie und hyophysistumor. Virchows Arch 176:115–168, 1904.

38. Epstein JA, Epstein BS, Molho L, Zimmerman HM. Carcinoma of the pituitary gland with metastases to the spinal cord and roots of the cauda equina. J Neurosurg 21:846–853, 1964.

39. Luzi P, Miracco C, Lio R, Malandrini S, Piovani S, Venezia SG, Tosi P. Endocrine inactive pituitary carcinoma metastasizing to cervical lymph nodes: A case report. Hum Pathol 18:90–92, 1987.

40. Mountcastle RB, Roof BS, Mayfield RK, Mordes DB, Sagel J, Biggs PJ, Rawe SE. Case Report: Pituitary adenocarcinoma in an acromegalic patient. Response to bromocriptine and pituitary testing: A review of the literature on 36 cases of pituitary carcinoma. Am J Med Sci 298:109–118, 1989.

41. Salassa RM, Kearns TP, Kernohan JW, Sprague RG, MacCarty CS. Pituitary tumors in patients with Cushing's syndrome. J Clin Endocrinol Metab 19:1523–1538, 1959.

42. Cavallero C. Sulla malignita dei tumori ipofisari. Tumori 16:256–289, 1942.

43. D'Abrera V St E, Burke WJ, Bleasel KF, Bader L. Carcinoma of the pituitary gland. J Pathol 109:335–343, 1973.

44. Cohen H, Dible JH. Pituitary basophilism associated with a basophil carcinoma of the anterior lobe of the pituitary gland. Brain 59:395–407, 1936.

45. Forbes W. Carcinoma of the pituitary gland with metastases to the liver in a case of Cushing's syndrome. J Pathol Bacteriol 59:137–144, 1947.

46. Sheldon WH, Golden A, Bondy PK. Cushing's syndrome produced by a pituitary basophil carcinoma with hepatic metastases. Am J Med 17: 134–142, 1954.

47. De S Queiroz L, Facure NO, Facure JJ, Modesto NP, De Faria JL. Pituitary carcinoma with liver metastases and Cushing's syndrome. Arch Pathol 99:32–35, 1975.

48. Kohlmeier W. Zur kenntnis der metastasierenden hyophysengeschwulste. Virchow Arch Pathol Anat 312:26–34, 1944.

49. Geroulanos ST. Chromophobes hypophysenkarzinom mit leber-und knoch enmetastasen. Schweiz Med Wochenschr 99:1817–1824, 1969.

50. Gilmour MD. Carcinoma of the pituitary gland with abdominal metastases. J Pathol Bacteriol 35:265–269, 1932.

51. Graf CJ, Blinderman EE, Terplan KL. Pituitary carcinoma in a child with distant metastases. J Neurosurg 19:254–259, 1962.

52. Scholz DA, Gastineau CF, Harrison EG. Cushing's syndrome with malignant chromophobe tumor of the pituitary and extracranial metastasis: Report of a case. Proc Staff Meet Mayo Clin 37:31–42, 1962.

53. Moberg A. A case of pituitary chromophobe adenoma with metastasis in the heart. Acta Pathol Microbiol Scand 45:243–249, 1959.

54. Nudleman KL, Choi B, Kusske JA. Primary pituitary carcinoma: A clinical pathological study. Neurosurgery 16:90–95, 1985.

55. Atienza DM, Vigersky RJ, Lack EE, Carriaga M, Rusnock EJ, Tsou E, Cerrone F, Kattah JG, Sausville EA. Prolactin-producing pituitary carcinoma with pulmonary metastases: A case report. Cancer 68:1605–1610, 1991.

56. Hoffman HJ, Duffner PK. Extraneural metastases of central nervous system tumors. Cancer 567:1778–1782, 1985.

57. Sadik AR, Port R, Garfinkel B, Bravo J. Extracranial metastasis of cerebral glioblastoma multiforme: Case report. Neurosurgery 15:549–551, 1984.

58. El-Gindi S, Salama M, El-Henawy M, Farag S. Metastases of glioblastoma multiforme to cervical lymph nodes. J Neurosurg 38:631–634, 1973.

12

METASTATIC NEOPLASMS TO THE PITUITARY GLAND

LONG JIN and RICARDO V. LLOYD

Metastatic tumors to the pituitary gland are relatively uncommon. Histological studies have revealed metastases in about 1% to 10% of pituitaries obtained at autopsy from patients with malignant tumors (1, 2). Higher incidences are seen when the entire gland is examined microscopically. Reported series in the literature are summarized in Table 12–1.

Various carcinomas can metastasize to the pituitary. However, metastatic sarcomas to the pituitary are rare. The breast in women and the lung in men are the most common primary sites (3). In the series of Teears and Silverman, the most common primary sites in women included breast (66%), lung (13.2%) and stomach (7.5%), while in men lung (62.9%), prostate (8.6%) and urinary bladder (5.7%) were the most common pri-

mary sites (3). Examination of pituitaries from autopsies and from hypophysectomy for treatment of disseminated breast carcinoma showed a 10% to 30% incidence of pituitary metastases (see Table 12–1). In addition, tumors from the prostate, colon, stomach, pancreas, kidney and thyroid; melanomas; and germ cell tumors are more often reported than others. The primary sites of 196 cases of tumors metastatic to the pituitary are shown in Figure 12–1. Pituitary metastases usually occur in patients with widespread systemic metastases involving many other organs (Figs. 12–2 and 12–3) (4, 5).

Metastases to the posterior lobe of the pituitary gland are more common than to the anterior lobe. The metastatic tumors are predominantly localized in the posterior lobe because of the direct systemic arterial blood

Table 12–1. Malignant Neoplasms With Pituitary Metastases

| | | Pituitary Metastases* | | |
| | | | | |
Report	Reference Number	*Metastases/Total No. Pituitaries*		*Percentage*
Gurling *et al* (1957)	9	11/44†	(S)	25.0
Duchen (1966)	6	12/155†	(S)	7.7
Hagerstrad and Schonebeck (1969)	4	34/214†	(A)	15.9
Abrams *et al* (1950)	27	18/1000	(A)	1.8
Hagerstrad and Schonebeck (1969)	4	29/763	(A)	3.8
Roessman *et al* (1970)	26	5/60	(A)	8.3
Kovacs (1973)	7	18/1857	(A)	1.0
Teears and Silverman (1975)	3	88	(A)	—
Max *et al* (1981)	5	18/500	(A)	3.6

*Material from autopsy cases (A) or surgical cases (S) after hypophysectomy.
†Breast carcinoma primary; all other cases are a mixture of various other primary neoplasms.

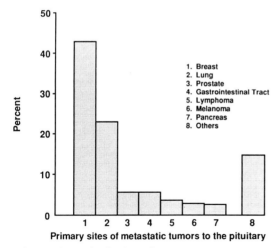

1. Breast
2. Lung
3. Prostate
4. Gastrointestinal Tract
5. Lymphoma
6. Melanoma
7. Pancreas
8. Others

Primary sites of metastatic tumors to the pituitary

Figure 12–1. Distribution of the most common sites of primary neoplasms with metastases to the pituitary gland.

supply. Metastases to the anterior lobe usually occur by direct extension from the posterior lobe or via the portal vessels (6). In some cases, the isolated metastatic foci may be reached by other routes, such as interlobar capillaries and capsular arteries, linking the anterior lobe with the arterial system (7, 8). In one study of 88 metastatic tumors to the pituitary gland, 56.8% were in the posterior lobe, while 13.6% were in the anterior lobe,

12.5% in the posterior and anterior lobes, 12.5% in the capsule and 2.3% in the stalk (3). Of a total of 192 reported cases of pituitary metastases, the posterior lobe alone was involved in 43.2%, the posterior and anterior lobes in 29.2%, the anterior lobe alone in 19.8% and the stalk and/or capsule in 7.8% (3, 4, 6, 7, 9).

Most metastases occur in grossly normal-appearing pituitary glands; only about a quarter of affected pituitaries are enlarged (3). A rich vascular network may be noted in metastatic lesions (10). Ischemic infarcts may develop secondary to the infiltration of the portal vessels by tumor cells.

Metastatic carcinomas may be misdiagnosed as pituitary adenomas (11–13) or overlooked if only small foci of metastases are present or if only a small specimen is obtained, especially at the time of frozen sections. In a study of 14 cases, patients with pituitary metastases commonly presented clinically with headaches/pain (69%), hypopituitarism (64%), visual field defects (50%), extraocular nerve palsy (43%) and diabetes insipidus (28%) (13). Immunohistochemistry can be a very useful tool in the differential diagnosis, using specific antisera against various pituitary hormones and other tumor markers. Cytokeratin or epithelial membrane antigen may not be helpful, since both meta-

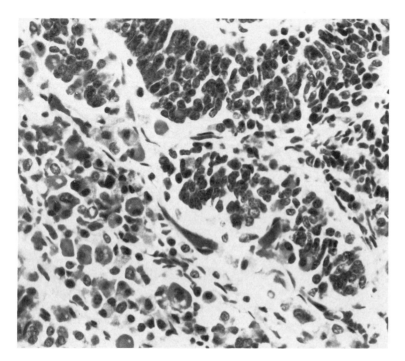

Figure 12–2. Metastatic small cell lung carcinoma to the pituitary gland in a patient with disseminated lung carcinoma (×350). (Courtesy of Dr. Lee Weatherbee, University of Michigan Medical Center, Ann Arbor, MI.)

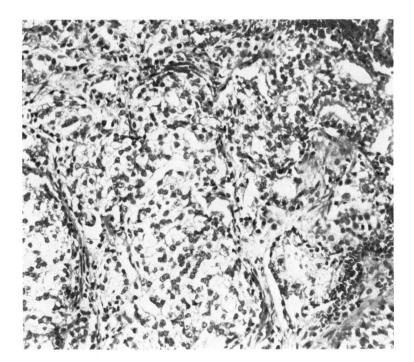

Figure 12—3. Metastatic prostate carcinoma to the sphenoid sinus. This 53-year-old man was thought to have a pituitary macroadenoma before the diagnosis of metastatic prostate carcinoma was made. Immunostaining was positive for prostate specific antigen (×350).

static carcinomas and pituitary adenomas may be positive. Undifferentiated carcinoma or renal cell carcinoma may look like pituitary null cell adenoma or oncocytoma (11). Broadspectrum endocrine markers such as chromogranin A and neuron-specific enolase (NSE) will help to distinguish these tumors in difficult cases (2). However, a few cases of metastatic neuroendocrine tumors to the pituitary with immunoreactivity for NSE or chromogranin A have been reported (14–16); careful clinicopathologic correlation is necessary. Electron microscopy has proven to be a useful diagnostic tool for plasmacytoma involving the pituitary (12, 17). In some cases of pituitary metastases, transsphenoidal surgery may provide the initial diagnosis of carcinoma (18, 19).

More than 10 cases of metastatic carcinomas to pituitary adenomas have been reported (8, 20–22). This rare tumor-to-tumor metastasis appears to be coincidental, although a higher incidence of this phenomenon may be found by examining more careful serial sections. Immunohistochemical studies have shown that the pituitary adenomas with metastatic carcinomas can be endocrine inactive or hormone-producing tumors such as those producing prolactin, growth hormone, follicle-stimulating hormone, luteinizing hormone or adrenocorti-

cotropic hormone. Possible mechanisms involved in tumor-to-tumor metastasis may include abnormalities in the capillaries and nonportal vessels or neovascularization in the areas adjacent to pituitary adenomas. Postoperative or radiation-induced vascular changes may also contribute to this rare development.

In most cases small pituitary metastases remain asymptomatic. Posterior pituitary insufficiency with diabetes insipidus is the most common clinical finding with metastases to the posterior lobe (23, 24). However, anterior pituitary failure caused by metastatic carcinoma, as the initial clinical manifestation, has been noted in some reports (13, 25). This may be a reflection of the availability of more sensitive endocrine tests. Diabetes insipidus and lateral extension of the neoplasm with nerve palsy are more common in sellar metastases when compared to pituitary adenomas, in which visual loss and anterior insufficiency are the common clinical signs (5). X-ray examination was found to be a relatively insensitive method for detecting metastatic lesions in the sella (5, 26, 27). Large foci of metastatic tumors that compress the pituitary stalk and destroy the hypothalamus may lead to hyperprolactinemia. The mean survival of patients with pituitary metastases is less than 1 year after diagnosis (24). This short period of survival is most likely a reflection of the extent of carcinoma at the time of diagnosis.

REFERENCES

1. Kovacs K, Horvath E. Tumors of the pituitary gland. In: Hartmann WH, Sobin LH (eds). Atlas of Tumor Pathology. 2nd Series. Fascicle 21. Washington, DC, Armed Forces Institute of Pathology, 1986.
2. Lloyd RV. Endocrine Pathology. New York, Springer-Verlag, 1990.
3. Teears RJ, Silverman EM. Clinicopathologic review of 88 cases of carcinoma metastatic to the pituitary gland. Cancer 36:216–220, 1975.
4. Hagerstrand I, Schonebeck J. Metastases to the pituitary gland. Acta Pathol Microbiol Scand 75:64–70, 1969.
5. Max MB, Deck MD, Rottenberg DA. Pituitary metastasis: Incidence in cancer patients and clinical differentiation from pituitary adenoma. Neurology 31:998–1002, 1981.
6. Duchen LW. Metastatic carcinoma in the pituitary gland and hypothalamus. J Pathol Bacteriol 91:347–355, 1966.
7. Kovacs K. Metastatic cancer of the pituitary gland. Oncology 27:533–542, 1973.
8. Ramsay JA, Kovacs K, Scheithauer BW, Ezrin C, Weiss MH. Metastatic carcinoma to pituitary adenomas: A report of two cases. Exp Clin Endocrinol 92:69–76, 1988.
9. Gurling KJ, Scott GBD, Baron DN. Metastases in pituitary tissue removed at hypophysectomy in women with mammary carcinoma. Br J Cancer 11:519–522, 1957.
10. Nelson PB, Robinson AG, Martinez AJ. Metastatic tumor of the pituitary gland. Neurosurgery 21:941–944, 1987.
11. Horikoshi T, Mitsuka S, Kimura R, Fukamachi A, Nukui H. Renal cell carcinoma metastatic to the hypophysis–case report. Neurol Med Chir (Tokyo) 28:78–82, 1988.
12. Poon MC, Prchal JT, Murad TM, Galbraith JG. Multiple myeloma masquerading as chromophobe adenoma. Cancer 43:1513–1515, 1979.
13. Branch CL Jr, Laws ER Jr. Metastatic tumors of the sella turcica masquerading as primary pituitary tumors. J Clin Endocrinol Metab 65:469–474, 1987.
14. Epstein S, Ranchod M, Goldswain PR. Pituitary insufficiency, inappropriate antidiuretic hormone (ADH) secretion, and carcinoma of the bronchus. Cancer 32:476–481, 1973.
15. Paulus P, Paridaens R, Mockel J, Coffernils M, Dhaens J, Baleriaux D, Rodesch G, Rutsaert J, Depierreux M, Flament-Durand J. Argysophilic breast carcinoma, single metastasis to the pituitary gland. Bull Cancer 77:377–384, 1990.
16. Rossi ML, Bevan JS, Fleming KA, Cruz-Sanchez F. Pituitary metastasis from malignant bronchial carcinoid. Tumori 74:101–105, 1988.
17. Sanchez JA, Rahman S, Strauss RA, Kaye GI. Multiple myeloma masquerading as a pituitary tumor. Arch Pathol Lab Med 101:55–56, 1977.
18. Dhanani A-NN, Bilbao JM, Kovacs K. Multiple myeloma presenting as a sellar plasmacytoma and mimicking a pituitary tumor: Report of a case and review of the literature. Endocr Pathol 1:245–248, 1990.
19. McClatchey KD, Lloyd RV, Schaldenbrand JD. Metastatic carcinoma to the sphenoid sinus. Case report and review of the literature. Arch Otorhinolaryngal 241:219–224, 1985.
20. Molinatti PA, Scheithauer BW, Randall RV, Laws ER. Metastasis to pituitary adenoma. Arch Pathol Lab Med 109:287–289, 1985.
21. Post KD, McCormick PC, Hays AP, Kandji AG. Metastatic carcinoma to pituitary adenoma. Report of two cases. Surg Neurol 30:286–292, 1988.
22. Zager EL, Hedley-Whyte ET. Metastasis within a pituitary adenoma presenting with bilateral abducens palsies: Case report and review of the literature. Neurosurgery 21:383–386, 1987.
23. Cox EV. Chiasmal compression from metastatic cancer to the pituitary gland. Surg Neurol 11:49–50, 1979.
24. Houck WA, Olson KB, Horton J. Clinical features of tumor metastasis to the pituitary. Cancer 26:656–659, 1970.
25. Markusse HM, Hekster REM, Velde J, Vecht CJ. Metastatic malignancy presenting as anterior pituitary failure. Neth J Med 30:135–143, 1987.
26. Roessmann U, Kaufman B, Friede RL. Metastatic lesions in the sella turcica and pituitary gland. Cancer 25:478–480, 1970.
27. Abrams HL, Spiro R, Goldstein N. Metastases in carcinoma: Analysis of 1000 autopsied cases. Cancer 3:74–85, 1950.

13

NEOPLASMS OF THE SELLAR REGION

Paul E. McKeever, Mila Blaivas and Anders A. F. Sima

The sellar region is fertile territory, producing a myriad of intriguing neoplasms. Their diversity arises from the variety of tissues susceptible to neoplastic transformation. Central and peripheral nervous, endocrine, germinal, meningeal, hematopoietic, epithelial and mesenchymal tissues converge in the region of the sella.

This chapter provides a detailed view of primary non-adenomatous neoplasms in the region of the sella turcica and is intended to be helpful in the daily practice of diagnostic pathology. The tables can be used as quick references for interpretation of unknown cases. They are organized according to categories of major characteristics of neoplasms, allowing construction of a differential diagnosis. These major characteristics are evident on initial inspection of hematoxylin and eosin (H & E)–stained sections and include fibrillary background of glial and neuronal neoplasms; prominent extracellular matrix of chordoma, fibroma, schwannoma and myxoma; cyst as a separate entity or as a feature of other neoplasm; and mixed tumors.

The most challenging problem is presented by the tendency of neoplasms to mimic pituitary adenomas or each other. For example, a meningioma in one case may resemble a pituitary adenoma, while in another it may look like a glioma or even a fibroma (Tables 13–1 through 13–7).

As described in Chapter 6, the majority of pituitary adenomas have a relatively uniform epithelioid structure with variable cytoplasmic granules barely perceptible by light microscopy. Glandular, epithelial and meningothelial neoplasms as well as oligodendroglioma and plasmacytoma can mimic these features (see Table 13–1). All these imitators, however, lack cytoplasmic granules which contain pituitary peptide hormones.

Fibrillary neoplasms, which include glial or neuronal components, are usually histologically low-grade neoplasms in the region of the sella (see Table 13–2). The fibrillarity of this group of tumors reflects cellular processes. The infundibuloma and optic nerve glioma are easily distinguished from collagenous neoplasms because these gliomas do not show reticulin or collagen when stained with Wilder's or Masson's stain. On the other hand, some of the ganglionic neoplasms and hamartomas contain substantial bands of collagen between their non-collagenous parenchyma, and recognition of their neuronal components becomes critical to their interpretation. This can be achieved by identification of neuronal Nissl substance with cresyl violet stain and neurites with silver stain (1, 2). Immunostaining for markers of central nervous system (CNS) parenchyma such as glial fibrillary acidic protein (GFAP), neurofilaments, synaptophysin, and S-100 protein will discriminate the more difficult cases from non-neuroectodermal neoplasms (see Tables 13–2 and 13–3) (1–3).

Neoplasms with prominent extracellular matrix (ECM) have significant parenchymal collagen and are most easily recognized with Wilder's stain for reticulin (which is especially sensitive

Text continued on page 146

Table 13–1. Epithelioid Neoplasms That Resemble Pituitary Adenomas

Neoplasm	Structures	Chemicals*	References
Meningioma	"Syncytial" cells; whorls; desmosomes	(Vimentin)† [S-100]‡	2,368,376, 388
Paraganglioma	Neurosecretory granules	Chromogranin; catecholamine	356,423,424
Granular cell tumor	Large, round cells; granular cytoplasm; autophagic vacuoles	PAS; S-100; (γ-enolase)	208,209, 212–215
Plasmacytoma	Round, discohesive cells; Golgi and RER	Ig	3,325,340 430,433,434
Oligodendroglioma	Perinuclear halo	S-100; Leu-7; [GC]	111,487,488
Ependymoma	Rosettes; cilia; elongated junctions	GFAP; (S-100); (Leu-7)	489

*List of the most useful special stains and immunoperoxidase methods. More comprehensive additional information is provided in the text.

†Markers in parentheses are not specific and are positive in many other neoplasms.

‡Markers in brackets are usually negative but still useful as described in text.

GFAP—Glial fibrillary acidic protein; GC—galactocerebroside; PAS—periodic acid–Schiff stain for vicinal hydroxyls; RER—rough endoplasmic reticulum.

Table 13–2. Neoplasms That Resemble Nervous Tissue

Neoplasm	Structures	Chemicals*	References
Gangliocytoma	Mature neurons; neurosecretory granules	NF; synaptophysin	1,127,135,136
Optic nerve glioma	Pilocytic astrocytes; Rosenthal fibers	GFAP	1,2,405,409,412
Infundibuloma	Pilocytic astrocytes	GFAP	1,2,309
Hamartoma	Clusters of mature neurons; glia; (neurosecretory granules)	Synaptophysin; GFAP; NF	222,225,226
Esthesioneuroblastoma	Fibrillary cells; round nucleus; neurosecretory granule	Synaptophysin; NF;[NT]‡; (S-100)	3,108–110,114–117

*List of the most useful special stains and immunoperoxidase methods. More comprehensive additional information is provided in the text.

†Markers in parentheses are not specific and are positive in many other neoplasms.

‡Markers in brackets are usually negative but still useful as described in text.

GFAP—Glial fibrillary acidic protein; NF—neurofilament; NT—neurotubulin.

Table 13–3. Neoplasms With Prominent Extracellular Matrix

Neoplasm	Structures	Chemicals*	References
Chordoma	Cords of physaliphorous cells; mitochondrial–RER complex	AFP; CEA; collagen II; CK; EMA; (S-100; vimentin)†	2,19–31 35-37
Histiocytosis X	Birbeck granules	S-100, MT1	285,292,298 302,303,307
Esthesioneuroblastoma	Fibrillary cells; round nucleus; neurosecretory granule	Synaptophysin; NF; NT; (S-100)	3,108–110,114–117
Fibroma	Spindled cells; fibrous collagen	Fibronectin; collagen; trichrome	123
Meningioma	Syncytial cells	Vimentin; EMA	2,368,376,388
Sarcoma	Malignant spindled cells; pleomorphism	Fibronectin; collagen; trichrome	462–465
Schwannoma	Fibrillary cells; continuous BL	Reticulin; S-100; Leu-7; [GFAP]‡	2,378,475,477,479
Myxoma	Stellate cells; mucinous background	Alcian blue, PAS	390,392
Giant cell tumor of bone	Benign multi-nucleated mononuclear cells	None	178
Osteosarcoma	Malignant cells producing osteoid		417,420
Hemangiopericytoma	Deformed vessels; thick pericellular BL	Reticulin; (vimentin)	2,265,266, 271–279
Hemangioblastoma	Vascular channels; foamy stromal cells	Lipid; erythropoietin; (vimentin; γ-enolase)	2,237,240–243,246–250
Sinus histiocytosis with massive lymphadenopathy	Histiocytes with cytoplasmic lymphocytes	S-100	291–293,304
Hemartoma with mesenchyme	Clusters of mature neurons; neurosecretory granules; glia	Synaptophysin; NF; GFAP	222,225,226

*List of the most useful special stains and immunoperoxidase methods. More comprehensive additional information is provided in the text.
†Markers in parentheses are not specific and are positive in many other neoplasms.
‡Markers in brackets are usually negative but still useful as described in text.
AFP—Alpha-fetoprotein; BL—basal lamina; CEA—carcinoembryonic antigen; CK—cytokeratin; EMA—epithelial membrane antigen; GFAP—glial fibrillary acidic protein; NF—neurofilament; NT—neurotubulin; PAS—periodic acid–Schiff stain for vicinal hydroxyls; RER—rough endoplasmic reticulum.

Table 13–4. Malignant Neoplasms

Neoplasm	Structures	Chemicals*	References
Endodermal sinus tumor	Hyaline droplet; Schiller-Duvall body	AFP	140,159,166
Esthesioneuroblastoma	Fibrillary cells; round nucleus; (neurosecretory granule)	Synaptophysin; NF; NT; (S-100)	3,108–110,114–117
Nasopharyngeal carcinoma	Epithelial; squamous; desmosomes	CK; EMA; (γ-enolase)	3,349,400
Sarcoma	Spindled cells	Fibronectin; collagen; trichrome	462–465
Osteosarcoma	Osteoid	DNA-ploidy	421
Lymphoma	Round, discohesive cells; vascular invasion	CLA; L26; UCHL-1	2,85,319–322, 328,331,342
Melanoma	Premelanosome; melanosome	Melanin; HMB45; (S-100)	2,343,352, 355,357
High-grade glioma	Fibrillary cells; endothelial proliferation	GFAP; (S-100; Leu-7)	2,180–184, 193,282,283

*Structures indicative of **malignancy** such as mitoses and necrosis are not listed individually for each neoplasm.
†List of the most useful special stains and immunoperoxidase methods. More comprehensive additional information is provided in the text.
‡Markers in parentheses are not specific and are positive in many other neoplasms.
AFP—Alpha-fetoprotein; CK—cytokeratin; CLA—common leukocyte antigen (CD45); EMA—epithelial membrane antigen; GFAP—glial fibrillary acidic protein; NF—neurofilament; NT—neurotubulin.

Table 13–5. Cysts

Neoplasm	Structures	Chemicals*	References
Rathke's cleft cyst	Epithelium on fibrovascular base	CK; GFAP; S-100; (vimentin)†	451–457
Epidermoid cysts	Squamous epithelium; keratinous material	Keratin; (vimentin)	2,94,97
Craniopharyngioma	Adamantinomatous tissue; cholesterol clefts; desmosomes	Keratin	2,67–69,71,72
Dermoid cyst	Keratinizing squamous epithelium; dermal adnexa; hair	Keratin	2,81,88

*List of the most useful special and immunoperoxidase methods. More comprehensive additional information is provided in the text.
†Markers in parentheses are not specific and are positive in many other neoplasms.
CK—Cytokeratin; GFAP—glial fibrillary acidic protein.

Table 13–6. Mixed Neoplasms

Neoplasm	Structures	Chemicals*	References
Ganglioglioma	Binucleated and disorganized neurons; neoplastic glia	Synaptophysin; NF; GFAP	127,128
Germinoma	Large neoplastic and small lymphoid cell; nucleolonema	ACE; CLA; PLAP	2,139,155–158,162–164, 167–169
Hamartoma	Clusters of mature neurons; glia; (mesenchyme; neurosecretory granules)†	Synaptophysin; NF; GFAP	222,225,226
Teratoma	Mature or immature elements of ectoderm, endoderm, mesoderm	Tissue dependent	2,6,480,481,485

*List of the most useful special stains and immunoperoxidase methods. More comprehensive additional information is provided in the text.
†Markers in parentheses are not specific and are positive in many other neoplasms.
ACE—Angiotensin I–converting enzyme; CLA—common leukocyte antigen (CD45); GFAP—glial fibrillary acidic protein; NF—Neurofilament; PLAP—placental-like alkaline phosphatase.

Table 13–7. Vascular Tumors and Malformations

Neoplasm	Structures	Chemicals*	References
Glomangioma	Uniform polygonal cells; vascular channels; BL	Desmin; myoglobin; actin	197
Hemangioma	Sinusoidal vascular channels; fibrous septae	FVIII-RA; UEA 1; (vimentin)†	255,257
Hemangioblastoma	Vascular channels; foamy stroma cells	Lipid; erythropoietin (vimentin; γ-enolase)	237,240–243, 246–250
Hemangiopericytoma	Deformed vessels; thick pericellular BL	(vimentin)	265,266, 271–279

*List of the most special stains and immunoperoxidase methods. More comprehensive additional information is provided in the text.
†Markers in parentheses are not specific and are positive in many other neoplasms.
BL—Basal lamina; FVIII-RA—Factor VIII related antigen; UEA—*Ulex europaeus* agglutinin.

for types III and IV collagen) and Masson's stain for collagen (see Table 13–3) (1).

Malignant neoplasms can be immediately distinguished from benign tumors, including pituitary adenoma, by virtue of the following malignant features:

1. High cellular density imparting a distinct blue macroscopic appearance to the sections stained with H & E.
2. High mitotic index and/or abnormal mitotic spindles
3. Spontaneous necrosis of regions and/or isolated neoplastic cells
4. Cellular and/or nuclear pleomorphism
5. Invasion of surrounding tissues

Malignant parasellar neoplasms have more than one of these features. Moreover, particular constellations of these features are suggestive of specific types of malignant neoplasms (2). Table 13–4 summarizes distinctive structures of different malignancies.

Numerous *cysts* occur in the region of the sella (see Table 13–5). Macroscopic examination *in situ* is the best way to examine a cyst. Careful attention must be directed toward sampling any solid regions of tissue to minimize the risk of interpreting a cystic craniopharyngioma, cystic prolactinoma or a transitional cell tumor as a simple epithelial cyst (2, 4, 5). The vast majority of simple epithelial cysts in this region are benign. When total removal without spilling cyst contents is anatomically feasible, an excellent prognosis is expected.

The category of *mixed neoplasms* consists of neoplasms with at least two different parenchymal tissue components (6). Only one component may be neoplastic, as in the germinoma. The tumor may be dimorphic, like the germinoma with two components, or oligomorphic, like the teratoma with tissues from three germ cell layers. The importance of this categorization is diagnostic rather than nosologic. Recognition of dimorphism or oligomorphism is critical to the diagnosis of germ cell neoplasms. Not all mixed neoplasms are germ cell tumors (see Table 13–6).

TYPES OF NEOPLASMS AND MALFORMATIONS

Chordoma

Chordomas are relatively common among non-adenomatous neoplasms in the region of the sella. In one study of 41 neoplasms in the region of the sella, two were chordomas of the clivus (7). Chordomas of the clivus and sphenoid region represent 30% to 40% of all chordomas (8, 9). This location corresponds to the most cranial portion of the notochord at the spheno-occipital synchondrosis, where notochordal remnants have been found in 2% of autopsies (10). Nearly all of the remainder arise in the spinal canal (8, 9). A chordoma can occur at virtually any age, but clival chordomas tend to occur in younger individuals than do chordomas in the spinal canal (9, 10). The most frequent clinical presentations of clival chordomas are diplopia and visual field abnormalities. Tumor compression of other cranial nerves can cause facial paralysis and dysphagia. Headaches and vomiting are also encountered (9, 10). Chordomas that involve the nasal region commonly show a nasopharyngeal mass (11).

In contrast to other primary parasellar tumors, chordomas commonly destroy bone of the clivus and sella (10, 11). Some clival chordomas destroy the clivus and cause a soft tissue mass in the sphenoid sinus or nasopharynx (11). Unilateral bone erosion occurs in nearly a third of the cases. Erosion of the tip of the clivus, sclerotic bone reactions and osteolytic changes can be detected early by radiography (9, 12, 13). Their presence is a significant feature to consider in the pathologic diagnosis. These early changes virtually rule out glioma and decrease the likelihood of meningioma and adenoma. Chordomas can narrow and deviate the path of the internal carotid artery (14). Spontaneous hemorrhage in clival chordomas is rare (12, 15).

The macroscopic appearance of chordomas can distinguish them from many other neoplasms. They are firmer than untreated pituitary adenomas. They are multi-lobular, gelatinous and myxoid. Their classic microscopic features are cords of physaliphorous cells that line up like beads on string (Figs. 13–1 through 13–5). The vacuoles of these cells are highly variable in size, ranging up to a whole cell diameter, and tend to be larger than macrophage vacuoles. Unlike perinuclear oligodendroglial vacuoles, they contain mucin and lie beside, rather than around, cellular nuclei. These cells lie within a substantial myxoid extracellular matrix, which stains with Alcian blue. While its staining characteristics are like mucin, this material is probably a highly glycosylated, acidic ground substance. Complete sampling of a

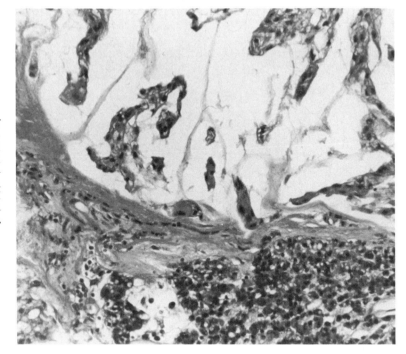

Figure 13–1. Dark cords of cells are highlighted by a transparent background formed where myxoid material dissolved during processing. This chordoma compresses adjacent dark, solid adenohypophysial cells (H & E; ×210). (Courtesy of Dr. Steven C. Bauserman, Temple, Texas.)

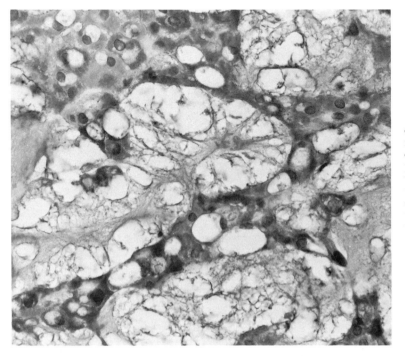

Figure 13–2. Section of a chordoma reveals typical pattern of marker expression (hematoxylin counterstains). Cords of physaliphorous cells express S-100 protein. Large intracytoplasmic vacuoles are S-100 negative. The cords surround a hematoxylinophilic myxoid extracellular matrix (immunoperoxidase anti–S-100 protein; ×420).

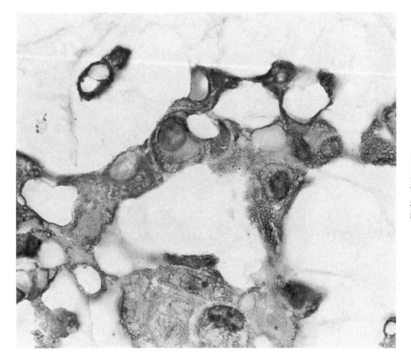

Figure 13–3. Chordoma section near that shown in Figure 13–2. Physaliphorous and epithelioid cells express cytokeratin. The large cytoplasmic vacuoles are CK negative (immunoperoxidase anti-CK; ×1040).

Figure 13–4. Chordoma section near those shown in Figures 13–2 and 13–3. Physaliphorous cells lack detectable levels of high-molecular-weight keratin (HMWK) (immunoperoxidase anti-HMWK; ×420).

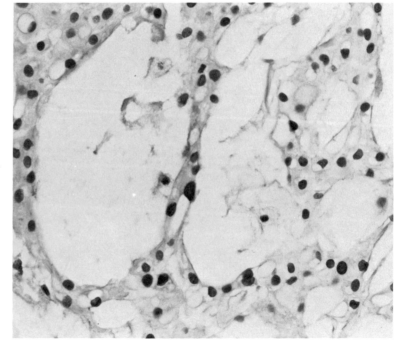

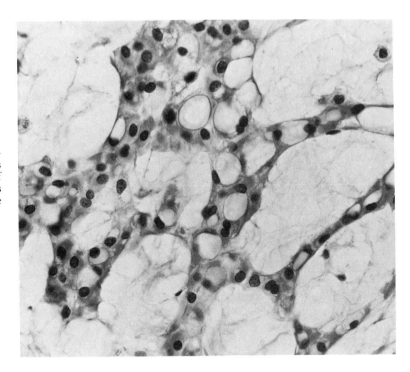

Figure 13–5. Chordoma section near those shown in Figures 13–2, 13–3, and 13–4. Cords of physaliphorous cells also express vimentin (immunoperoxidase anti-vimentin; ×420).

chordoma specimen is important, since other portions of a chordoma may not show this typical appearance. Some portions may be very epithelioid with less matrix and resemble a meningioma or low-grade carcinoma, while other portions may contain spindle cells resembling a fibroblastic neoplasm (8–10).

The physaliphorous cells are sufficiently distinctive to be recognized on fine-needle aspiration or cerebrospinal fluid cytology specimens in individual cases (16–17). However, some specimens closely resemble well-differentiated adenocarcinoma (18), making sole reliance on cytologic criteria hazardous. Immunocytochemistry and electron microscopy augment interpretation of cytologic specimens (16, 19).

Chordomas contain S-100 protein (see Fig. 13–2), but this marker is present in many parasellar neoplasms that are likely to be confused with chordoma. These include chondroma, chondrosarcoma, histiocytosis, schwannoma, melanoma, and some carcinomas (Fig. 13–6) (16, 20–31). On the other hand, lack of S-100 reactivity suggests a neoplasm other than chordoma.

A panel of antibodies is needed in complex cases. Cytokeratins (see Figs. 13–3 and 13–4), epithelial membrane antigen, and 5'-nucleotidase in chordomas distinguish some chordomas from chondrosarcomas, which lack these features, but confusing transitional forms include chondroid chordomas, dis-

cussed later (6, 23–27, 29, 31, 32). Histiocytosis, fibromatosis, and melanoma also lack cytokeratin. Strong immunoreactivity with vimentin (see Fig. 13–5) and α-fetoprotein, and especially the type II procollagen reactivity of chordomas, distinguish them from most carcinomas (18, 31). The use of tissue polypeptide antigen and monoclonal antibody ICR.2 in such panels is an exciting possibility. However, their range of reactivity with other parasellar tumors remains to be determined (33, 34).

Electron microscopy reveals that the large vacuoles of physaliphorous cells contain sparse, short microvilli protruding into their lumens from their limiting membrane (35). These large vacuoles contain matrix material similar to the prominent extracellular matrix of chordomas. Smaller cytoplasmic vacuoles appear to be dilated rough endoplasmic reticulum (RER) in continuity with mitochondria (26, 35). Still other vacuoles contain glycogen (37, 38). The presence of these vacuoles of various sizes and contents distinguishes chordomas from most other parasellar tumors. Vacuoles of macrophages and histiocytic cells are phagocytic vacuoles that differ from RER. Pituitary adenomas and plasmacytomas have abundant RER but lack large cytoplasmic vacuoles lined with microvilli and containing matrix material.

Mitochondrial-RER complexes are typical of chordomas (37). These are sandwiches of

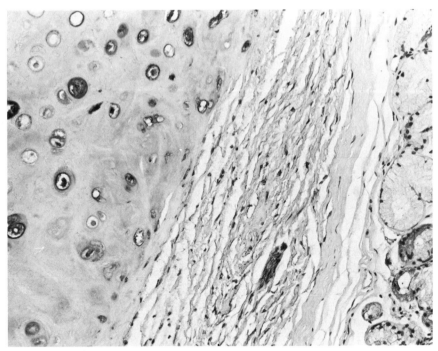

Figure 13–6. This neoplasm of the skull base has invaded the nasopharyngeal region despite numerous resections over more than a decade. Tumor from this resection is invading fibrous tissue (*center*) near olfactory glands of Bowman in the lamina propria (*edge opposite tumor*). The myoepithelial cells of these glands, a peripheral nerve twig in fibrous tissue, and the neoplastic cells express S-100 protein. Single cells and doublets are distributed within a hematoxylinophilic matrix of the chondroid tumor (immunoperoxidase anti-S-100, hematoxylin counterstain; ×210).

alternating layers of RER and elongated mitochondria. The mitochondria have bulbous ends, producing a dumbbell configuration. The entire complex suggests considerable need for energy close to the protein production facilities of these cells.

Distinguishing among chordoma, chondroid chordoma, chondroma, and low-grade chondrosarcoma presents a particularly difficult diagnostic problem (39, 40). This distinction may be of considerable clinical importance, since the survival of patients with chondroid chordomas is actually five times as long as patients with typical chordoma (39, 41). In seven neoplasms with structural features of chondrocytes resembling chondroid chordomas, epithelial membrane antigen markers, which were present in six typical clival chordomas (39), led to the interpretation of these seven tumors as low-grade chondrosarcomas.

However, a different clival chordoma has shown a mixture of chondromatous and chordomatous histologic features and a mixed pattern of epithelial staining (40). During multiple partial excisions, the tumor progressed toward the structural appearance and epithelial antigenicity of a typical chordoma. This tumor exhibited ultrastructural features of monoparticulate glycogen, seen in chordomas, and also microtubular inclusions within the endoplasmic reticulum, seen in chondrosarcomas. The patient lived for only 14 months following diagnosis (40). While this case does not exemplify a longer prognosis for those with chondroid chordoma, it suggests that typical chordoma may not be distinguished from low-grade chondrosarcoma by the presence or absence of both cytokeratin and epithelial membrane antigen. It remains to be determined whether true transitional tumors exist, and whether more decisive markers will facilitate their detection. Transitions between conventional chordomas and malignant spindle cell tumors have also been noted (42).

Chordomas of the clivus eventually kill patients by invasion of surrounding structures, including bone, and compromise of critical neuroanatomic structures. Invading chordomas occasionally compromise the internal carotid artery (14). However, many chordomas have a low proliferative rate and grow very slowly (43). The incidence of metastases varies between studies, ranging from rare to up to 43% (9, 44). Average survival for a patient with a typical chordoma is 4 years (41). Studies of proliferative capacity may eventually be of greater prognostic value than immunophenotyping in the assessment of clival chordomas (39–43, 45). Patients with well-differentiated chondroid tumors tend to survive longer.

Craniopharyngioma

Craniopharyngioma is a common epithelial tumor arising in the region of the sella turcica. It is the second most frequent neoplasm in the sellar region and the most common suprasellar neoplasm in children (47). In a series of 74 children with parasellar tumors, 21 had craniopharyngiomas (48). Of 41 neoplasms in this region from patients of all ages, five were craniopharyngiomas (7). About 94% of craniopharyngiomas are found in the suprasellar location, with 18% situated within the sella turcica at the time of the diagnosis (49). Later in the course of the disease, the tumor expands, and at the time of autopsy, intrasellar involvement may increase to 31% (49). Twenty-one intrasellar craniopharyngiomas had been reported by 1989 (50–53).

Craniopharyngiomas are primarily tumors of *young adults* and *children,* but neonatal or congenital tumors are very rare (54, 55). However, no age group is immune from craniopharyngioma—the oldest patient reported was an 83-year-old woman (56). Occasional neoplasms in children or young adults assume giant proportions involving vast regions of adjacent brain (57, 58).

The major presenting clinical symptoms are headache and visual disturbances. Diplopia may be the initial symptom (52). Hydrocephalus and mental changes, as well as autonomic and focal neurologic disturbances, are less frequent. Endocrinopathy occurs with intrasellar location of the tumor (53).

Craniopharyngiomas rarely coexist with other tumors and conditions. These rare concomitant lesions include pinealoma and a complex of parathyroid adenoma, two cerebral arteriovenous malformations and persistent vena cava (59, 60). It has also been associated with moyamoya disease, subependymoma and centronuclear myopathy (61, 63).

Grossly, craniopharyngioma is an irregular, nodular mass 3 to 4 cm in average diameter and usually cystic. The cysts vary in size and in the appearances of their lining and content. The latter can be yellow or brown, resembling motor oil; clear; or grumous and blood stained (Fig. 13–7). Calcifications are frequent and can be found in both solid and cystic regions. Histologically, the epithelial cells of the tumor form an *adamantinomatous pattern* in which a layer of pseudostratified columnar cells rests on thin

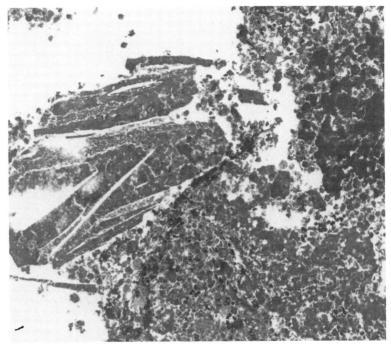

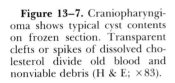

Figure 13–7. Craniopharyngioma shows typical cyst contents on frozen section. Transparent clefts or spikes of dissolved cholesterol divide old blood and nonviable debris (H & E; ×83).

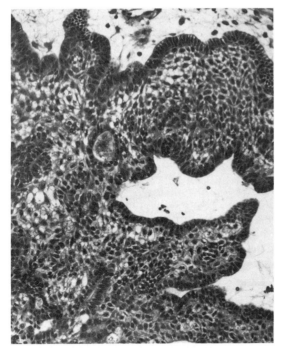

Figure 13–8. Craniopharyngioma with an adamantinomatous pattern. A basal epithelial layer at the edges of tumor projections surrounds stellate cells of lower density (H & E; ×165).

basement membrane and palisades around loose aggregates of stellate cells (Fig. 13–8). Another pattern is formed by solid nests of squamous cells, which often exhibit keratini-

zation and occasionally possess keratohyalin granules (Fig. 13–9). Both patterns form cysts lined by columnar basal cells resting on basement membrane or by flattened, stratified, squamous epithelium. In this latter case the lumina contain exfoliated squamous cells and keratin debris. Typical keratoid nodules are prominent in some cases. The irregular nests of tumor cells are embedded in a vascular stroma that may exhibit prominent gliosis with or without Rosenthal fibers. Foreign body giant cell reaction and chronic inflammatory infiltrates triggered by *irritative cystic contents* are sometimes quite prominent (Fig. 13–10). In the cerebrospinal fluid spaces, these and cholesterol can produce a severe chemical meningitis (64, 66).

Craniopharyngioma has the described adamantinomatous pattern, a squamous pattern, or a combination of the two. The demonstration on a frozen section of adamantinomatous epithelium renders the diagnosis of craniopharyngioma. In the absence of epithelium, a specimen from a calcified suprasellar mass that shows fibrous tissue, necrotic debris, and cholesterol clefts provides a strong suspicion of craniopharyngioma (67). The presence of only a thin epithelial lining raises the issue of the *epidermoid cyst* (Fig. 13–11). However, the validity of separating craniopharyngioma from epidermoid cyst was questioned by Petito *et al.* (49), since

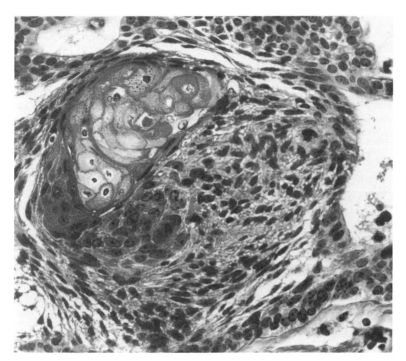

Figure 13–9. The squamous nodule of this craniopharyngioma contains keratohyalin granules (H & E; ×330).

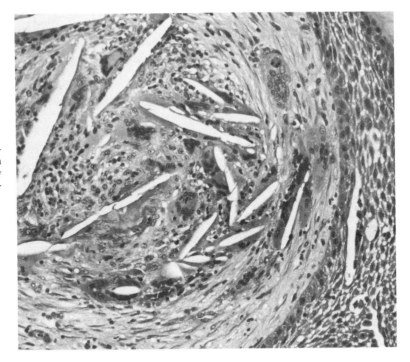

Figure 13–10. Giant cells highlight a granulomatous reaction in this craniopharyngioma. They contain cholesterol clefts and cellular debris (H & E; ×165).

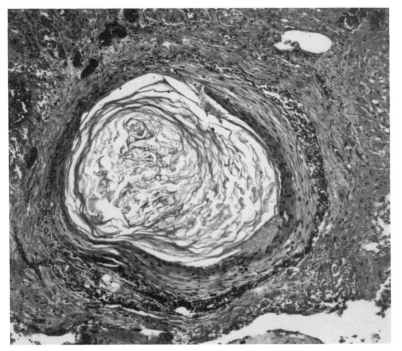

Figure 13–11. This portion of a craniopharyngioma reveals only a cyst lined by squamous epithelium and filled with squamous debris (H & E; ×85).

it was found that histological distinction between the two tumors often cannot be made. About one third of 245 cases reviewed by these authors showed transition between adamantinomatous and squamous epithelium with the presence of keratin and keratohyalin granules.

A peculiar combination of typical histological features of craniopharyngioma with ciliated and mucin-containing cells was observed in a suprasellar craniopharyngioma, suggesting a close relationship with *Rathke's cleft cyst* (68). *Papillary craniopharyngioma* is a distinctive suprasellar neoplasm that differs from the classic adamantinomatous craniopharyngioma by predominant, if not exclusive, occurrence in adulthood, frequent radiologic solidity and a well-differentiated papillary squamous epithelium. It lacks calcification, palisaded cells, keratoid nodules, cholesterol clefts, and foreign body giant cells (69, 70).

Ultrastructurally, craniopharyngioma is characterized by numerous desmosomes, tonofilaments and glycogen particles within the epithelial portion and by fenestrated capillary endothelium within the connective tissue stroma. Mineralized precipitates are calcium and phosphorus, which initially appear among the disintegrated keratinized cells, with collagen fibers, elastic fibers and cytoplasmic fibrils serving as supportive skeletons in forming large calcific nests (71). Using the immunoperoxidase technique, the epithelial cells of the neoplasm stain intensely for keratin (72).

Mitotic figures are inconspicuous in craniopharyngioma. This emphasizes the potential prognostic value of the more sensitive labeling index assay calculated by determining the percentage of bromodeoxyuridine (BUDR)-labeled cells (73). *In vitro* $_3$H-thymidine labeling index demonstrated a peculiar topographic arrangement of cells in S phase within the epithelium of the cystic walls. This is now under investigation with regard to intracavitary treatment with bleomycin or radiocolloids (74).

Craniopharyngiomas are histologically benign neoplasms that may frequently behave aggressively, invading the bone and compressing adjacent nervous structures. Arterial compression is less common (14).

Malignant transformation in a craniopharyngioma had not been described until 1988. A recurrent craniopharyngioma in a 46-year-old woman disclosed nuclear pleomorphism, hyperchromatism, nuclear molding and prominent eosinophilic nucleoli within the epithelial cells. It had increased mitotic activity, occasional bizarre cells and foci of tumor necrosis (75).

Craniopharyngiomas are curable after radical excision. However, because of the difficulty of total resection, *recurrence is common*. A few residual cells are sufficient to seed recurrence. In fact, seeding of epithelial cells into the brain substance has occurred along the needle tract after needle biopsy (76).

The recurrence rate and clinicopathologic correlations in surgically treated craniopharyngiomas have been reviewed by Adamson *et al.* (77). This study addresses the validity of separating craniopharyngiomas into two histological groups: predominantly solid, noncalcified, squamous, papillary tumors that occur mostly in adults and the usually cystic, calcified, adamantinomatous tumors that occur in adults and children (69, 78). In contrast to other reports, adult adamantinomatous tumors were found to be associated with a worse postoperative outcome and a slightly higher risk for recurrence than the childhood type. Otherwise, the study was supportive of previous findings, including the fact that the patients with tumors lacking calcifications on skull x-ray films had a significantly better 5-year survival rate. No correlation between survival rates and age of the patients, ratio of adamantinomatous to squamous regions or ratio of solid to cystic tumors was found. Increased survival was associated with absence of calcifications on plain skull films, negative results on analysis of cerebrospinal fluid (CSF), tumor size under 3.0 cm, diagnosis after 1955, and radiotherapy, as concluded by Petito *et al.* after studying 245 craniopharyngiomas (49).

Craniopharyngioma patients treated with external beam radiotherapy are susceptible to radiation-induced malignant astrocytomas (discussed in "Glioma Associated With Radiation"). Recurrent craniopharyngiomas are especially suitable for radiation treatment using yttrium 90 (^{90}Y) silicate or phosphorus 32 (^{32}P) colloid injected directly into the tumor cavity, since the recurrent neoplasms are most often cystic. The observations by Szeifert *et al.* indicate that the radiation of ^{90}Y destroys the lining squamous epithelium of cysts, thus preventing further expansion of the tumor (79). The limited range of penetration of radiation from these colloids might reduce the hazard of radiation-induced astrocytomas.

Dermoid Cyst

Parasellar dermoid cysts are very rare. They can be intrasellar, suprasellar, or both (80). Multiple dermoid cysts in the pituitary and ovary have been described (80). A dermoid cyst has also been found in the great wing of the sphenoid bone (81).

Clinical symptoms of dermoid tumors are variable. Among the reported cases, two patients had diabetes insipidus (80). One patient had hyperprolactinemia, probably due to pituitary stalk compression (80); another had precocious puberty (82). Visual symptoms sometimes occur (81). A dermoid cyst has also been implicated in the production of atypical angina pectoris by disturbing the hypothalamic function of one patient (83).

Bromocriptine has replaced surgical treatment of some prolactinomas. Since bromocriptine is ineffective against a dermoid cyst, differentiation of dermoid cysts from prolactinoma is important (80). Computed tomography (CT) scans distinguish the dermoid as a cyst, rather than a solid adenoma. The surrounding capsule may enhance with CT contrast media. Magnetic resonance imaging (MRI) may demonstrate a low intensity on T1-weighted images (80). Pathologic confirmation of such images is recommended.

With proper sampling of the cyst wall and macroscopic observation of cyst content, the diagnosis of dermoid cyst is straightforward. Dermoid cysts contain hair and adnexa, immediately distinguishing them from epidermoid cysts, cystic craniopharyngioma and nearly every other abnormality. One exception is the teratoma, which may generate a dermoid cyst as part of its multiple germ cell layers of neoplastic tissue (80, 84, 85). Teratoma is excluded from the differential diagnosis when complete sampling fails to demonstrate additional tissue elements. Dermoid cysts tend to occur in the midline, possibly reflecting embryonic origin during neural groove closure (86).

Ruptured dermoid and epidermoid cysts can cause sterile meningitis and inflammation resembling an abscess (87). Clues to proper identification of the cause are squamous epithelial cells or cholesterol clefts within the inflammation. Surgical removal of cysts should be done carefully to avoid spillage of contents.

Epidermoid Cyst

Parapituitary epidermoid cysts are more common than dermoid cysts and constitute 2% to 10% of all tumors in this region in

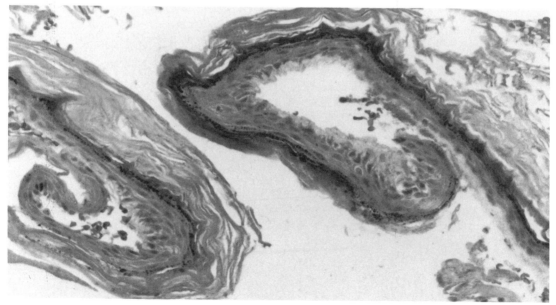

Figure 13–12. A squamous cell carcinoma arising in a suprasellar epidermoid cyst. The epidermoid cyst is composed of keratinizing squamous epithelium on a fibrous base (H & E; ×145). (From Lewis AJ, *et al.* Squamous cell carcinoma arising in suprasellar epidermoid cysts. J Neurosurg 59:538–541, 1983.)

adults (7, 88–90). In an autopsy series of 41 parasellar tumors, four were epidermoid cysts (7). In contrast to craniopharyngiomas, which are most commonly observed in childhood and adolescence, epidermoid cysts show a peak incidence during the fifth decade (91). They may occur intra- or extradurally with erosion of underlying bone. They tend to occur in the midline and have been associated with defects of neural tube closure (92), suggesting that epithelial rests may be involved in the genesis of epidermoid cysts (92, 93). Others attach to main arteries (14). About one third of all cranial and spinal epidermoid cysts occur in the parasellar region. The cysts are irregular or nodular, encapsulated and may reach considerable size. They may show areas of calcification, and they contain a waxy or fluid content rich in cholesterol. Microscopically the epidermoid cyst is lined by a squamous epithelium covered by keratinous material exfoliating toward the cyst center (Fig. 13–12). The cysts are benign non-neoplastic lesions, which rarely may dedifferentiate into squamous cell carcinomas (Figs. 13–13 and 13–14) (94, 95).

Epidermoid cysts resemble the cystic portion of craniopharyngiomas (4, 96). Neuroradiographic correlation and sampling are critical factors. A solitary cyst with a thin collagenous capsule lined with well-differentiated keratinizing squamous epithelium and having no mass of adamantinomatous cells is typical of an epidermoid cyst (4). However, a cystic craniopharyngioma sample may be histologically identical. Their histological identity and similar embryologic origin from Rathke's pouch have stimulated the view that epidermoid cysts and craniopharyngiomas are indistinguishable (96).

Rare epidermoid tumors grow *en plaque* along the base of the skull into the pituitary region. These are difficult to diagnosis radiographically and are prone to recurrence. It is unclear whether this peculiar growth pattern reflects extravasation and seeding of basal epithelial cells.

Esthesioneuroblastoma (Olfactory Neuroblastoma)

Esthesioneuroblastomas probably arise from the olfactory sensory cells lining the superior portion of the nasal cavity. They occur in patients of all ages, but peak incidences are during the second and sixth decades (97). They usually arise in the nasal cavity and present with epistaxis and nasal obstruction (98).

Esthesioneuroblastomas are rare in the parasellar region (98). Intracranial involvement is usually secondary to local extension from its origin near the cribriform plate. Clinical presentation depends on the extent of involvement of surrounding structures.

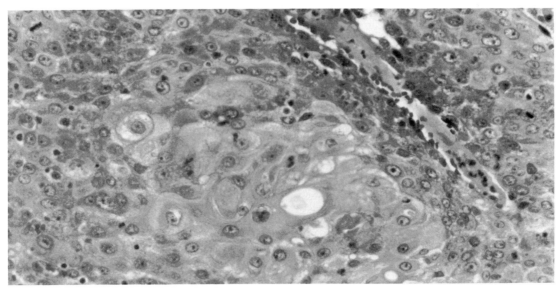

Figure 13–13. From the same case shown in Figure 13–12. Mitosing pleomorphic squamous cells produced this mass (H & E; ×240). (From Lewis AJ, *et al.* Squamous cell carcinoma arising in suprasellar epidermoid cysts. J Neurosurg 59:538–541, 1983.)

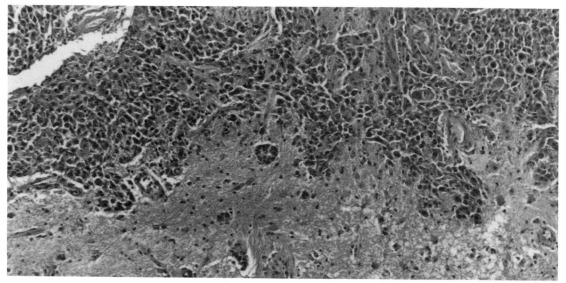

Figure 13–14. From the same case shown in Figures 13–12 and 13–13. The margin of this mass invades surrounding brain parenchyma in a manner typical of metastatic carcinoma. (H & E; ×95). (From Lewis AJ, *et al.* Squamous cell carcinoma arising in suprasellar epidermoid cysts. J Neurosurg *59*:538–541, 1983.)

Cranial nerve signs and symptoms are common (98–104).

CT reveals large tumors of mixed density (99–102). Erosion of the cribriform plate, sinus walls and other bones of the skull base is common (102, 105). The bone lesions are more apparent on CT images than on MRI images, but MRI is of great value when the tumor is within the cranial fossa (105).

Esthesioneuroblastoma occasionally metastasizes into the cranial vault (106). However, it can produce paraneoplastic Cushing's syndrome without invading the hypothalamus or pituitary (107).

The neoplastic parenchyma of esthesioneuroblastoma is moderately to highly cellular. Esthesioneuroblastoma cells extend fibrillary cellular processes. This fibrillarity is critical to the diagnosis and is evident on more than four fifths of cases stained with H & E (Fig. 13–15) (108). Silver stains for neurites or immunostains for neurofilaments or S-100 protein will accentuate these filaments, but equivocal cases should be examined ultrastructurally. Homer Wright rosettes with fibrillary cores or Flexner rosettes with central lumens rimmed by distinct pink borders are valuable diagnostic features but are often not evident. Perinuclear cytoplasm is minimal. Nuclei are small and round, with minimal to moderate pleomorphism. Mitotic indices vary substantially between cases. The amount of fibrovascular stroma is highly variable. In some tumors, it is very thick and resembles desmoplasia in carcinoma (102); in other cases, it is minimal (3).

Esthesioneuroblastomas express neuroectodermal and neural antigens (3, 103, 104, 109–112). Many esthesioneuroblastomas contain S-100 protein and Leu-7 reactivity, and all contain γ-enolase (neuron-specific enolase, or NSE) (3, 109, 110). While these particular antigens can be helpful as part of a diagnostic panel of immunostains, their relatively broad specificity includes other neoplasms in the region of the sella that may be confused with esthesioneuroblastoma.

Neuronal markers such as neurofilament, β-tubulin, and microtubule-associated protein 2 have more restricted specificity that can help identify esthesioneuroblastoma. However, immunostaining does not detect these markers on all esthesioneuroblastomas (3, 109, 110). Synaptophysin is expressed by virtually all esthesioneuroblastomas (110). Synaptophysin is relatively specific for neuronal cells but will not distinguish an esthesioneuroblastoma from a cerebral neuroblastoma or a medulloblastoma. Like primitive neuroectodermal tumors, esthesioneuroblastomas occasionally express cytokeratin (109) and rarely contain melanin pigment (113).

Tyrosine hydroxylase is a marker with promise in the differential diagnosis of esthesioneuroblastoma (112). However, its frequency of expression by esthesioneuroblas-

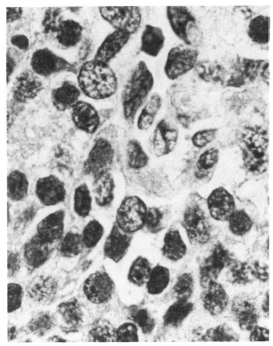

Figure 13–15. Fibrillary cells with round and oval nuclei and a high nucleus-to-cytoplasm ratio characterize this esthesioneuroblastoma. Clusters of fibrils surrounded by nuclei vaguely resemble Homer Wright rosettes. This neoplasm invaded the cribriform plate and ethmoid region of a middle-aged man (H & E; ×1300).

toma and lack of expression by other malignant neoplasms need to be more fully evaluated.

Fibrillar cellular processes are frequently found in esthesioneuroblastomas by electron microscopy (98, 101–104, 112, 114, 115). Some of these cellular processes contain microtubules and filaments in a neuritic pattern (115, 116). Neurosecretory granules with an average size of 180 nm occur in many cases (102, 112–115, 117). Occasionally, more specific structures that resemble immature olfactory vesicles are evident (102).

Other neoplasms that might be confused with esthesioneuroblastoma include lymphoma and melanoma (118–120). Both of these neoplasms lack the true neuronal markers described earlier (see Table 13–2). Lack of cellular fibrils and the presence of lymphocytic markers should distinguish lymphomas. Ultrastructural morphometry differentiates between esthesioneuroblastomas and lymphomas (118), but neuronal and lymphoid markers are sufficient in nearly all cases (see Table 13–4). Melanomas can be more problematic, since they share with es-

thesioneuroblastomas S-100 reactivity and the capability of melanin production (109, 113). However, most melanomas have larger cells, nuclei and nucleoli than esthesioneuroblastomas. Demonstration of neurosecretory granules or neuronal markers by immunoperoxidase distinguishes the esthesioneuroblastoma.

As a result of their origin in the nasal cavity and their propensity toward local invasion, most esthesioneuroblastomas have been recognized by the time they enter the region of the sella. The differential diagnosis is simpler in the nasal cavity than in the sella, since the nasal cavity seeds few neuroectodermal tumors other than esthesioneuroblastoma (119, 120). The most frequently confusing neoplasm in the nasal cavity is the sinonasal undifferentiated carcinoma (SNUC). Distinguishing the esthesioneuroblastoma from SNUC is clinically important, since patients with esthesioneuroblastoma have a better prognosis. Interval cures of up to 75% have been recorded (108). Esthesioneuroblastomas are less likely to invade vessels than SNUC (Fig. 13–16). Careful assessment of cellular shape may distinguish the fibrillar cells of the esthesioneuroblastoma from the clusters and ribbons of small epithelioid cells in the SNUC (3, 102, 114, 121, 122). Unfortunately, these neoplasms are so crowded with cells with very high nucleus-to-cytoplasm ratio that cellular borders are hard to discern. Homer Wright or Flexner rosettes identify esthesioneuroblastoma but may not be evident.

Immunocytochemistry for neuronal markers is recommended to distinguish esthesioneuroblastoma from SNUC. Some esthesioneuroblastomas stain for neurofilaments or neurotubules, which SNUC lack (109, 110). Synaptophysin is the most sensitive and specific marker for esthesioneuroblastoma in this context and should be employed in difficult cases (110). Difficult cases may also be recognized as esthesioneuroblastomas if they express S-100 protein, which is lacking in SNUC (3).

Fibroma

Few intracranial fibromas have been reported (123, 124). Frank and collaborators reported a case of chondromyxoid fibroma arising from the sphenoid bone with extension into the sella (125). An interesting case

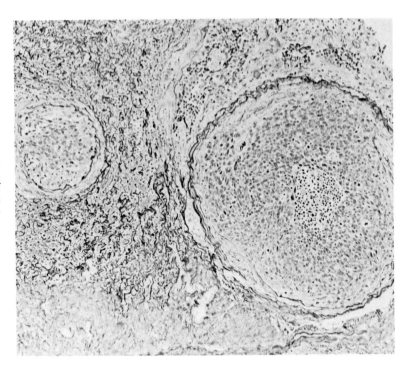

Figure 13–16. Vascular invasion is a typical feature of sinonasal undifferentiated carcinoma (SNUC). The central portion of the larger intravascular tumor is necrotic (Wilder's stain for reticulin; ×105).

of a pseudotumor arising from sphenoid sinuses with subsequent spread to the sella causing bony erosion was reported by Gartman and colleagues (126). The latter lesion demonstrated chronic inflammatory changes and dense fibrosis.

Ganglioglioma and Gangliocytoma (Ganglioneuroma)

Gangliocytomas (ganglioneuromas) generate mature neuronal components. Gangliogliomas contain a neoplastic glial stroma. These tumors often contain calcospherites. They can be regarded as being in the middle of a spectrum of tumors, with neuronal hamartomas at one extreme and the rare malignant ganglioglioma at the other extreme. Gangliocytomas are tumors of children and young adults, with 80% of cases occurring in patients younger than 30 (127). They are commonly located in the temporal lobe or the floor of the third ventricle. They are usually small, firm and well circumscribed but may occasionally reach considerable size, particularly in infants (127).

Histologically they are composed of irregularly oriented mature neuronal elements, which frequently include binucleated forms. Occasionally the neoplastic ganglion cells may display features of degeneration such as paired helical filaments (128). In pure gangliocytomas the glia are reactive and inconspicuous, whereas in gangliogliomas the glia are neoplastic.

Gangliocytomas often show calcospherites and calcification of the vascular walls. Occasionally more primitive neuronal precursors form small perivascular clusters of mononuclear cells (129). The true nature of these cells can be demonstrated by the immunocytochemical identification of neurofilament proteins (127).

Important to the differential diagnosis are subependymal giant cell astrocytomas, some of which accompany tuberous sclerosis. They display large astrocytes with large vesiculated nuclei and prominent nucleoli (130). These giant astrocytes can be differentiated from ganglion cells of a gangliocytoma by their positivity for GFAP (131). However, it should be noted that some subependymal giant cell "astrocytomas" express neural markers, while others lack GFAP (132). This underscores the importance of clinical, morphological and neuroanatomic criteria to the current diagnosis.

Malignant change of gangliogliomas is rare and occurs in 10% of cases (127). In such cases, the glial component is responsible for the malignant transformation. This may ultimately produce a glioblastoma.

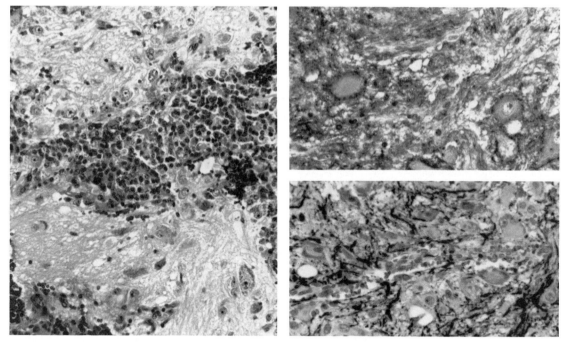

Figure 13–17. Mixed gangliocytoma-pituitary adenoma (*left*) contains axosomatic synapses (*top right*) and a diffuse network of neurites (*bottom right*) demonstrated by immunohistochemistry for synaptophysin and neurofilament antigen (left: ×125; top right: ×250; bottom right: ×125). (From Kamel OW, *et al.* Mixed gangliocytoma-adenoma. A distinct neuroendocrine tumor of the pituitary fossa. Hum Pathol *20*:1198–1203, 1983.)

A number of reports describing the coexistence of gangliocytomas or neuronal hamartomas, particularly with growth hormone–producing pituitary adenomas (133–136), are discussed in the section, "Hamartomas" (Figs. 13–17 and 13–18).

Germinoma

Germinomas are one of a number of primary intracranial germ cell tumors (137). Others include teratomas, embryonal carcinomas, endodermal sinus tumors and chorio-

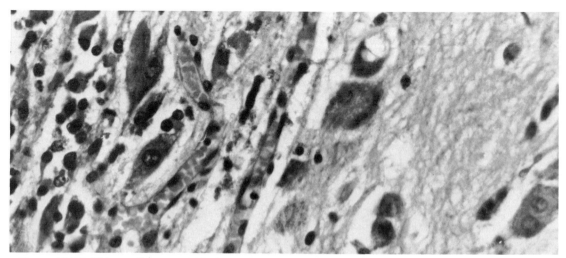

Figure 13–18. This gangliocytoma (*right*) is associated with a growth hormone–producing pituitary adenoma (*left*) in a patient with acromegaly. Occasional binucleated ganglion cells are seen (H & E; ×360).(From Asa SL, *et al.* A case of hypothalamic acromegaly: A clinicopathological study of six patients with hypothalamic gangliocytomas producing growth hormone-releasing factor. J Clin Endocrinol Metab *58*:796–803, 1984, © by the Endocrine Society.)

carcinomas. Teratomas are discussed separately. Germ cell tumors other than germinoma are rare as homogeneous entities in the suprasellar region (1, 2, 11).

Germinomas represent from 4% to 6% of parasellar tumors in various studies (141). In a series of 74 parasellar tumors in patients up to 20 years old, five tumors were germinomas (48). Ninety-five percent of intracranial germ cell tumors arise along the midline from the suprasellar cistern to the pineal gland (138). The percentage that arise in the suprasellar cistern varies from 18% to 37% in different populations (138, 139). Most of these suprasellar germ cell tumors are germinomas. An additional 6% to 13% of intracranial germinomas involve both the pineal and suprasellar regions (138, 139, 142). One fifth of hypothalamic germinomas involve the sella (143, 144). This is usually secondary to spread from an original suprasellar mass.

Although cases occur in children to middle-aged adults, two thirds of patients are diagnosed in adolescence (138, 139). This age distribution suggests that pubertal changes activate growth of germinomas (138).

Diabetes insipidus is the most common clinical manifestation of patients with suprasellar germinoma, present in nearly all cases (145, 146). Signs of hypopituitarism are almost as common. These include hypogonadism, hypocortisolism, hypothyroidism, growth delay and pubertal delay. Visual disturbances, headache or vomiting are present in about half of the cases. A minority of patients have cranial nerve paresis, papilledema or ataxia (145, 146).

Germinomas have been reported to be associated with discrete clinical syndromes. One of these is Klinefelter's syndrome. One reported patient had a mediastinal teratocarcinoma in addition to a hypophyseal stalk germinoma (147). Another patient who had Cornelia de Lange's syndrome with mental retardation and characteristic facial features had a suprasellar germinoma at 18 years of age (148). Another patient developed multiple tumors, including a third ventricular germinoma, and a hypothalamic cystic mixed astrocytoma and oligodendroglioma (149).

The majority of suprasellar germinomas displace the third ventricle, but not the optic chiasm or carotid artery (48, 141). Most suprasellar germinomas do not calcify and do not erode the dorsum sellae (141, 146, 150). Germinomas produce a soft tissue density or hyperdense mass that enhances with contrast dye on CT scans (146). Germinomas are usually isodense on T1-weighted MRI images and hyperintense on T2-weighted images (141, 146).

Intrasellar germinomas are less common than suprasellar germinomas. Their radiographic features are different from those of suprasellar germinomas (151, 152). The clinical and radiographic features of an intrasellar germinoma can mimic those of a prolactinoma. A tissue diagnosis is recommended to avoid inappropriate pharmacologic therapy (151). Some intrasellar germinomas expand the sella turcica (152).

Histological features of germinoma duplicate testicular seminoma and ovarian dysgerminoma. There are two distinct cell populations. Large, neoplastic, epithelioid cells contain large, round vesicular nuclei with prominent nucleoli (Figs. 13–19 and 13–20). The nucleoli are irregular and pleomorphic. The second cell population is composed of small lymphocytes. Some germinomas are complicated with granulomatous inflammation (153).

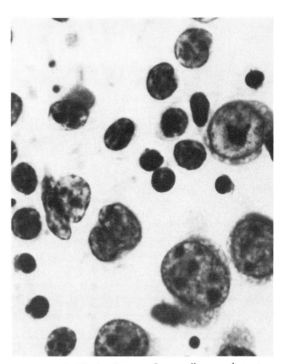

Figure 13–19. A mixture of two cell types characterizes this tumor from the infundibulum of an adolescent male. Large epithelioid neoplastic cells with huge nuclei and large irregular nucleoli contrast with surrounding small lymphocytes (touch preparation of germinoma, H & E; ×1300).

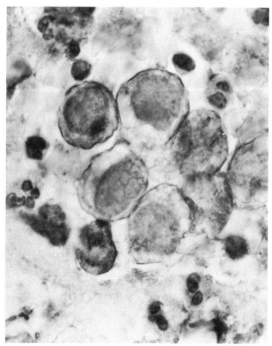

Figure 13–20. Large epithelioid cells with large, vesicular nuclei mixed with small lymphocytes characterize this germinoma. Placental-like alkaline phosphatase (PLAP) immunoreactivity is conspicuous on the plasma membranes of the large cells (immunoperoxidase anti-PLAP; ×1300).

Germinomas require careful tissue handling to preserve their histological features. Small tissue samples may show only the lymphocytes creating the appearance of a lymphoid proliferation. The lymphocytes smear easily, producing streaks of hematoxylinophilic material that obscure fine histological detail.

Histological features of nongerminomatous germ cell tumors differ from those of germinoma. Lymphocytes are not prominent in pure choriocarcinoma, embryonal carcinoma or endodermal sinus tumors. Choriocarcinoma is a mixture of huge syncytial and smaller trophoblastic cells (syncytiotrophoblasts and cytotrophoblasts.) Schiller-Duval bodies are characteristics of endodermal sinus tumors (Fig. 13–21). Foci of these other germ cell tumors occur in some parasellar germinomas.

Most germinomas contain placental-like alkaline phosphatase (PLAP), which can be localized by immunoperoxidase in their large cells (154, 155). Membranous reactivity is stronger than cytoplasmic reactivity. One study showed that 93% of germinomas were positive for PLAP (139). In contrast, 25% of

embryonal carcinomas and no choriocarcinomas were positive. Unfortunately, a minor percentage of metastatic carcinomas also express PLAP (156), compromising its specificity as a germ cell tumor marker.

A second new marker of germinomas that appears relatively specific is angiotensin I–converting enzyme (ACE). ACE is detectable in germinomas tissues as well as in the plasma of affected patients (157, 158). Virtually all germinomas from various organs express ACE (159). The labeling may be specific for germinomas, since embryonal carcinomas and teratocarcinoma are negative (157). However, a wider variety of neoplasms need testing to gauge the specificity of ACE.

Human chorionic gonadotropin (hCG) and alpha-fetoprotein (AFP) are uncommonly expressed by germinomas (139, 146, 159). In contrast, the majority of endodermal sinus tumors and embryonal carcinomas are positive for AFP (139, 140, 159). The majority of choriocarcinomas express hCG (139, 159). Occasional hCG-positive cells in what otherwise resembles a germinoma do not by themselves indicate a different prognosis (160).

There is surprising evidence of regional

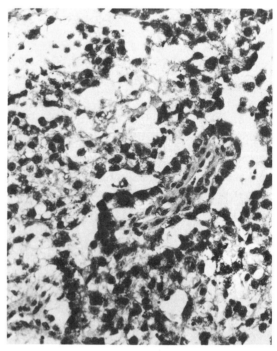

Figure 13–21. Small vascularized papillae project into channels. Papillae and channels are lined by cuboidal epithelium forming Schiller-Duval bodies. This region of endodermal sinus tumor (EST) formation was evident in a mixed germinoma/EST in an adolescent male (H & E; ×210).

difference in antigen expression by intracranial germinomas. Although the number of cases studied is small, suprasellar germinomas appear to lack epithelial and intermediate filament markers expressed by some pineal and brain germinomas (161). These include epithelial membrane antigen (EMA), cytokeratin (CK) and vimentin (161).

The second population of small cells in germinomas is a polyclonal collection of T lymphocytes, B lymphocytes, and natural killer (NK) cells (162, 165). These antigens can be stained with the monoclonal antibodies described in the lymphoma section (see Table 13–4). These cells express major histocompatibility complex (MHC) class I and II antigens (164).

A distinctive ultrastructural feature of germinomas are intranuclear membranous profiles and fenestrated nucleoli (167–169). The ultrastructural features of parasellar germinomas, including nucleolonemae, are similar to those of pineal germinomas, as well as to gonadal seminomas and dysgerminomas (160, 170). Other ultrastructural features of germinomas, including tubuloreticular structures, annulate lamellae, glycogen and distended rough endoplasmic reticulum are relatively nonspecific (167–169).

Histological type and extent of disease are both important prognostic factors in germ cell tumors (138). Patients with germinomas survive significantly longer than those with nongerminomatous germ cell tumors. Tumor involvement of the hypothalamus, third ventricle or spinal cord significantly decreases survival (138). Systemic metastases are more common from pineal than from suprasellar germinomas (138, 171). Ten percent of patients who require ventriculosomatic shunts developed abdominal or pelvic metastases (138, 165). Ki-67 is a nuclear antigen used to estimate proliferation. More is known of the Ki-67 proliferative potential of pineal germinomas than that of suprasellar germinomas (172).

Giant Cell Tumor of Bone

Giant cell tumor of bone (GCTB) rarely occurs in the skull. However, the sphenoid and temporal bones are the most frequently affected sites. More than 30 cases of GCTB of the sphenoid bone with or without sellar erosion have been reported (173–175).

Frontal headaches and visual impairment with or without field defects and oculomotor palsy are the most frequent symptoms, whereas pituitary dysfunction is rare. Radiographically, *destruction of the dorsum sellae* and erosion of the floor of the sella are invariably found. This early destruction of bone with no mass in soft tissue narrows the differential diagnosis. With the spread of the tumor, the destruction of various adjacent bony structures, such as the ethmoid, sphenoid wings, the floor of the temporal fossa, the apex of the petrous bone and the clivus, occurs. This corresponds to the assumption that the tumor originates from the floor of the sella in relation to the zone of enchondral ossification of the sphenoid body and spreads inferiorly, laterally and caudally (173).

Preoperative diagnosis is rarely possible, since radiologic destruction of the sella occurs in many other conditions. The tissue obtained at surgery is usually gray-brown, soft, friable and hemorrhagic. Microscopically, the tumor is composed of oval or spindle-shaped cells and variable numbers of *evenly dispersed benign multinucleated cells* and sheets of benign mononuclear cells with similar nuclear features (Fig. 13–22) (175). The nuclei are usually hypochromatic, and mitotic figures are not uncommon. Some of the tumors may show prominent hemorrhages with iron-pig-

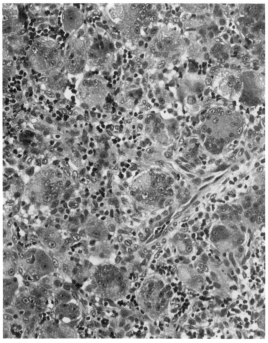

Figure 13–22. This mixture of giant cells and small cells typifies giant cell tumor of bone (H & E; ×165).

ment deposition and distinct areas of collagenization along with myxomatous changes. The differential diagnoses include giant cell reparative granuloma, aneurysmal bone cyst, fibrous dysplasia and "brown tumor" of hyperparathyroidism.

GCTB are histologically benign lesions. However, their location in the sellar region and their capacity for local destruction may produce clinically devastating results. The usual modes of therapy are surgical excision and radiotherapy. Malignant transformation of a GCTB of sphenoid bone has been reported following radiotherapy (176). A peculiar case of multicentric GCTB originating in the sphenoid bone and sella turcica of a 17-year-old girl was reported with a subsequent 23-year period of observation (177).

GCTB is usually diagnosed by its characteristic histological features. However, its negative staining for S-100 protein was found useful in the differential diagnosis of GCTB from chondroblastoma, since the latter is positive for S-100 protein (178). While its dimorphic populations of large and small cells vaguely resemble those of germinoma, the larger cells of GCTB are multinucleated (Fig. 13–23). The small cells are neither as polymorphic nor as epithelioid as those seen in granulomatous inflammation. The DNA

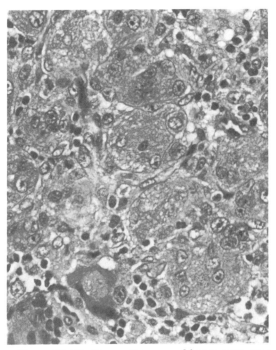

Figure 13–23. Giant cell tumor of bone; same case shown in Figure 13–22 (H & E; × 330).

analysis of GCTB of bone has limited utility for predicting the tumor's biological behavior (179).

Glioma

Pilocytic astrocytomas are discussed in the sections, "Infundibuloma" and "Optic Nerve Glioma." Malignant gliomas are discussed in the sections, "Glioma Associated With Radiation" and "High-Grade Glioma." Mixed neoplasms are discussed in the sections, "Gangliocytoma and Ganglioglioma" and "Hamartoma."

GFAP is the most decisive marker of parasellar gliomas. Gliomas with astrocytic or ependymal components contain GFAP (Fig. 13–24).

While they originate above the sella, ependymomas may grow ventrally and simulate pituitary adenoma. Modern clinical detection and neuroradiographic localization have minimized this hazard of former years. The distinguishing feature of ependymomas is their paraventricular location. Histologically, the ependymoma has fibrillar regions that may be limited to perivascular regions in the most epithelioid ependymomas. They can be highlighted with GFAP stains, which distinguish them from nonglial neoplasms (see Table 13–1). Cilia, microvillous cytoplasmic inclusions, basal bodies and elongated intercellular junctions are typical of ependymoma (Fig. 13–25).

Oligodendroglioma is another glioma that simulates pituitary adenoma. It can virtually always be distinguished by its extrasellar location. While oligodendrogliomas contain Leu-7 and S-100 protein, many neoplasms share these markers. More specific markers like galactocerebroside (GC) are compromised by paraffin embedding but may be useful on frozen sections.

Glioma Associated With Radiation

The majority of neoplasms that have occurred after therapeutic radiation of the sellar region have been either sarcomas or gliomas. Post-radiation sarcomas are described in the section, "Sarcomas." Gliomas that have occurred after radiation of this region are discussed here.

Accepted criteria to be fulfilled before consideration of a correlation between radiation

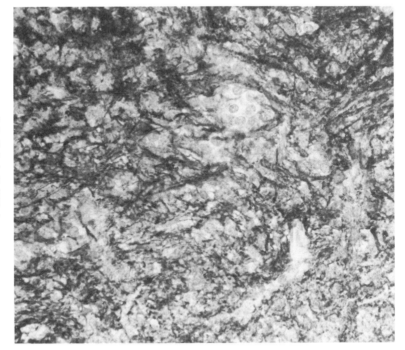

Figure 13–24. Extensive immunoreactivity for glial fibrillary acidic protein (GFAP) reflects neoplastic astrocytes in this low-grade glioma. Its precise neuroanatomic origin could not be determined, since it involved the hypothalamus, thalamus and basal ganglia (immunoperoxidase anti-GFAP; ×420).

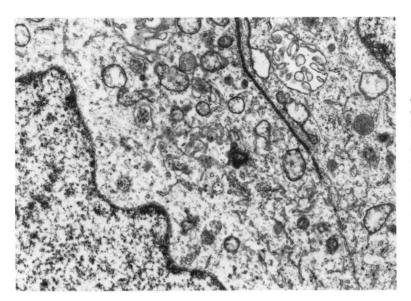

Figure 13–25. Elongated intercellular junction and cytoplasmic cilia, basal body and microvillous inclusions identify this tumor from outside of the sellar region as an ependymoma (lead citrate and uranyl acetate; ×10,100). (From McKeever PE, Blaivas M. In: Sternberg S, et al. (eds). Diagnosis in Surgical Pathology. Vol 1. New York, Raven Press, 1989, pp 339–343.)

exposure and a second tumor were originally proposed by Cahan and associates (180, 181) and have been modified many times, including here. These include the following:

1. The second tumor is located within the irradiated region.
2. The first and second tumors are histologically confirmed to be different types.
3. Asymptomatic latency was sufficiently long to indicate that the second tumor was not present at the time of irradiation.

Unlike some others, we do not automatically exclude cases that arise in the context of a phakomatosis if the preceding criteria are met. Neglected in most reports are epidemiological and statistical evaluation of appropriate populations and time intervals at risk to determine the likelihood of correlation between parasellar radiation and second glioma. One study provides data from a Japanese institution suggesting an incidence of 1% of the irradiated patient population at risk (181). Since this was an 18-year study (Dr. N. Shitara, personal communication), this extrapolates to an estimated yearly incidence of over 50 gliomas per 100,000 from this radiated population. This would be more than 15 times the incidence of 2.8 gliomas per 100,000 in the general population of Japan (National Epidemiologic Study, 1982). Thus, an association between previous radiation and these gliomas is suggested.

High-grade astrocytic gliomas (glioblastomas and anaplastic astrocytomas) are the most common gliomas in patients with previous parasellar radiation. Of a reported total of 14 patients who had parasellar radiation, six had subsequent glioblastomas and six had anaplastic astrocytomas, together accounting for 85% of all such gliomas (180–192). One other case was an anaplastic oligodendroglioma (180, 191). Half of these patients had received previous radiation of pituitary adenomas as adults; the other half had been radiated for craniopharyngiomas when younger. Their total radiation doses ranged between 45 and 66 Gy.

The latency period between parasellar radiation and diagnosis of malignant glioma varied between 4 and 25 years (180–192); average latency was 10 years. Both sexes were equally affected. Since the total survival of treated anaplastic astrocytoma was less than 3 years and glioblastoma less than 1 year during the time these data accrued, these grades of glioma were probably not present

at the time of radiation. This does not rule out possible lower grade glial proliferation present during radiation with subsequent tumor progression.

High-grade gliomas that occur within fields of previous parasellar radiation are not always confined to the sella. Many involve the temporal and/or ventral frontal lobes of the cerebrum, the diencephalon or the optic chiasm (180–192). As more focused radiotherapy beams are employed in future decades, it will be of interest to compare the neuroanatomic distributions of subsequent gliomas.

The histological features of high-grade gliomas occurring after parasellar radiation are like those in gliomas in patients who have never received therapeutic radiation (193) (see "High-Grade Glioma"). It is of interest that no "radiation-specific" histological feature has been proven. This is in contrast to the effects of radiation on preexisting neoplasm (193, 194).

Virtually all post-radiation gliomas in the sellar region occur after radiotherapy of craniopharyngioma or pituitary adenoma (180–192). Thus, clinical circumstances and tumor biology establish the differential diagnosis. The pituitary adenoma and craniopharyngioma are epithelioid tumors that lack the fibrillary cytoplasmic processes of astrocytic gliomas and are negative for GFAP. Parasellar sarcomas also occur subsequent to radiation. Sarcomas are more difficult to distinguish from high-grade gliomas, since glioblastomas produce spindle cells that resemble those of sarcoma. GFAP is usually sufficient to identify the glioma and differentiate it from GFAP-negative sarcomas. Cytologic and nuclear anaplasia of GFAP-positive cells is critical in distinguishing them from gliosis trapped by tumor. Since some glioblastomas do not express large quantities of GFAP, a sensitive immunocytochemical detection system with appropriate positive and negative controls is recommended (195, 196).

Glomus Tumor (Glomangioma)

The first case of a glomangioma in the sellar region was reported in 1984 (197). Glomus tumor is a neoplasm that is most commonly found in the nail beds and pads of the fingers and toes, where it arises in a glomus body. The latter is a specialized form of arteriovenous anastomosis that serves in thermal regulation. Extracutaneous locations of the glomus tumor are unusual and include muscles and tendons, nasal cavity, trachea, mediastinum, gastrointestinal tract and vagina (198–200). These tumors are usually solitary and well circumscribed. They are rarely multiple and in such cases are likely to be familial and inherited almost exclusively via the paternal line (201). Glomus tumor should not be confused with the *glomus jugulare tumor,* which is a highly vascular paraganglioma in the petrous bone and middle ear (200).

The proportion of glomus cells, vessels and smooth muscle varies from one tumor to another, providing a basis for subclassification in three groups: standard glomus tumor, glomangioma and glomangiomyoma (2). Glomus tumor is considered to be benign. However, it can be locally infiltrative or even malignant cytologically (202, 203). Gould and associates divided the aggressive glomus tumors into three categories: locally infiltrative; cytologically malignant, arising and merging with a typical glomus tumor, which they named "glomangiosarcoma arising in a benign glomus tumor"; and *de novo* glomangiosarcoma, which should be distinguished from other round cell sarcomas (203). One of their cases involved the base of the skull, and in a case reported by Harvey and Walker, glomus tumor extended near the skull base (202, 203).

The sellar glomangioma of Asa and associates was composed of sheets of uniform round and polygonal cells interrupted by vascular channels lined by flat endothelial cells (Fig. 13–26). The nuclei of the tumor cells were round or oval, with fine chromatin and inconspicuous nuclei. Mitotic figures were rare. The cytoplasm was homogeneous and acidophilic; the cell borders were indistinct. Occasional serotonin-positive mast cells were present. All pituitary hormones as well as GFAP and S-100 protein were negative by the immunoperoxidase technique. Factor VIII was present only in endothelial cells, whereas actin, desmin and myoglobin were identified within the cytoplasm of the tumor cells. These were surrounded by abundant basement membrane.

Two studies reiterated the question of a possible relationship between glomus tumor and *hemangiopericytoma.* In a series of 40 glomus tumors, two hemangiopericytomas and two glomus bodies analyzed immunohisto-

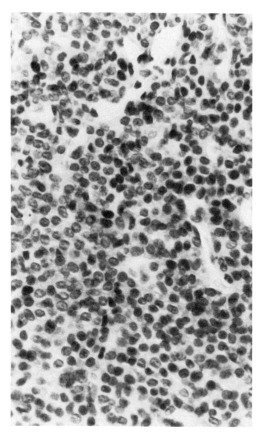

Figure 13–26. Glomangioma of sella turcica. Cells have round and oval nuclei with indistinct cytoplasmic borders (H & E; ×128).

chemically, Nuovo and associates found that virtually all glomus tumors and hemangiopericytomas were positive for vimentin and muscle-specific actin. None of the tumors expressed cytokeratin or S-100 protein. Desmin was positive in 73% of glomus tumors and negative in hemangiopericytomas and glomus bodies. This prompted the proposal that desmin activity may help distinguish glomus tumor from hemangiopericytoma. However, the authors conclude, "attempts to rigorously separate these lesions may prove to be artificial" (204). In another series of 16 glomus tumors and 11 hemangiopericytomas, no evidence for analogous smooth muscle differentiation was found in hemangiopericytoma (205).

The ultrastructural appearance of glomus tumors consists of epithelioid cells with features of *smooth muscle* differentiation (Fig. 13–27). The cell cytoplasm contains numerous myofibrils showing focal condensation onto dense bodies and pinocytotic vesicles near the cell periphery. Abundant basement mem-

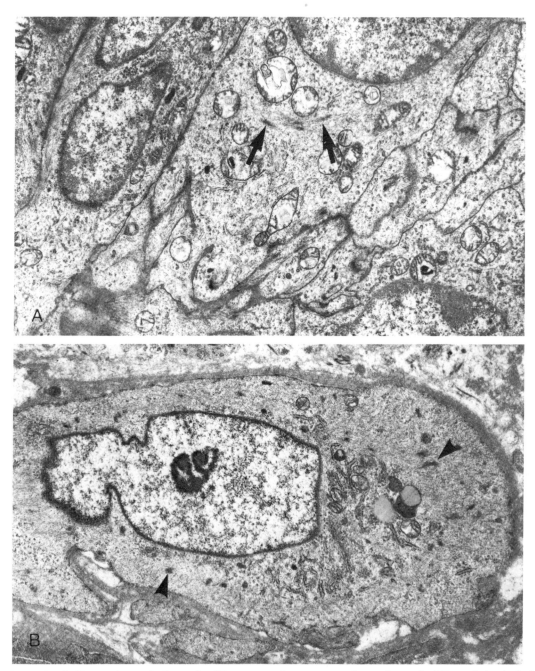

Figure 13–27. Glomangioma of sella turcica. Ultrastructural appearance of smooth muscle differentiation includes cytoplasmic myofibrils (*arrows*). Myofibrils focally condense (*arrowheads*) (UALC; *A:* ×10,400; *B:* ×10,200). (From Asa SL, *et al*. Sellar glomangioma. Ultrastruct Pathol 7:49–54, 1984.)

brane surrounds individual tumor cells, which, in turn, encircle vessels lined by fenestrated endothelium (197).

Granular Cell Tumor (Granular Cell Myoblastoma, Choristoma)

Granular cell tumor (GCT) or, as known in the older literature, myoblastoma, choristoma, tumorett or pituicytoma, most frequently arises in the neurohypophysis and infundibulum and is found incidentally in 1% to 6.5% of autopsies (206, 207). The incidence becomes higher (6% to 17%) if serial sections of hypophysis are examined (208).

These incidental aggregates of granular cells, approximately 1 to 2 mm in diameter, are commonly found in the posterior lobe of the hypophysis and less frequently in the lower portion of the pituitary stalk (206). They are usually well circumscribed in contrast to poorly circumscribed GCT elsewhere in the body (209). GCT is slow growing and, as long as it remains small, asymptomatic. If it enlarges to compress the pituitary, optic chiasm or hypothalamus, then headaches, visual disturbances or hypopituitarism occur. Less commonly, hydrocephalus and diabetes insipidus ensue. With this clinical presentation, GCT can easily be mistaken for an adenoma, craniopharyngioma or optic glioma. Symptomatic GCT is found most frequently in the 4th and 5th decade and in women twice as often as in men (210). The occurrence of an asymptomatic GCT showed positive correlation with age and no correlation with gender (208).

CT and angiography are helpful in distinguishing GCT from adenomas, gliomas and craniopharyngiomas. GCT is a dense, noncalcified, homogeneous, well-delineated, vascular intrasellar or suprasellar mass that produces contrast enhancement on CT and a vascular blush on angiogram (211). Pituitary adenomas, craniopharyngiomas and gliomas are less vascular and usually do not produce as much contrast enhancement. Craniopharyngiomas are, in addition, nonhomogeneous and frequently calcified. At operation, GCT is a "characteristically tough, nonsuckable, vascular tumor" (211).

A pathologist sees GCT tissue as a firm, gray or tan, spherical or lobulated nodule. Histologically, a sharply demarcated but not encapsulated mass is composed of closely

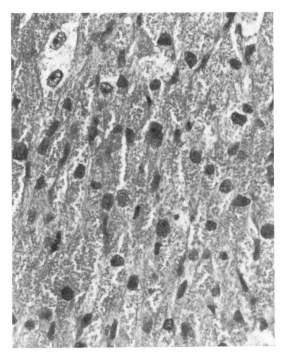

Figure 13–28. Granular cell tumor showing cells with granular cytoplasm (H & E; ×530).

placed, large granular cells (Fig. 13–28). Luse and Kernohan recognized *three cellular patterns*. The predominant pattern seen in GCT of the neurohypophysis was a sharply circumscribed nodule composed of cells arranged in irregular columns, frequently positioned about thin walled vessels, which were plentiful in some tumors (208). The large and irregularly polygonal cells had abundant eosinophilic cytoplasm filled with fine and coarse granules. The cell outlines were either well delineated or quite indistinct. The small, round to oval, uniform nuclei contained small nucleoli. This pattern is similar to the one in GCT of the peripheral nervous system (212). Another, less frequent pattern was remarkable for poor demarcation of the tumor nodules and arrangement of the cells in irregular strands. The elongated cells with indistinct plasmalemmal outlines created a syncytial appearance. The nuclei were large and irregular in shape, with coarse chromatin and prominent nucleoli. The third pattern was only seen in two tumors of the pituitary stalk. The large nodules, sharply circumscribed, were made of slender elongated granular cells with blurred cytoplasmic margins, and small elongated nuclei were arranged in a whorled fashion around small vessels. Mitotic figures were not observed in any of these patterns.

The cytoplasmic granules, especially the large ones, are positive for periodic acid–Schiff (PAS) and are diastase resistant (see Table 13–1). In some cases, they also stain with phosphotungstic acid–hematoxylin. Immunohistochemical studies yielded results similar to the ones obtained for GCT elsewhere in the body (209, 212–214). Tumor cells are positive for S-100, NSE and, rarely, GFAP when located in the central nervous system; they are positive for S-100, NSE and the NT-Leu-7 (HNK-1) monoclonal antibody when located in the peripheral nervous system. The described immunoreactivity supports their much-debated origin from Schwann cells. Astrocytes are suggested cells of origin in the central nervous system (212). An immunohistochemical and ultrastructural study of a giant GCT of the suprasellar region by Liwnicz and associates brought about a possibility of still another cell of origin: microglia (215). The plethora of plausible candidates suggests a multicellular origin of GCT.

Rare intracerebral tumors are identified as GCT. One such case reported by Gambini contained typical PAS-positive granules, the ultrastructure of which corresponded to various vacuoles, dense bodies and multivesicular bodies (216). The cells were strongly positive for S-100 protein but negative for GFAP and neurofilaments. Dickson and associates reported an intracerebral GCT that was composed of two cell types: granular cells and filament-rich cells (217). GFAP was demonstrated in both cell types, but it was not as prominent in the granular cells as in astrocytes. In contrast to extracerebral GCT, neither S-100 protein nor vimentin was detected in intracerebral GCT, whereas peanut lectin labeled both cerebral and non-cerebral GCT. On electron microscopy, these authors found the tumor to be composed of several cell types: lipid-laden macrophages, which predominated and tended to congregate around blood vessels; cells with cytoplasm rich in GFAP-positive filaments; less frequent astrocytes located in the perivascular region; and granular cells, which were the least common type. The latter were filled with heterogeneous, membrane-bound dense bodies consistent with autophagic vacuoles ranging in size from 20 to over 200 nm in diameter, as well as multivesicular bodies, empty vacuoles, phagocytosed mitochondria, filaments and

other organelles. The nuclei had similar ultrastructural appearance in both filamentous and granular cells. The case of Dickson and associates was different from many other reported cases of GCT. The features of the neoplasm were reminiscent of a *pleomorphic xanthoastrocytoma,* as pointed out by the authors.

In fact, a rare astrocytoma shows GCT-like changes (218). This neoplasm was positive for GFAP and vimentin and negative for S-100 protein, which is a highly unusual staining pattern. Autophagic vacuoles were not conspicuous. However, granular cells in this neoplasm existed alongside typical astrocytes, again suggesting an astrocytic origin of the granular cells.

GCT is considered a *benign* neoplasm. However, rare malignant cases in the neck and peritoneum have been reported (219, 220). None have yet been reported from the sella. Morphological and staining characteristics of *malignant* tumors are indistinguishable from those of benign tumors.

GCT was previously considered to be radioinsensitive, but one report claims effective treatment with radiation of an extracranial GCT (221).

Hamartoma (Neuronal Choristoma)

Hypothalamic neuronal hamartomas are rare lesions. They present as a well-defined mass attached to the tuber cinerum or the mammillary bodies; some are attached by a thin stalk. They occur more commonly in males. Situated behind the pituitary stalk, hypothalamic hamartomas often present with endocrinologic disturbances and visual field defects (226, 227). They are often accompanied by precocious puberty.

A few cases of neuronal hamartomas or neuronal choristomas have been accompanied by acromegaly and growth hormone–producing pituitary adenomas confirmed by immunohistochemistry. The first such case was reported by Asa and associates (225), who suggested that the neurosecretory activity of the hamartoma promoted the development of the growth hormone-producing adenoma. This interesting possibility was expanded by Scheithauer and associates (226) and Slowik and collaborators (227), who demonstrated cytoplasmic secretory granules within neuronal processes of hamartomatous cells and their expanded terminals, which, in

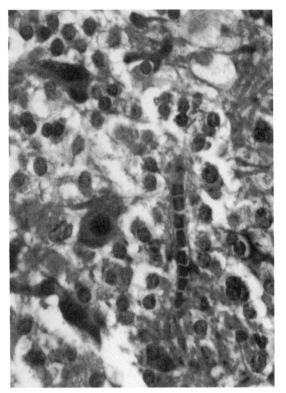

Figure 13–29. Adenohypophysial neuronal choristoma associated with a pituitary adenoma. Growth hormone–producing pituitary adenoma exhibits scattered neuronal elements (neuronal choristoma) (H & E; ×640.) (From Scheithauer BW, *et al.* Hypothalamic neuronal hamartoma and adenohypophyseal neuronal choristoma: Their association with growth hormone adenoma of the pituitary gland. J Neuropathol Exp Neurol 42:633–648, 1983.)

turn, were intimately associated with adenoma cells via cellular junctions (Figs. 13–29 and 13–30). These authors suggested that a paracrine effect of growth hormone releasing factor synthesized by the neurogenic tumor could be responsible for the development of the adenoma.

Occasionally other tissues, such as lipomatous tissue (227) or the anlage of the retina, have been described within hamartomas (228). Hypothalamic hamartomas in infants may be associated with congenital malformations of the olfactory bulbs, absent pituitary, syndactyly, and renal and cardiac abnormalities (229, 230).

The hamartoma is a round, commonly firm mass. It reveals a pale cut surface. Microscopically the lesion is characterized by mature neurons that may vary in size and may be either uni- or multi-polar. The neurones often occur in clusters or aggregates separated by unmyelinated axons (223, 224).

Some terminal axons resemble Herring bodies (226). Their ultrastructural and immunohistochemical features reflect their glial and neuronal constituents (see Table 13–1).

Hemangioblastoma

Hemangioblastomas comprise about 1% to 2% of all intracranial neoplasms and in about 10% of cases are associated with *von Hippel-Lindau disease*. Among over 300 cases of hemangioblastoma reported in the literature, almost 94% were located in the posterior fossa, and less than 3% were supratentorial. Three cases of hemangioblastoma involving the pituitary have been reported: hemangioblastoma of the anterior lobe of the pituitary in an 84-year-old man (231), in a 26-year-old man (232), and in a 28-year-old woman. The woman presented with a *Chiari-Frommel syndrome* of 3 years' duration, complaining of bilateral galactorrhea and fronto-orbital headaches that were accompanied by obesity and mild loss of hair (233). The first two cases were associated with von Hippel-Lindau disease, and the third had no sign of phakomatosis. Rarely, obstructive hydrocephalus due to hemangioblastoma involves the sella (234).

Hemangioblastomas are rarely seen in children or in patients older than 70, with most symptomatic cases occuring in patients in their 2nd, 3rd or 4th decade. On CT scan, the tumor appears as a sharply demarcated isodense mass with no calcifications and little or no surrounding edema. About half of all cases are solid tumor, and the other half are cystic with a mural nodule. This ratio may also apply to the sellar region, where cystic and solid forms are reported, but the scarcity of described cases limits confirmation (231, 233). The mass or nodule enhances significantly after contrast medium injection. *Angiography* is the most helpful procedure and reveals a highly vascularized lesion with persistent blush and feeding vessels.

Macroscopically, about half of the tumors contain cysts that are filled with clear fluid characterized by high protein content. The tumors are not encapsulated and have a reddish tan color. Histologically, hemangioblastomas are composed of capillary-sized vascular channels lined with endothelial cells and large, polygonal, *foamy stromal cells* (Figs. 13–31 and 13–32). The endothelial cells are uniform and rather flat, while the stromal

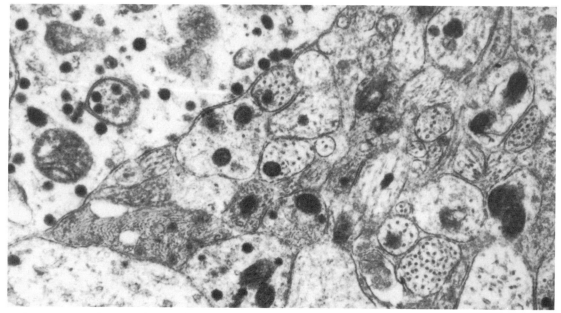

Figure 13–30. Electron micrograph of the same case shown in Figure 13–29 demonstrates expanded nerve terminals closely associated with an adenoma cell (*center*) (H & E; ×650). (From Scheithauer BW, *et al.* Hypothalamic neuronal hamartoma and adenohypophyseal neuronal choristoma: Their association with growth hormone adenoma of the pituitary gland. J Neuropathol Exp Neurol *42*:633–648, 1983.)

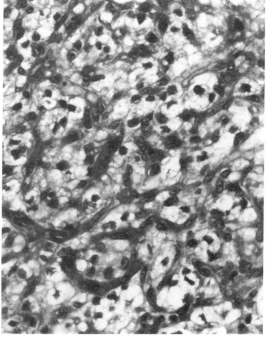

Figure 13–31. Capillary-sized vascular channels are prominent in this region of a hemangioblastoma (H & E; ×330).

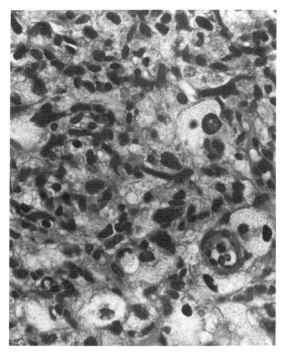

Figure 13–32. Foamy stromal cells have lost their cytoplasmic lipid during paraffin embedding of this hemangioblastoma (H & E; ×330).

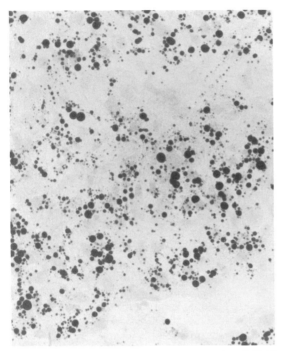

Figure 13–33. Oil red O stain shows cytoplasmic lipid on a frozen section of a hemangioblastoma (×330).

mesenchymal origin (243). Kepes and associates suggested that the stromal cells on light microscopy are a heterogeneous group of cells including astrocytic as well as other elements, and they resemble each other because of the "equalizing" effect of cell lipidization (235). Since some of the cells expressed GFAP positivity, it was suggested that they could have been of *astrocytic* origin. Deck and Rubenstein proposed four hypotheses accounting for the presence of GFAP-positive stromal cells, one of them being that these cells express an artifactual GFAP positivity borrowed from neighboring astrocytes (236). In Ironside and associates' series, all stromal and endothelial cells were positive for vimentin, most of the stromal cells were positive for NSE and aldolase C4, all stromal cells were positive for α-enolase and process-bearing stromal cells were positive for GFAP and histiocytic markers. Only endothelial cells were positive for factor VIII–related antigen and *Ulex europaeus* 1 lectin. These results support the view that the stromal cells are a heterogeneous population that includes entrapped reactive astrocytes and locally derived non-vascular cells of *neuroectodermal (pial)* origin (241).

The problem of differentiation of hemangioblastoma from a metastatic *renal carcinoma* is an acute diagnostic question faced by the surgical pathologist (Fig. 13–34). Cytological and histological features of malignancy (see "Malignant Neoplasms") distinguish some, but not all, renal cell carcinomas. Fortunately, advances in immunohistochemical techniques provide reliable confirmation of previously used PAS and lipid stains. *Epithelial membrane antigen* (EMA) was positive in all tested renal cell carcinomas and negative in all hemangioblastomas (246, 247). Hemangioblastomas also expressed diffuse vimentin positivity, whereas renal cell carcinoma showed focal vimentin positivity in perivascular tumor cells and weak or negative staining in the cells not adjacent to vessels (246).

A series of special stains and immunoperoxidase techniques helps in differentiating hemangioblastoma from *angioblastic meningioma*, highly vascular *astrocytoma* and *oligodendroglioma*. Reticulin stains accentuate the vascular network of the tumors, and the lipid stains such as Sudan black and oil red O bring out the lipid within the stromal cells. The presence of a fourth type of cell (in addition to capillary endothelial cells, pericytes and stromal cells) was suggested within a capillary hemangioblastoma (248). These

cells vary in size and shape and the amount of sudanophilic and oil red O–positive lipid granules within their cytoplasm (Fig. 13–33). Nuclei of the stromal cells may exhibit some hyperchromasia and pleomorphism, even multinucleation, but mitotic figures are inconspicuous. Based on the difference in the vascular network and the lipid content of the stromal cells, the tumors are subclassified into three types: capillary, cellular and cavernous. This subtyping bears no prognostic value.

The question of the origin of stromal cells has generated numerous papers over the years (235–243). Positive fibronectin reaction and negative GFAP reaction in some series suggested derivation of the stromal cells from *angiogenic mesenchyme*, as proposed previously based on ultrastructural studies of hemangioblastomas (238, 244, 245). However, Feldenzer and associates found a distinct difference between stromal and vascular cells for a number of markers, including NSE and factor VIII (240). Their findings were interpreted as supportive for a *neuroendocrine* origin of stromal cells. *Endothelial* origin was also proposed (20, 244). Frank and associates concluded that the stromal cell is not endothelial, neural, epithelial, pericytic or neuroendocrine in origin but instead is of *undifferentiated*

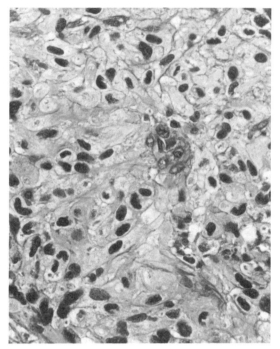

Figure 13–34. Hemangioblastoma resembles renal cell carcinoma (H & E; ×330).

small granular cells stained positively for erythropoietin and renin. The same cells also stained positively for alpha$_1$-antitrypsin. Alpha$_1$-antitrypsin was also found in eosinophilic intracytoplasmic hyaline globules noted in stromal cells and in the extracellular space in 8 of 10 cerebellar hemangioblastomas. Few primary tumors of the central nervous system contain alpha$_1$-antitrypsin, which is a glycoprotein regularly found in macrophages, hepatocytes and other cells.

Both stromal and endothelial cells of hemangioblastoma were found to be proliferative by the AgNOR technique (249). Ultrastructurally, hemangioblastomas contain three types of cells: endothelial, pericytes and stromal cells (250). The vascular channels are lined by fenestrated endothelium, and a discontinuous periendothelial cell layer is surrounded by basement membrane. The stromal cells contain membrane-bound lipid responsible for their "foamy" appearance (251).

Hemangioma

Cavernous hemangioma is a hamartomatous lesion that occasionally may grow in size (252). Intracranial cavernous hemangiomas are more common in females. The majority located near the middle cranial fossa involve women over 30 years of age, with an overall *female-to-male ratio of 7:1* (252). Of the patients reported by Kawai and associates, one presented with one-sided blindness, decreased vision in the other eye, oculomotor palsy with ptosis and amenorrhea (253). The second patient had headaches, double vision and one-sided ptosis due to the oculomotor paralysis. One Japanese patient presented with hyperprolactinemia (254). A large pituitary cavernous hemangioma was found incidentally at the autopsy of a 72-year-old woman who died of a metastatic breast carcinoma (255). This clinically silent lesion was a dumbbell-shaped mass filling the sella and extending upward to the left hypothalamic region, displacing the left oculomotor nerve. A crescent-shaped pituitary gland was flattened over the hemangioma. Of interest in this particular case was the coexistence of two hamartomatous lesions in the kidneys that did not fulfill the criteria for phakomatoses. Vascular malformations of the CNS are associated with visceral *hamartomas* in Sturge-Weber and von Hippel-Lindau disease (255).

Angiography reveals an avascular mass with remarkable *blush* and without visualization of feeding arteries or draining veins, apparently due to the very small caliber of the feeding artery and slow circulation, which is further compromised by extensive thrombosis (253, 256). CT demonstrates a lesion isodense with the normal brain and extreme homogeneous enhancement (256). Erosion of the bone of the sella turcica with thinning of the sellar floor or ballooning of the sella without calcification is characteristic (252, 253, 256).

Histologically, cavernous hemangiomas contain multiple *large sinusoidal spaces* filled with blood or thrombi at various stages of organization. The sinusoids are separated by fibrous septa with no intervening glial tissue (5). Cavernous hemangiomas stain for factor VIII–related antigen, *U. europaeus* agglutinin 1 and vimentin by immunoperoxidase. They are negative for carcinoembryonic antigen, EMA and cytokeratin (257).

Hemangiopericytoma (Hemangiopericytic Meningioma)

Primary hemangiopericytomas of the pituitary are rare (258–264). Many hemangiopericytomas arise in the meninges of the skull base, the orbital region and the sinonasal region (259, 265–270). Hemangiopericytomas tend to recur persistently and to invade locally (260, 265, 267, 270), eventually reaching parasellar and sellar regions. Such tumors are often recognized in their primary location as hemangiopericytomas. Review of previously resected portions of the neoplasms can facilitate interpretation of such cases.

Partial loss of visual fields is the most consistent abnormality of parasellar and suprasellar hemangiopericytomas (260, 262, 263). Individual patients have developed headaches, ptosis, amenorrhea and acromegaly (262, 263).

CT scans reveal higher density than surrounding brain and pituitary. Enhancement of the tomographic image with contrast is usual, possibly reflecting the tumor vasculature. The tumor margins on CT scans are often surprisingly distinct (260–263).

The most prominent features of hemangiopericytomas are high cellular density and monotonous appearance (271–273). Cells with round to oval nuclei compress and distort vascular lumens, producing odd shapes (Fig. 13–35) (271, 272). Regions of tumor parenchyma contain extensive pericellular reticulin, producing a microscopic appearance like cell walls in a plant (Fig. 13–36). Local invasion contributes to their 80% re-currence rate. The most common pathway for invasion is along the penetrating vessels. Mitotic figures are always present but are quite variable in number.

The common immunohistochemical pattern of staining of hemangiopericytomas is seen in Table 13–3 (265–269, 274–279). Consistent reactivity for vimentin and scarcity of other common markers are typical of hemangiopericytomas. Specific lack of EMA and cytokeratins in hemangiopericytomas differentiates them from most carcinomas and many meningiomas (265, 266, 268, 270, 277). Lack of desmin and smooth muscle actin reactivity in hemangiopericytomas distinguishes them from tumors of muscular origin (265, 266, 274–276, 278). Lack of these markers also suggests that the pericyte may not be the cell of origin of hemangiopericytomas (278). However, it should be noted that rare hemangiopericytomas express focal muscle–specific actin and EMA reactivity (268, 276). EMA reactivity is not surprising, since transitional forms between hemangiopericytoma and meningioma occur (273).

Their distinct ultrastructural features, combined with the lack of reactivity for many immunoperoxidase markers, makes hemangiopericytomas especially amenable to identification by electron microscopy. The most common features of the neoplastic cells are

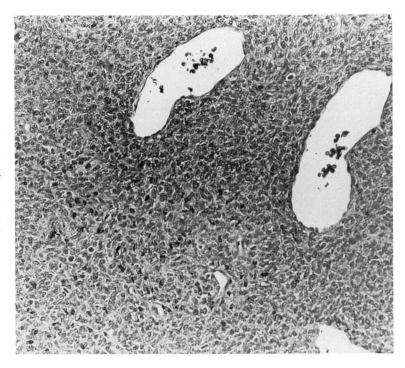

Figure 13–35. Monotonous collection of cells with round and oval nuclei compress and distort vascular lumens into reniform shapes. This specimen is one of numerous resections of a hemangiopericytic meningioma from the base of the skull where it invaded the region of the sella (H & E; ×210).

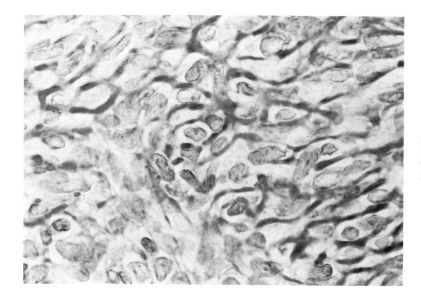

Figure 13–36. Extensive pericellular reticulin approaches the thickness of a cell wall in this extracellular matrix of a hemangiopericytoma (PAS; ×1040).

basal lamina, extracellular matrix materials, thick cytoplasmic processes and intermediate filaments distributed diffusely throughout the cytoplasm (276). Only one third of hemangiopericytomas contain neoplastic cells differentiated like pericytes. Large collagen fibers are present in some cases. In certain cases, the basal lamina is thick and multilaminated (276).

Hemangiopericytomas tend to recur relentlessly. Since many vital structures around the sella are at risk to local invasion, the ultimate prognosis is poor for patients with tumors in this region, despite such tumors' relatively low "official" histological grade of II on a scale of IV (280). New treatment modalities with high-activity radioiodine offer the hope of better prognosis (281).

High-Grade Glioma

High-grade gliomas are rare in the region of the sella. Many reported cases occur after sellar radiation. These are described in the section, "Glioma Associated With Radiation."

Cardinal histological features of astrocytic gliomas are stellate cells, which extend fibrillar cytoplasmic processes in numerous directions, and a glial parenchyma. There is little or no collagen in the glioma parenchyma, and most of it is associated with vessels.

High cellularity, nuclear pleomorphism, mitoses and endothelial proliferation indicate a high grade of malignancy (193, 282). Ana-

plastic astrocytomas manifest these features, which are more extreme in glioblastomas. Characteristically glioblastomas also contain regions of coagulation necrosis (283). The coagulation necrosis contains a rim of hypercellularity called "pseudopallisades" in some cases.

Histiocytosis

When histiocytosis affects the brain, it often involves the parasellar region. There is a tendency to affect children and young adults, although a case involving the pituitary in a 63-year-old woman has been reported (284). In a series of 74 parasellar tumors in children, there is one case of histiocytosis X (48).

Histiocytosis of the parasellar region commonly presents with all or a portion of the classic triad of diabetes insipidus, pituitary insufficiency and visual deterioration (285–290). Lesions with distal optic extension may present with proptosis (291).

CT images vary from unremarkable to isodense (48, 291). Enhancement with contrast medium is typical, and this improves detection (291). While anterior or posterior fossa or brain stem may be affected, the hypothalamic-pituitary axis and optic regions are particularly susceptible (48, 284, 285, 291–295). About half of the patients who present with primary histiocytosis X of the hypothalamus subsequently develop secondary lesions in other CNS locations (286–291, 295). In other cases, a parasellar lesion is one of multiple systemic lesions (284, 285, 293).

Firm consistency is typical of the histiocytic lesion and aids in its recognition and handling. It is firm due to the admixture of fibrous tissue with the cells (284, 285, 291, 292). Fibrous tissue is important in distinguishing the lesions from gliomas at biopsy, where frozen section alone may be misleading. This collagen hinders stereotactic biopsy. Lesions involving the diaphragma sellae, dura or skull base may be particularly difficult to resect (291, 292).

The microscopic appearance of histiocytosis is a mixture of histiocytes, inflammatory cells and collagen. The histiocytes are typically larger than microglia. Their oval to kidney-shaped nuclei may be deeply invaginated by cytoplasmic clefts. Their cytoplasm is prominent and hyaline to finely granular.

New lesions of histiocytosis are less fibrotic than older lesions (285, 292). Exceptional cases are noncollagenous and filled with phagocytic cells with or without lipid (295, 296). One reason for this variation is that histiocytic lesions comprise a variety of disorders, including histiocytosis X (Langerhans' cell histiocytosis) (48, 284, 285, 295), eosinophilic granuloma (294), extranodal sinus histiocytosis with massive lymphadenopathy (SHML) (291–293) and xanthoma disseminatum (296). Xanthoma disseminatum is rare. By definition it is widespread, involving more than the sella. There are numerous foamy histiocytes and occasional Touton giant cells (296). Some cases of eosinophilic granuloma have abundant eosinophils mixed with histiocytes and lymphocytes (294). The hallmarks of extranodal SHML are lymphocytes within the cytoplasm of large histiocytes (Fig. 13–37) (291–293).

Histiocytosis can be confused with reactive and chronic inflammatory processes and meningioma (285, 292, 294, 297). When routine light microscopic examination is inconclusive, a panel of immunostains is recommended to rule out other possibilities and establish the diagnosis of histiocytosis. The panel should include markers that demonstrate histiocytic properties such as alpha$_1$-antichymotrypsin, lysozyme, KP1, peanut agglutinin, and the MT1 marker (298–303). Numerous markers are positive in individual cases, but these markers are positive in a high percentage of the histiocytoses (298–300, 304). Various histiocytoses express other histiocytic markers

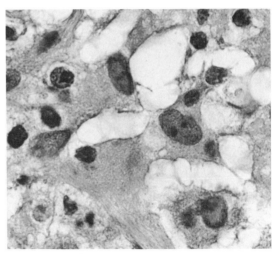

Figure 13–37. Large histiocytes with prickly cellular margins, large oval nuclei and cytoplasmic inflammatory cells characterize this tumor as extranodal sinus histiocytosis with massive lymphadenopathy (SHML) (H & E; × 1040).

(299, 300, 304, 305), a T-cell marker with probable macrophage specificity (298), a Hodgkin's cell marker (306) and S-100 protein (298–304).

S-100 protein should be included in the panel to eliminate the possibility of a reactive process, which is more common than histiocytosis in the base of the skull. S-100 protein is interesting, since it is present in the Langerhans' cell histiocyte and absent in many other types of histiocytes, in addition to being absent in the foamy macrophages of xanthoma disseminatum (291, 296, 298). The S-100 reactivity of SHML cells contrasts with their apparent lack of Birbeck granules and raises the question of their lineage. In the parasellar region, many types of neoplasms, including schwannomas, gliomas and a few meningiomas, are S-100 positive. Here S-100 staining is more useful to distinguish histiocytosis from S-100–negative macrophages or Gitter cells reacting to injury than to distinguish histiocytosis from other neoplasms (291).

When the lesion is suspected to be multicentric, malignant or a true histiocytic lymphoma, additional markers should be included in the panel. Histiocytic lymphomas and the immature component of malignant histiocytosis are stained with monoclonal anti-human monocyte 1 (Mo1) marker (305). Malignant histiocytic cells also contain ferritin (299). While presumed to be less, the extent of expression of these two markers by solitary and more self-limited forms of histiocytosis requires more precise determination.

Different types of histiocytosis have different ultrastructural features (see Table 13–3). Histiocytosis X is composed of abnormal Langerhans' cells, which can be identified by their content of Birbeck granules on electron microscopic examination (307). Currently, the presence of Birbeck granules appears to be a property of histiocytosis X that distinguishes it from the related disorder, SHML (284, 292, 295, 296). However, some specimens of histiocytosis X contain Birbeck granules in as few as 2% of their cells (285). The rarity of Birbeck granules in classic histiocytosis X diminishes their diagnostic impact when they are not found. For this reason, the diagnosis of related disorders reported to be negative for Birbeck granules should not rely solely on their absence in electron micrographs. In the case of SHML, routine light microscopic evidence of lymphocytes within the cytoplasm of large histiocytes is more definitive evidence of SHML than lack of Birbeck granules. The large histiocytes of SHML may also contain other types of blood cells (293).

Most cases of histiocytosis X are euploid by flow cytometric analysis (308). Since these tumors contain a mixture of morphologically diverse cells within a collagenous stroma, a more discriminating analysis of ploidy of these cell types might be accomplished with cytophotometric image analysis.

Infundibuloma

The glial elements of the posterior pituitary and infundibular stem, the so-called "pituicytes," are of astroglial derivation. Gliomas arising in this region are of the pilocytic variety. They resemble cerebellar pilocytic astrocytomas and show no distinguishing features from other pilocytic gliomas arising in the area (see "Optic Nerve Glioma"). Gliomas involving the infundibulum often show spread and involvement of neighboring structures such as the optic chiasm, hypothalamus and the third ventricle, making it impossible to ascertain their origin. Tumors localized to the posterior pituitary and/or the infundibulum are rare, and as pointed out by Rubinstein (309), only a few can be accepted as true infundibulomas (310). Hypothalamic gliomas are somewhat more common. In a series of 74 children with parasellar

tumors, two had hypothalamic gliomas (48). A neoplastic transformation of mature pituicytes or pituicytoma (see also "Granular Cell Tumor") was described by Liss and Kahn (311).

Lymphoepithelioma

Lymphoepithelioma (undifferentiated carcinoma) is discussed in the section, "Nasopharyngeal Carcinoma."

Lymphoma (Reticulum Cell Sarcoma-Microglioma)

Primary parasellar lymphomas usually involve the hypothalamus, either directly or by invasion from the thalamus or basal ganglia (312–317). Characteristic presenting symptoms signal various hypothalamic dysfunctions. Diabetes insipidus is most common (313, 314). Other endocrine defects, including hypoglycemia and weight loss, have heralded hypothalamic invasion by lymphomas (315–318). Suprasellar lymphomas are close to isointense on T1-weighted magnetic resonance images and consistently hyperintense on spin density and T2-weighted images (141). Sinonasal lymphoma may also invade the parasellar region. This is accompanied by destruction of bone (3). Sinonasal lymphomas typically involve multiple regions of the nasal cavity (3).

Most primary CNS lymphomas are B-cell lymphomas (319–321). Their B-cell immunoglobulin marker expression is a critical early clue to their identification as lymphomas rather than sarcomas (320). Sinonasal lymphomas are also predominantly B-cell lymphomas in the United States (3). The morphology of these lymphomas varies from small cell and plasmacytoid to large cell and immunoblastic (321, 322). While the reported number of parasellar lymphomas with proper immunophenotyping is too small to be definitive, histiocytic lymphoma may be more common in hypothalamic lymphomas than in other primary CNS locations (312, 321, 322).

The incidence of primary CNS lymphomas is increasing, partly due to its occurence among immunosupressed individuals and those infected with human immunodeficiency virus (HIV) (319). Despite this, primary intrasellar lymphomas associated with

HIV infection are rare. In a study of pituitary lesions of 49 autopsied patients with acquired immunodeficiency syndrome (AIDS), no lymphomas invaded the pituitary despite the occurence of 12 CNS lymphomas (323).

Many primary CNS lymphomas are multicentric (324). Multiple brain masses associated with signs of hypothalamic dysfunction raise suspicion of CNS lymphoma with hypothalamic involvement.

Recognition of a primary parasellar lymphoma depends on consideration of the possibility and procurement of adequate specimens at biopsy. A crowded accumulation of small- to medium-sized malignant cells that are non-fibrillar and non-cohesive suggests lymphoma. Perivascular distribution of neoplastic cells with vascular wall invasion also suggests CNS lymphoma (Fig. 13–38). If these are encountered during intraoperative frozen section examination, additional frozen sections for markers should be cut from the block prior to fixation and embedding the frozen section control. Whenever possible, portions should be fixed in glutaraldehyde for electron microscopy and a portion frozen for possible analysis of DNA. Careful touch preparations without smearing may be critical in delineating isolated, round neoplastic cells without processes (Fig. 13–39). Unfortunately, the critical functions of the hypo-

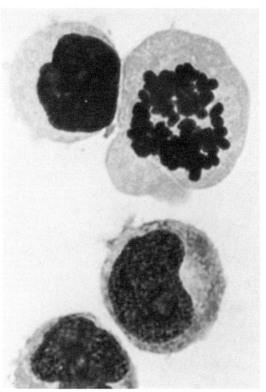

Figure 13–39. High nucleus-to-cytoplasm ratio, nuclear pleomorphism and mitoses reflect the malignancy of these neoplastic cells. Lack of cellular cohesion and no extended cell processes are typical of lymphoma (whole cells; Wright's stain; ×2100).

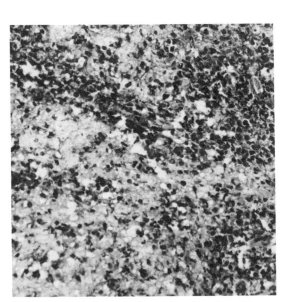

Figure 13–38. Perivascular cuffs of small malignant cells that infiltrate the surrounding brain parenchyma resemble clods of dirt on concrete in this frozen section of a stereotactic biopsy specimen. This primary lymphoma infiltrated brain parenchyma above the hypothalamus (H & E; ×210).

thalamus usually preclude accession of the desired amount of tissue. The advent of reliable immunophenotypic markers for paraffin sections of routine formalin-fixed tissues allows identification of straightforward B-cell lymphomas from small samples of tissue (325).

The deep location of lymphomas in clinically sensitive neuroanatomic regions has stimulated recommendations for stereotactic biopsies (326–328). While adequate for straightforward cases, this approach does not provide sufficient tissue for complete analysis of complex cases by present methods (329–332). Present Southern blot DNA analytical methods for B-cell immunoglobulin or T-cell receptor gene rearrangements require more tissue than is available from stereotactic biopsy. Future combination of polymerase chain reactions with Southern blot analyses may make these studies feasible (330, 331, 333).

An important morphological feature of CNS lymphomas is their tendency to invade vascular walls (332). Stains that distinguish vascular walls from parenchyma and simultaneously demonstrate neoplastic features of nuclei highlight this vascular invasion. Masson's trichrome, Mallory's phosphotungstic acid hematoxylin (PTAH) or anti-NSE with hematoxylin counterstain are recommended for the parasellar region (196, 240, 319). In contrast to endothelial proliferations of malignant gliomas and desmoplasia of carcinomas, the cytologic features of neoplastic cells within vascular walls and parenchyma are identical in lymphomas (319).

Confirmation of lymphoma and immunophenotyping can be accomplished simultaneously with an appropriate immunostaining panel (see Table 13–4). The minimal panel should include common leukocyte antigen (CLA; LCA; CD45), L26 marker of B cells and UCHL-1 (CD45R) marker of T cells (334–340). These three markers survive paraffin embedding well. The most common pattern shows all lymphoid cells positive with CLA, lymphoma cells additionally positive with L26 and smaller focal reactive lymphocytes, some of which are L26 positive but most of which are UCHL-1 positive (Figs. 13–40 through 13–43).

Not all parasellar lymphomas express the common lymphoma phenotype. A few CNS lymphomas are CLA or L26 negative. Histiocytic lymphoma has been reported in the hypothalamus (312). The immunostaining panel should be expanded with additional markers to accommodate such refractory cases. MB1, MB2, MT2 and KP1 (CD68) are recommended (322, 325). Monoclonal antibodies LN-1, LN-2 and LN-3 are also useful in diagnosing B-cell lymphomas.

Immunostaining for subtypes of immunoglobulin heavy and light chains has been largely superceded by the forementioned markers. It is less useful for lymphomas than myelomas. This is due in part to a low signal-to-background ratio of these stains when applied to routine surgical pathology tissue specimens. Preservation of epitopes with mercuric fixatives such as B-5 or with zinc chloride formalin improves staining if this method is to be used.

Immunophenotyping is more specific for diagnosis of lymphomas than ultrastructural examination. Primary CNS lymphomas show rounded cells with scanty cytoplasm and no specific organelles (341, 342). Their vasculature is fenestrated (336).

Melanoma

Primary melanomas are rare within the pituitary itself (343–345). Headaches and deterioration of vision have been presenting complaints. Other clinical abnormalities have

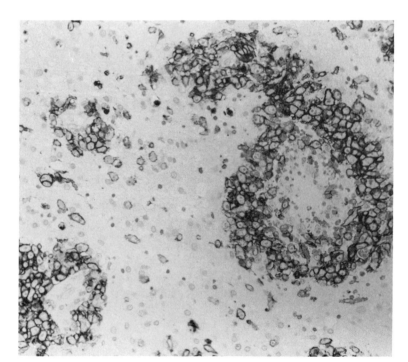

Figure 13–40. Primary lymphoma with a typical immunophenotype. Perivascular cuffs of malignant cells express B-cell phenotype (immunoperoxidase anti-L26; ×210).

Figure 13–41. Same case shown in Figure 13–40. Lack of S-100 reactivity in the perivascular cuffs and staining of the surrounding brain parenchyma reverse the staining pattern in another section of this primary lymphoma. Figures 13–40 and 13–41 are different sections of the same lymphoma. Malignant cells invade the wall of the vessel (*center*) (immunoperoxidase anti–S-100 protein; ×420).

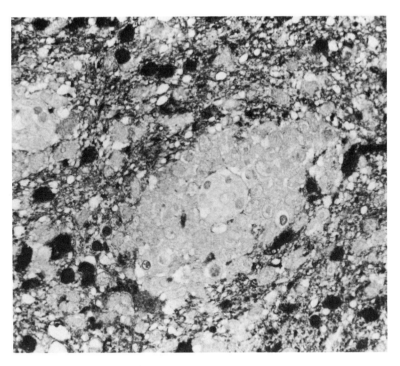

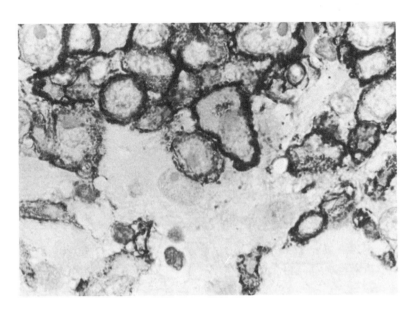

Figure 13–42. Same case shown in Figures 13–40 and 13–41. The L26 B-cell antigen localizes to the plasma membrane of malignant lymphoma cells. These cells have large and pleomorphic nuclei and nucleoli and are considerably larger than the surrounding reactive lymphocytes, few of which are positive (immunoperoxidase anti-L26; ×1040).

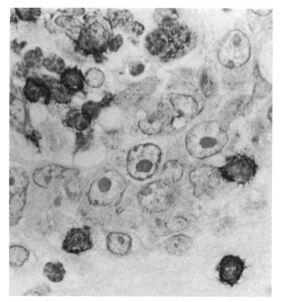

Figure 13–43. Same case shown in Figures 13–40 through 13–42. In contrast to the lymphoma cells, only small reactive lymphocytes express T-cell surface antigen (immunoperoxidase anti–UCHL-1; ×1040).

included memory impairment, optic disc atrophy and hypopituitarism (343, 345).

Radiographic abnormalities include expansion of the pituitary fossa and erosion of the dorsum sellae (343). CT scans demonstrate a mass of heterogeneous density. Individual cases involve different surrounding structures, producing different radiographic images (346–349).

The origin of intrasellar melanomas is unknown. Possible sites include pigmented cells in the pars nervosa, Rathke's pouch remnants and meninges (343, 345). In view of the rarity of their occurrence, thorough dermatological examination is necessary to rule out the possibility that the intrasellar melanoma is actually a metastasis from a cutaneous or mucosal primary.

Melanomas locally invade and spread along the meninges (348–351). When this includes the sella, it may produce confusion with pituitary carcinoma. Parasellar growth in sinonasal regions may resemble olfactory neuroblastoma or sinonasal undifferentiated carcinoma (116, 121, 349).

Most parasellar tumors identified as melanomas have been pigmented. Their macroscopic appearance has been gray to black, with soft regions of necrosis (343–347).

The classic histological features of melanoma are those of a malignant neoplasm composed of epithelioid to spindled cells (352, 355). Melanomas that contain melanin show tiny cytoplasmic granules that are more uniform and darker than hemosiderin. Nuclei are pleomorphic with prominent chromatin. Nucleoli are pleomorphic and conspicuously large in individual tumors. Regional coagulation necrosis, individual cell necrosis and pyknotic nuclei are common. Pleomorphism and heterogeneity characterize melanomas. Consequently, individual sellar melanomas display papillae and fewer mitoses than most melanomas (343).

Confronted with a new case or differential diagnosis, fine granules of dark brown pigment reactive with the Fontana stain substantially increase suspicion of melanoma (353). However, occurrences of other pigmented parasellar tumors, including melanotic schwannoma and meningioma, and of amelanotic melanomas complicate sole reliance on pigmentation as a discriminator. Combined structural and chemical criteria must be evaluated to produce the diagnosis.

Melanomas contain S-100 protein (349, 354, 355). This marker is more useful in dermatopathology than pathology of the sellar region, since many other neoplasms around the sella are S-100 positive. Individual melanomas grow as cords between reactive and fibrous tissue in a manner resembling chordoma and particularly carcinoma (Fig. 13–44) (352). The combination of strong S-100 and vimentin immunoreactivity and lack of cytokeratin distinguish melanoma from carcinoma and chordoma (356).

The HMB-45 monoclonal antibody detects an antigen within lipoid cytoplasmic vacuoles (352). The specificity of HMB-45 is more restricted than S-100. It recognizes melanocytic cells, including cells of melanoma. HMB-45 helps when pigment cannot be discerned on standard H & E or Fontana stains. However, most available HMB-45 antibodies are not strongly reactive with their epitopes, and minimal positivity may be overlooked. Avidin-biotin or immunoglobulin bridge enhancement is recommended (196) (Fig. 13–45). The combined use of the melanocytic marker HMB-45 and the neural marker antisynaptophysin to distinguish HMB-45–positive melanoma from synaptophysin-positive esthesioneuroblastoma has been recommended (see Table 13–1) (349). However, the spectrum of reactivity of parasellar and pigmented neuroectodermal tumors for HMB-45 remains to be comprehensively evaluated.

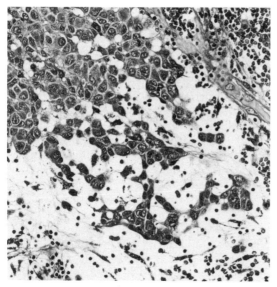

Figure 13–44. Epithelioid cells occasionally form cords within a myxoid matrix. Tumors like this melanoma then resemble carcinoma and chordoma (H & E; ×210).

The antibody ME 1-14 reacts with alpha-chondroitin sulfate proteoglycan. It reacts with 60% of melanomas stained as whole cells (354). Its reactivity with other parasellar neoplasms also remains to be fully explored.

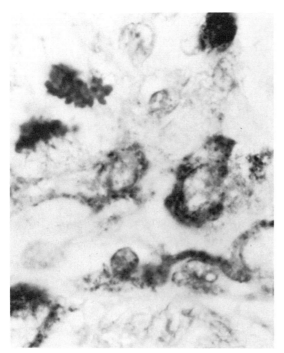

Figure 13–45. HMB-45 reactivity of neoplastic cells in another section of this tumor indicates the melanocytic nature of its malignant cells. One cell is in mitosis (avidin-biotin immunoperoxidase anti–HMB-45, counterstained with hematoxylin; ×1660).

The most important ultrastructural feature of melanoma is the premelanosome. While aggregates of mature melanosomes are visible light microscopically, amelanotic melanomas lack these visible aggregates. Ultrastructural confirmation of an amelanotic melanoma requires identification of the lamellar or spiral premelanosome (357). These 100-nm × 400-nm ellipsoidal, membrane-bound structures contain striated cores of parallel filaments. These are lamellar premelanosomes. The spiral premelanosome of similar size and shape contains coils of zigzag filaments (357). Mature melanosomes are densely black. While other tumors with pigmented variants may contain these structures, nonpigmented tumors lack them.

Meningioma

Meningiomas of the sellar region are common nonadenomatous neoplasms with an incidence comparable to craniopharyngioma (7, 358). According to their location they can be separated into olfactory, suprasellar or parasellar meningioma (359–364), and together they make up approximately 14% of parapituitary tumors (358). The olfactory meningiomas arise in the region of the cribriform plate and along the olfactory grove; parasellar ones arise from the medial sphenoid wing or the lateral portion of the sella turcica; and the suprasellar meningiomas arise from the tuberculum sella. The last type constitutes between 5% and 10% of all meningiomas (365–367).

Among meningiomas of the sellar region, the suprasellar mengingiomas have attracted special attention (361–367). They are believed to originate from arachnoid cells of the villous processes of the venous sinuses (368), which surround the hypophysis under the diaphragm sellae. Hence, they may originate at the tuberculum sellae, under the optic nerve or laterally or behind the infundibulum anterior to the dorsum sellae.

Meningiomas in general show a significant female predominance of about 3:2 (376–377). The predominance has been attributed to female steroid hormone receptors. This is even more pronounced in suprasellar meningiomas, with several series reporting a female preponderance of 4:1 (361, 365, 367). Furthermore, the peak incidence of suprasellar meningiomas occurs earlier in females (between 30 and 39 years of age) than in males (50 to 59 years of age) (364).

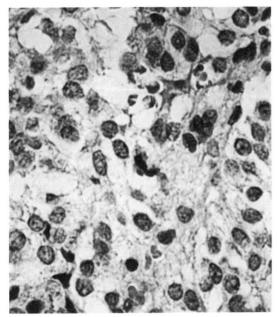

Figure 13–46. Neoplasm from the sellar region. Chromophobe adenoma shows poor cytoplasmic stainability with H & E (×370). (From Yamada K, *et al.* Coincidental pituitary adenoma and parasellar meningioma. Case report. Neurosurgery *19*:267–270, 1986.)

A coincidental occurrence of parasellar meningiomas and pituitary adenomas has been reported repeatedly (379–385). In five cases the two neoplasms were juxtaposed (Figs. 13–46 and 13–47). Some authors have suggested that this may reflect a paracrine effect brought about by the topographical relationship to the adenohypophysis. This notion has not been proven.

Suprasellar meningiomas present in 75% to 98% of cases with the typical chiasmal syndrome, first described by Cushing, consisting of primary optic atrophy and bitemporal hemianopia with normal sella turcica and no endocrinopathy (361, 362, 365, 366). Visual abnormalities are less common with olfactory and parasellar meningiomas, in which anosmia and involvement of cranial nerves III, IV, V and VI, as well as mental changes, are more prominent (359, 361, 363). Parasellar meningiomas are more prone to involve neighboring structures. Bonnal and associates (360) reported in a series of 24 meningiomas of the lateral sella turcica that 14 had invaded the cavernous sinus, and eight showed invasion into the sella turcica. Vascular obstruction can be significant (14). Accompanying hyperostosis of underlying bone is a common feature of suprasellar meningiomas (49%) and olfactory meningiomas (62%) (364).

Meningiomas are histologically heterogeneous. Transitional and fibroblastic subtypes have prominent extracellular matrices (see Table 13–3). Epithelioid or endotheliomatous mengingiomas resemble pituitary adenomas (see Table 13–1). The histological types of parasellar meningiomas have been compared with their anatomic sites. In a

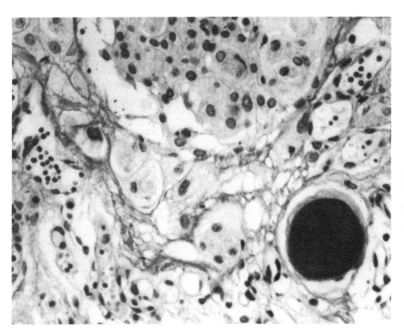

Figure 13–47. Second neoplasm from the sellar region of the same patient shown in Figure 13–46. Meningotheliomatous meningioma occurred coincidentally with the adenoma. The patient never received radiation (H & E; ×280). (From Yamada K, *et al.* Coincidental pituitary adenoma and parasellar meningioma. Case report. Neurosurgery *19*:267–270, 1986.)

Danish series of 30 suprasellar meningiomas, the authors reported 13 syncytial (endotheliomatous, meningothelial), 11 transitional and six fibroblastic meningiomas (365). In a similar series of 55 suprasellar meningioma, Solero and associates (361) reported 44 transitional (fibroendotheliomatous), 10 psammomatous and one angioblastic mengingioma. In a series of 98 olfactory meningiomas by the same authors, 90 were of the transitional type and eight were psammomatous meningiomas (361).

Five suprasellar meningiomas have been reported to have arisen from the diaphragm sellae (363, 369, 370, 371). Papo and associates (372) described five extradural parasellar tumors with their base at the anterior clinoid process. All patients presented with slowly developing oculomotor disorders. Four tumors showed highly vascular meningotheliomatous meningiomas.

Three cases of intrasellar meningiomas have been reported; this lesion understandably may be confused with pituitary adenoma on preoperative diagnosis (373, 374). Surprisingly, none of these cases demonstrated any endocrinologic abnormalities. On the other hand, Shah and associates described parasellar meningiomas in two women who presented with galactorrhea and amenorrhea, suggesting a hypothalamic-pituitary dysfunction with inhibition of the prolactin inhibitory factor (375).

Meningiomas are notorious for mimicking a variety of intracranial neoplasms (376, 377). Transitional and/or fibroblastic meningiomas with a streaming cellular pattern may be mistaken for schwannoma, and meningotheliomatous meningiomas exhibiting an epithelioid cellular morphology may mimic the appearance of a pituitary adenoma (Figs. 13–46 and 13–47). In such cases, electron microscopy or immunohistochemistry aids in arriving at the correct diagnosis. Meningiomas are positive for both vimentin and EMA, variably positive for S-100 protein and negative for GFAP. So-called "secretory meningiomas" express keratin positivity (268, 388). Schwannomas are highly immunoreactive for S-100 protein and are also vimentin positive and variably EMA positive (378, 388). Thus, a panel of appropriate antigens may be helpful; however, significant overlap in expression of antigenic markers makes electron microscopy the most decisive way to distinguish these two neoplasms. Meningiomas have interdigitating cellular processes, desmosomes and tonofilaments (Fig. 13–48), in contrast to schwannomas, which have continuous basement membranes around their plasmalemmae. One also should keep in mind that occasional astrocytomas may express vimentin positivity.

Pituitary adenomas can be differentiated from meningiomas either by electron microscopy or by employing the appropriate immunohistochemical techniques for the demonstration of hormone products. Meningiomas displaying nests of neoplastic cells may be confused with a paraganglioma. The latter diagnosis is established by chromogranin and neurotransmitter expression.

A unique example of a suprasellar granular meningioma was reported by Friede and Yasargil (386) that demonstrated clusters of granular cells that were negative for both GFAP and S-100 thus excluding a glial or Schwann cell derivation. Interestingly, as described by Mitsumori and associates (387), granular meningioma is the most common spontaneously occurring meningeal tumor in rats.

The occurrence of meningiomas consequent to irradiation is described following low-dose radiation to the scalp for fungal infection (368). An orbital roof meningioma with infiltration into the orbit was described in a 54-year-old woman by Meyrignae and associates 20 years following radiation of a chromophobe adenoma (389).

The majority of parasellar meningiomas can be surgically removed, and patients subsequently have a good prognosis. Exceptions are patients with *en plaque* meningiomas and meningiomas that encase or invade critical neuroanatomic structures (Fig. 13–49). These tend to recur repeatedly until they eventually compromise a critical vascular or neuroanatomic region.

Myxoma

The only report of a primary myxoma in the pituitary fossa was published in 1987 (390). The patient was a 38-year-old Japanese man who developed a sudden and rapid deterioration of right visual acuity. A CT scan showed a normodense mass in the right side of the pituitary fossa with a suprasellar extension that was slightly and homogeneously enhanced by contrast. Pituitary function was not affected. A non-functioning adenoma was suspected clinically, and at

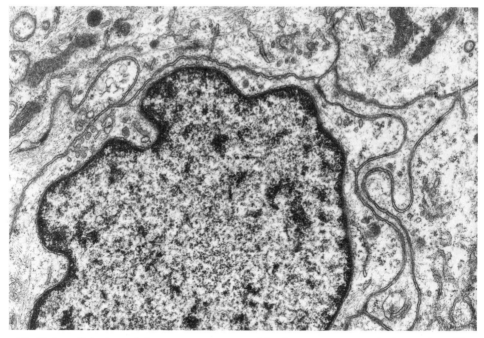

Figure 13–48. Interdigitating cellular processes punctuated by desmosomes create the impression of barges on a meandering river between cells of this recurrent meningioma growing *en plaque* along the dura over the base of the skull (uranyl acetate and lead citrate; ×16,300). (From McKeever PE, Blaivas M. In: Sternberg S, *et al.* (eds). Diagnosis in Surgical Pathology. Vol 1. New York, Raven Press, 1989, pp 357–359.)

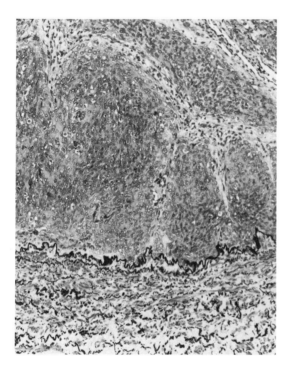

Figure 13–49. Vascular invasion by aggressive meningiomas and meningiomas *en plaque* is a more significant problem in the skull base than over the cerebral convexities. This meningioma has occluded the vascular lumen while leaving the vascular wall and its dark undulated elastin relatively intact (Movat's pentachrome stain; ×105).

surgery a gray, gelatinous, semi-transparent, well-circumscribed tumor was found occupying the right side of the sella.

Microscopically, the tumor was composed of stellate, spindled and bipolar cells with hyperchromatic nuclei and a mucinous background. The cells were organized in lobules separated by connective tissue trabeculae. The myxomatous stroma was Alcian blue positive, hyaluronidase digestible, and PAS positive. The tumor cells were more intensely PAS positive than the stroma. The neoplasm was excised, and the patient was tumor free 5 years later. Other reported intracerebral myxomas are metastases and emboli from cardiac myxomas (391).

Myxomas are benign neoplasms that probably originate from fibroblasts that produce excessive amounts of glycosaminoglycans and inhibit polymerization of normal collagen (392). They are rare and can be found in various tissues of the body, including skeletal muscle, heart, bones and peripheral nerves. Perineurial, or nerve sheath, myxoma is a peculiar neoplasm of dermis that is S-100 positive; it is also known as "*neurothekoma*" (393). Myxoma involving skull bones and orbit was described by Stout, who considered these neoplasms to be tumors originating from primitive mesenchyme (394). When a myxoma involves the jaw bones it is known as "*odontogenic myxoma*" and can develop in the maxilla or in the mandible, frequently associated with unerupted or missing teeth. The neoplasm is histologically benign. However, it has the potential of local invasion of the underlying bone and, if not completely excised, may recur (395). Myxomas of the jaw do not usually metastasize, in contrast with myxomas of soft tissue.

Nasopharyngeal Carcinoma

Nasopharyngeal carcinoma (NPC) is a rare neoplasm in most countries of the world but occurs with exceptionally high frequency among the Chinese. There is an epidemiological link to prior *Epstein-Barr virus* exposure and prevalence of certain human leukocyte antigens (396). Approximately 15% to 25% of malignant tumors of the nasopharynx have invaded the base of the skull when first diagnosed (397). The neoplasm in this location is difficult to visualize and operate on. Miura and associates analyzed 29 NPC patients with skull base or intracranial involve-

ment and outlined six major directions of the primary tumor spread from the nasopharynx (398). The superior and supralateral extensions, which involve the sphenoid sinus, cavernous sinus and middle cranial fossa, were found to be less common than anterior and postero-lateral directions of the spread.

NPC derives from nasopharyngeal surface epithelium and, according to the World Health Organization, is classified into three major types: *squamous cell carcinoma*, nonkeratinizing carcinoma and undifferentiated carcinoma. The undifferentiated carcinoma, or *lymphoepithelioma*, may have a prominent inflammatory component, making it indistinguishable from lymphoma on H & E–stained slides (3). Further classification based on correlations of histological subtypes of the neoplasm and survival rate was offered in a study of 494 patients (399).

Histologically, the squamous variants present no problems to the surgical pathologist. The undifferentiated carcinoma is another matter. The tumor, which is also called SNUC, consists of polygonal cells that form nests, trabeculae, ribbons or sheets. Round or oval nuclei are surrounded by a moderate amount of eosinophilic cytoplasm. Chromatin is diffuse or coarsely granular, the nucleoli are usually large and mitotic figures are numerous (3). Vascular invasion is common (Fig. 13–16).

Immunohistochemical techniques help to differentiate NPC from *olfactory neuroblastoma*, which possesses synaptophysin and intercellular fibrils that NPC is lacking (see "Esthesioneuroblastoma"). *Lymphoma*, small cell undifferentiated *carcinoma*, malignant *melanoma* and *rhabdomyosarcoma* have different antigenic phenotypes (Table 2–4). Undifferentiated NPC is positive for cytokeratin and epithelial membrane antigen and frequently for NSE. It is negative for HMB-45, S-100 protein, synaptophysin and myogenous markers (3, 349, 400). Ultrastructurally, undifferentiated NPC demonstrates desmosomes and tonofilaments in most of the cases. The absence of tonofilaments does not preclude positive immunologic staining for keratin (400).

Two other neoplasms that can infiltrate the sella from the nasopharynx are worth mentioning: *angiofibroma* and *adenocarcinoma resembling colonic carcinoma* (ARCC) (10, 401, 402). Twenty percent of cases of juvenile angiofibroma reportedly extended into the parasellar sphenoid and petrous portions of the temporal bones, resulting in the involvement of the anterior and middle cranial fossae (401). ARCC is a distinctive neoplasm that is most frequent in men in their 5th and 6th decades and is associated with occupational exposure to *hardwood dust* (10). Franquemont and associates analyzed 15 cases, only four of which involved woodworkers. They classified this neoplasm into papillary tubular cylinder cell type, grades I and II; alveolar goblet cell type; signet-ring type; and a mixed pattern. Median survival was 9 years for papillary tubular grade I, 3 years for papillary tubular grade II, and 7 years for alveolar goblet cell type (402).

Optic Nerve Glioma

The overall incidence of optic gliomas is approximately 1% of all intracranial neoplasms, and since these tumors usually affect the younger population, the incidence in pediatric specimens is approximately 4% (403).

Gliomas occurring in the optic nerve and chiasm involve mostly young subjects and are present in at least 10% of cases associated with von Recklinghausen's disease (404, 405). In a series of 74 children with parasellar tumors, two had optic gliomas (48). These lesions often show a favorable clinical course, particularly if they are confined to the intraorbital optic nerve (406–408). Histologically they are pilocytic astrocytomas of the juvenile type, with spindle cell–shaped cellular elements forming parallel bundles of fibrils. Mitotic figures are usually not seen. A feature of these tumors is the presence of Rosenthal fibers. Occasionally they may demonstrate microcystic areas with myxomatous changes (409). The latter feature has been interpreted as an oligodendroglial participation in the neoplasm (405). Only rarely have malignant forms been reported, and when these occur, they appear to evolve from optic gliomas associated with von Recklinghausen's disease (406, 410).

In contradiction to the relatively benign juvenile form of optic gliomas, optic gliomas occurring in adults usually exhibit more aggressive characteristics with rapid growth and infiltration of the hypothalamus and temporal lobes and may histologically display the features of malignant astrocytomas. The clinical outcome of this adult form is naturally less favorable (411, 412).

Tumors involving the optic chiasm, both the juvenile and adult forms, may show extension into the hypothalamus and third ventricle. In such cases it may be impossible to determine whether the tumor originated in the optic pathway or in the hypothalamus, since gliomas arising in the hypothalamus generally show the same character as optic gliomas. Involvement of the internal carotid or opthalmic artery is not common (14).

Special attention should be drawn to optic gliomas associated with von Recklinghausen's disease, since these may be multiple. Davis (413) reported that approximately 40% of the cases manifested bilateral involvement. Furthermore, in von Recklinghausen's disease optic gliomas tend to be associated with pronounced arachnoidal hyperplasia and more extensive tumor infiltration of the leptomeninges (406, 413).

Osteogenic Sarcoma

Osteosarcoma is the most frequent primary malignant bone tumor, secondary only to multiple myeloma (414). It may occur at any age; however, in about half of the cases, it arises in the first two decades of life. In older patients it is usually associated with other pre-existing bone disorders such as Paget's disease, fibrous dysplasia, aseptic necrosis or previous irradiation. Roentgenographically, osteosarcoma is a poorly defined, osteolytic (or osteoblastic or mixed osteolytic-sclerotic) lesion that frequently produces a characteristic "sunray" or "sunburst" appearance that is lacking in the skull lesions. Less than 9% of all osteosarcomas originate in the craniofacial bones, of which the mandible is the most common site (415).

Two cases of primary osteogenic sarcoma of the sellar region, in a 48-year-old woman and a 22-year-old man, were characterized by a history of headache and diplopia (416, 417). A CT scan in the latter case showed a homogeneous enhancing mass in the region of the tuberculum sellae encroaching on the anterior part of the sphenoid sinus. Three osteosarcomas of sphenoid bone have also been reported: two primary, and one 15 years after radiation therapy for a craniopharyngioma (418, 419).

By definition, osteogenic sarcoma is a malignant primary tumor of bone, the malignant cells of which produce *osteoid* substance

(415). The major histological subdivisions of the neoplasm are osteoblastic, chondroblastic and fibroblastic types, all with similar survival rates.

The value of immunohistochemistry and electron microscopy is rather limited in the differential diagnosis of osteosarcoma from chondrosarcoma or malignant fibrous histiocytoma. Class II histocompatibility antigen expression in bone and soft tissue sarcomas was also found not to be helpful (420). DNA analysis has been used to differentiate an osteosarcoma from myositis ossificans and typical giant cell tumor of bone, since over 80% of osteosarcomas exhibit DNA aneuploidy with a large proportion of cells in S phase (421).

Paraganglioma

Paragangliomas rarely pose a problem in the differential diagnosis of sellar and parasellar tumors, because they occur in different locations. Paragangliomas arise in association with sympathetic and parasympathetic ganglia. Only one case has been reported within the sella, and this was of uncertain cellular origin. An intrasellar paraganglioma accompanied by hypopituitarism was described by Bilbao and associates (422).

Paragangliomas arising in the carotid bodies and glomus jugulare tumors may rarely extend into the cranial cavity, and the former may involve the parasellar region. These could be confused with an extrasellar pituitary adenoma. However, the immunopositivity of paraganglioma for catecholamines or methionine-enkephalin establishes the diagnosis (423). Paragangliomas are typically immunoreactive for chromogranin, NSE and catecholamines (423, 424). Their lack of cytokeratin immunoreactivity distinguishes them from many other neuroendocrine tumors (356). Since the cells resemble pituitary adenoma cells, their lack of pituitary hormone immunoreactivity is key to their recognition (422, 425). The neurosecretory granules of paragangliomas are barely visible on H & E–stained paraffin sections. They are best seen in Epon plastic sections (Fig. 13–50) (426).

Plasmacytoma (Myeloma)

The solitary sellar plasmacytoma is a rare entity that is difficult to diagnose by light microscopy (428–432). Only those confronted by a solitary plasmacytoma or first presentation of multiple myeloma in the sella can fully appreciate how much this unrelated neoplasm can mimic a pituitary adenoma. This simulation of endocrine by hematopoietic neoplasia seems improbable due to major differences in cellular lineages. How-

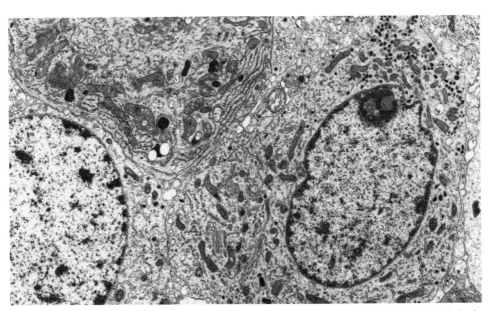

Figure 13–50. Round nuclei and nucleoli, neurosecretory granules and cellular processes are typical of paraganglioma (uranyl acetate and lead citrate; ×7200).

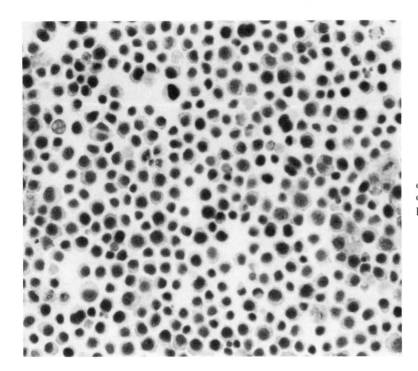

Figure 13–51. Monotonous collection of discohesive cells compose this myeloma of the soft palate (H & E; × 1300).

ever, both neoplasms share secretory apparati designed for large-scale export. This produces similarities in appearance.

The term "plasmacytoma" is used here to describe the solitary neoplasm composed of plasma cells. If time or additional clinical studies reveal multiple lesions of systemic involvement, the neoplasm is then called "multiple myeloma."

About 90% of extramedullary plasma cell neoplasms occur in the head and neck region (Fig. 13–51) (3, 427). Since at least 75% of these involve the sinonasal region (Fig. 13–52), direct extension to the parasellar region is a concern. Careful review of the previous studies of such cases will often confirm the diagnosis.

The majority of intrasellar plasmacytomas evolve into multiple myeloma (428, 429). Primary intrasellar plasmacytomas may be a larger group than recognized. Two cases were initially diagnosed as pituitary adenomas. The subsequent systemic course of the illness did not occur until 3 to 5 months later, stimulating a reevaluation of the initial diagnosis (428, 429). A more indolent solitary plasmacytoma that has not progressed to multiple myeloma might elude correct diagnosis in the sella, since its light microscopic features resemble pituitary adenoma.

Different secretory products and biological behavior provide keys to distinguish plasma-

cytomas from pituitary adenomas, which are exceedingly more common in the sella. The importance of clinical and laboratory data to the pathologist who encounters such a plas-

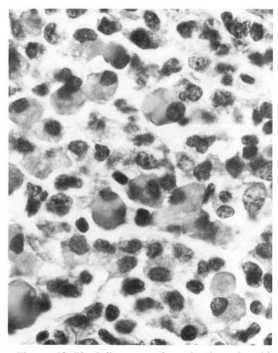

Figure 13–52. Solitary neoplasm in the sphenoid bone. Discohesive cells have eccentric nuclei; some contain cytoplasmic Russell bodies (H & E; × 1040).

macytoma is paramount. The sellar lesion can be lytic with a sharp margin in bone. Radiologic evidence of other "punched-out" lesions in the skull or other bones may suggest multiple myeloma (428, 429). Serum or urinary protein abnormalities may indicate a monoclonal gammopathy (52, 429). The majority of multiple myelomas presenting as a sellar or parasellar mass will have a systemic manifestation (428). Thus, a second tumor, lytic lesion or protein abnormality should immediately raise suspicion.

The majority of diagnoses of these solitary plasmacytomas have been established by electron microscopy, a procedure eminently suited to distinguish plasmacytoma from adenoma. Myeloma cells lack hormone storage granules, intercellular junctions and basement membrane. All of these are present in pituitary adenomas (430).

If definitive electron microscopy is not feasible in a given case, immunocytochemistry is recommended. Monoclonal expression of an immunoglobulin (Ig) heavy chain subtype and κ or λ light chain distinguish myeloma from pituitary adenoma (Figs. 13–53 and 13–54) (430).

Immunostaining provides the additional advantage of distinguishing myeloid neo-

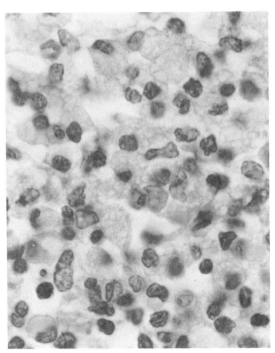

Figure 13–54. Solitary neoplasm in the sphenoid bone. Lack of IgM reflects the monoclonal nature of this plasmacytoma (immunoperoxidase anti-IgM, counterstained with hematoxylin; ×1040).

plasms from lymphomas, histiocytoses and inflammatory lesions (see Table 13–4). Plasma cell immunoreactivity for EMA and frequent lack of activity for CLA distinguish myelomas from lymphomas (340, 433). Primary brain lymphomas have high nucleus-to-cytoplasm ratios and infiltrate in and around vessel walls, producing prominent perivascular cuffs (312, 319, 322). These features help distinguish lymphomas from plasmacytomas. Plasmacytomas recognized in the sella have substantial heterochromatin, multiple lamellae of well-developed rough endoplasmic reticulum and Golgi apparatus, ultrastructurally distinguishing them from lymphomas and histocytoses (341, 428, 430). However, the ultrastructural distinction between plasmablastic myelomas and lymphomas is more subtle (341, 434). Immunocytochemistry is recommended to distinguish equivocal cases. Myelomas do not immunostain with some monoclonal antibody markers of B cells such as L26, LN1, LN2, MB1, MB2 or MB3 (325). While myelomas tend to have more immunoglobulin in their cytoplasm than lymphomas, immunoglobulin secretion is their most characteristic feature. Therefore, when it is positive, serum protein electrophoresis is a more reliable assay than

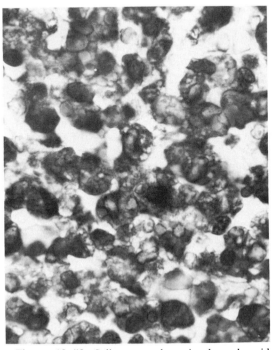

Figure 13–53. Solitary neoplasm in the sphenoid bone. All cells contain cytoplasmic IgG (immunoperoxidase anti-IgG, counterstained with hematoxylin; ×1040).

staining for Ig to distinguish myeloma from lymphoma.

Plasmacytomas differ from inflammatory processes by their monoclonal nature. Numerous other inflammatory cells in addition to plasma cells suggest inflammation. In more difficult cases, examination of heavy and light chain subclasses for neoplastic expression of monoclonality may be useful (325).

Emphasis has been placed on distinguishing plasmablastic myelomas and myelomas positive for common acute lymphoblastic leukemia antigen (CALLA) (434). On the other end of the spectrum of malignancy, indolent plasma cells associated with monoclonal gammopathy of undetermined significance (MGUS) lack the antibody against natural killer cells CD56 and have weak to negative staining with the MB2 monoclonal antibody to an intracytoplasmic B-cell antigen (435–437). Stains for myeloma phenotype and proliferative activity are being applied to MGUS and other myelomas to estimate the prognosis of patients (438–445). These markers remain to be applied to myelomas of the sella.

Rathke's Cleft Cyst

Rathke's cleft cysts are common within the sella, with their incidence depending on the cyst diameter considered large enough to be abnormal. Common locations of Rathke's cysts include the intermediate lobe of the pituitary, suprasellar region, anterior sella turcica or anterior suprasellar cistern (446). Larger cysts span more than one of these locations. Many Rathke's cleft cysts cause no symptoms and are incidental radiographic or necropsy findings. Most are less than 2 cm in diameter (446). When symptomatic, cysts near the optic chiasm cause disturbances in vision, including visual field defects and chiasmatic syndrome. Suprasellar cysts cause headaches and hypopituitarism (447, 448).

Individual Rathke's cysts vary from homogeneous low density to slight hyperdensity relative to brain parenchyma in CT scans (446). When present, contrast enhancement usually occurs in a ring near the capsule of the cyst and not in the nonvascular center. The variability in CT contrast enhancement among individual cysts may reflect variable inflammation or squamous metaplasia in the wall (86). Extravasation of cyst contents

within the cranial wall is known to inflame affected structures (6). Cysts near the pituitary stalk may enlarge it. This structure can be evaluated by comparison with surrounding structures. In children, a stalk-to–basilar artery ratio of 1 or more should be further evaluated for cyst or other abnormality (449).

Nearly half of Rathke's cysts examined by MRI have the same intensity as cerebrospinal fluid on T1 - and T2 - weighted images. The remainder are focally hyperintense on T1-weighted images, with diminished focal signal intensity on T2-weighted images (446).

Rathke's cleft cyst located solely in the suprasellar region can be difficult to distinguish from craniopharyngioma (4). The radiographic interpretation is enhanced by metrizamide cisternography (450). However, decisive tissue confirmation of Rathke's cyst requires careful macroscopic inspection and sampling to prove the absence of solid tumor.

The histological features of Rathke's cleft cysts are relatively distinctive. The wall of the cyst is composed of a thin epithelial layer of cells that lies directly on fibrovascular connective tissue. The epithelium is usually composed of a single layer of cells, but pseudostratification occurs. The cuboidal to columnar epithelium is composed of goblet cells with mucin and other cells with cilia and microvilli (Fig. 13–55). Squamous cells and small basal cells contain numerous tonofilaments and desmosomes. These cell types are most easily appreciated by electron microscopy (447, 448). This epithelium resembles the mucosa in the sphenoid sinus and some cystic craniopharyngiomas (447, 451).

Rathke's cysts coexpress three types of intermediate filaments: GFAP, cytokeratins and, to a lesser extent, vimentin (452, 453). Their immunohistochemical profile is similar to squamous nests of the pars tuberalis, suggesting a common origin (452). One provocative study of asymptomatic Rathke's cleft cysts shows negative GFAP and vimentin staining and reactivity of all 10 asymptomatic cysts for two or more pituitary peptide hormones (455). This study requires confirmation and explanation of differences in intermediate filament phenotypes. These staining patterns may relate to transitional cell tumors of the pituitary.

The differential diagnosis of Rathke's cleft cysts includes the arachnoid cysts. The arachnoid cyst often has a thinner lining than the epithelium of a Rathke's cyst, and the arachnoid cyst lining cells are syncytial. S-100 reac-

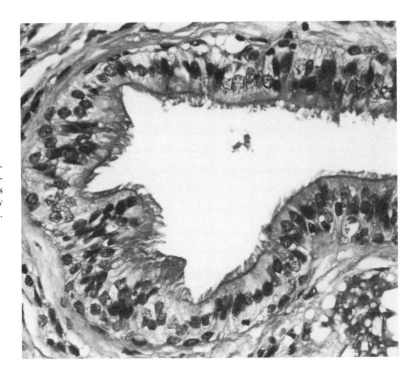

Figure 13–55. Ciliated columnar epithelium lining a fibrovascular capsule. The lumen of this Rathke's cleft cyst has partially collapsed (*center*) (H & E; ×420).

tivity favors a Rathke's cyst but is not completely reliable (454, 455).

Choroidal epithelial cyst may mimic a suprasellar Rathke's cyst in the region of the third ventricle. The choroidal cyst is usually attached to choroid plexus and will be positive with immunostaining for prealbumin (454). Colloid cysts of the third ventricle are located in a neuroanatomic position near the foramina of Monro and may be distinguished from Rathke's cysts by their more dorsal location.

Transitional cell tumors of the pituitary are rare mixtures of pituitary adenoma and Rathke's cleft cells (5, 456). They are similar to cystic prolactinomas (456). There is a high incidence of S-100 protein–positive cells and mucus-secreting cells among these mixed tumors (457, 458).

Keratinous debris within epidermoid cysts usually distinguishes them from Rathke's cysts filled with mucin. However, exceptional cysts have features of both Rathke's and epidermoid cysts (459). Dermoid cysts contain keratinized material, hair and adnexa.

A cyst that resembles the Rathke's cleft cyst but arises in the sphenoid sinus is the mucocele. Sphenoid sinus mucoceles may be multiple and bilateral (460). Some are secondary to other neoplasms (461). Sphenoid sinus

mucoceles are more hyperintense on T1- and T2-weighted images than Rathke's cleft cysts (141).

Sarcoma

Sellar or parasellar sarcomas are rare tumors. The vast majority of sarcomas represent a late complication of therapeutic radiation to preceding pituitary adenomas (462–464). Post-radiation pituitary sarcomas typically do not metastasize but show aggressive local behavior affecting the optic nerves, eroding overlying brain and compressing brain stem structures (464, 465). Approximately 20% of cases are histologically osteogenic sarcomas (see "Osteogenic Sarcoma"), and the rest are made up of fibrosarcomas (464, 466). The former show varying cellularity with striking pleomorphic spindle-shaped or polyhedral cells with eosinophilic cytoplasm. The amount of osteoid and bone tissue may vary (467). Fibroblastic sarcomas are often of the spindle cell type (Fig. 13–56) or the pleomorphic type, with considerable pleomorphism and numerous mitosis (462–464). The fibrosarcomas commonly show nests of the preexisting adenomas (Fig. 13–57) within the fibrocollagenous stroma demonstrable with the appropriate antisera.

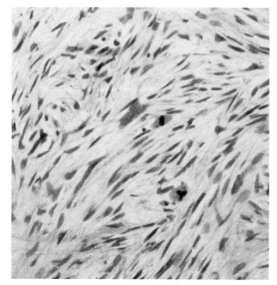

Figure 13–56. Fibrosarcoma that occurred following radiation of a pituitary adenoma. Spindled cells have pleomorphic nuclei and abnormal mitoses (H & E; × 195). (From Powell HC, *et al.* Post-irradiation pituitary sarcoma. Acta Neuropathol (Berl) *39*:165–167, 1977.)

Such adenomatous rests seldom demonstrate malignant differentiation (468, 469). In patients with post-radiation sarcomas, approximately half had received 30 to 50 Gy to the sellar area and half had received in excess of 50 Gy. The latent period from time of therapeutic irradiation to manifestation of sarcoma varies from 2.5 to more than 20 years. However, death occurs within months from the time symptoms manifest themselves (464).

Spontaneous sarcomas of the sellar area in which radiation has not been implicated as an etiological factor are extremely rare. Willis reported a case of fibrosarcoma arising in the pituitary (470). A case of pituitary leiomyosarcoma localized to the sellar and parasellar region was reported by Anderson and associates (471). The latter was believed to have arisen from vascular smooth muscle cells. In contrast to post-radiation sarcomas, primary sarcomas tend to metastasize (470).

Schwannoma

Intracranial schwannomas make up 8% to 10% of primary intracranial neoplasms and originate most frequently from sensory cranial nerves, with the eighth nerve being by far the most common source, followed by the trigeminal nerve (472, 473). Occasionally schwannomas have been reported to arise from the facial (473) and oculomotor nerves (474). Intracranial schwannomas unrelated to cranial nerves are exceedingly rare in the absence of von Recklinghausen's disease.

Four cases of schwannomas of the sellar region have been reported in patients without any stigmata of von Recklinghausen's disease (475–478). In two instances the tumors arose in the sella (475, 476); one was located on the tuberculum sella (477), and one originated from the trigeminal nerve with suprasellar extension (478). One of the intrasellar cases was associated with panhypopituitarism (475), whereas the second intrasellar case showed no endocrinologic compromise (476).

In two cases, detailed histological descriptions were given (475, 477) that revealed the characteristic pattern of Antoni A and B areas, as well as the presence of characteristic Verocay bodies in one case (477) (Figs. 13–58 and 13–59). It is believed that these rare schwannomas arise from sensory nerve twigs in the meninges or autonomic vasomotor nerves (476, 477) or possibly from ectopic Schwann cells (479).

Schwannomas of the sellar region could be misinterpreted as meningioma with a streaming cellular pattern or as a chordoma or myxoma if the Antoni type B component is prominent. A few schwannomas demonstrate

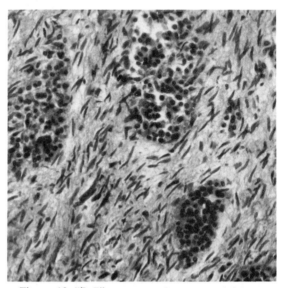

Figure 13–57. Fibrosarcoma that occurred following radiation of a pituitary adenoma, from the same case shown in Figure 13–56. Sarcoma surrounds nests of residual adenoma (H & E; × 160). (From Powell HC, *et al.* Post-irradiation pituitary sarcoma. Acta Neuropathol (Berl) *39*:165–167, 1977.)

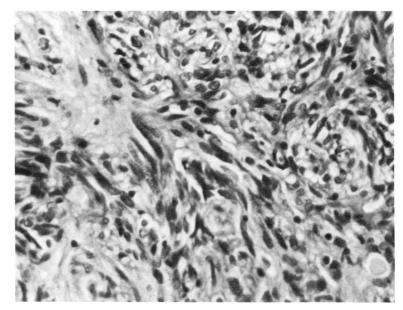

Figure 13–58. Intrasellar schwannoma displays Antoni type A differentiation (H & E; ×220). (From Wilberger JE Jr. Primary intrasellar schwannoma. Case report. Surg Neurol *32*:156–158, 1989.)

GFAP, distinguishing them from these other tumors (378). Immunopositivity for S-100 protein distinguishes schwannoma from myxoma. The other neoplasms have a distinct ultrastructure that differs from that of schwannoma (Fig. 13–60) (see Tables 1 and 3).

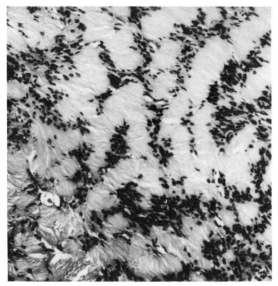

Figure 13–59. Schwannoma of the sellar region shows repeating pallisades of Verocay bodies (H & E; ×130). (From Goebel HH, *et al.* Schwannoma of the sellar region. Acta Neurochirurg *48*:191–197, 1979.)

Sinonasal Undifferentiated Carcinoma

See "Esthesioneuroblastoma" and "Nasopharyngeal Carcinoma."

Teratoma

Teratomas of the sellar region are rare neoplasms and usually occur in children or young adults. In a series of 74 patients from birth to 20 years old with parasellar tumors, two had malignant intrasellar teratomas (48). In an autopsy series that included patients of all ages, 2 of 41 parasellar tumors were teratomas (7).

In five cases of suprasellar teratomas reported by Tekeuchi and associates, the clinical symptoms consisted of *diabetes insipidus, visual disturbance* and *hypopituitarism* along with occasional increased intracranial pressure (480). The age of these five patients varied from 5 to 10 years, and histologically only one neoplasm, that in the youngest patient, was a benign teratoma. The other four cases were a *combination* of teratoma with carcinoma, adenocarcinoma or germinoma and choriocarcinoma. An immature teratoma mixed with germinoma that arose from the pituitary gland was reported in a 19-year-old man whose skull radiographs and tomography of the sella turcica demonstrated mild

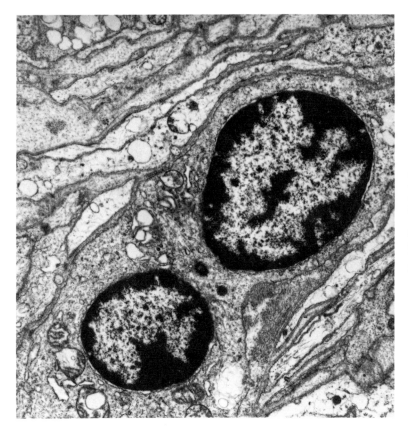

Figure 13–60. Basal lamina completely surrounds each flat cellular process of this acoustic schwannoma (lead citrate and uranyl acetate; ×10,100). (From McKeever PE, Blaivas M. In: Sternberg S, *et al.* (eds). Diagnosis in Surgical Pathology. Vol 1. New York, Raven Press, 1989, pp 361–365.)

enlargement of the sella with irregular demineralization and thinning of the sellar floor and the dorsum sellae (481). CT demonstrated an enhancing intrasellar mass. Similar findings were described in an intrasellar tumor in a 33-year-old man whose tumor was classified as teratoid rather than a teratoma, since only endodermal and mesodermal tissues were present and no ectodermal elements were detected (482).

There have been two reports in the literature of peculiar cases in which the sellar region was secondarily involved with a teratoma in two *neonates with facial teratoma* associated with the presence of a craniopharyngeal canal (483, 484).

Teratomas are complex neoplasms that contain a variety of well-differentiated tissues derived from all three germinal layers. Russell and Rubinstein separate them into *mature teratomas* formed by well-differentiated representatives of all three layers, including neuroectodermal, and *immature teratomas* made of less differentiated elements derived from all or any of the three germinal layers (485). In the mature forms, solid or cystic foci of squamous epithelium are mixed with glandular or tubular structures lined by columnar or cuboidal epithelium separated by mesenchymal stroma. Glial and neuronal tissue is found, and cartilage is occasionally present (Fig. 13–61). Immunoperoxidase staining depends on which tissues are present.

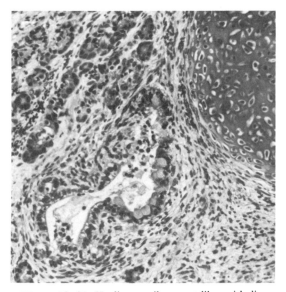

Figure 13–61. Hyaline cartilage, gut-like epithelium, glandular acini and mesodermal stroma characterize this teratoma (H & E; ×130).

Teratomas are not usually confused with other tumors when elements of all three germinal layers are present. Confusion arises primarily from *inadequate sampling*. As with all germ cell tumors, surgical sampling should be complete for an adequate diagnosis.

Histologically immature elements that are prognostically important most frequently belong to embryonal neuroepithelial structures of medulloepithelioma, neuroblastoma, retinoblastoma or ependymoblastoma (485).

The survival rate for patients with immature teratomas was found to be similar to those with embryonal carcinomas and endodermal sinus tumors. Half of the patients died within the first year (486).

REFERENCES

1. McKeever PE, Balentine JD. Histochemistry of the nervous system. In: Spicer SS (ed). Histochemistry in Pathologic Disease. Vol 22. In: Schwartz MK (ed). Clinical and Biochemical Analysis. New York, Marcel Dekker, 1987, pp 873–881.
2. McKeever PE, Blaivas M. Surgical pathology of the brain, spinal cord and meninges. In: Sternberg S, Antonioli D, Kempson R, Carter D, Eggleston J, Oberman H (eds). Diagnosis in Surgical Pathology. Vol 1. New York, Raven, 1989, pp 320–327.
3. Mills SE, Fechner RE. Undifferentiated neoplasms of the sinonasal region: Differential diagnosis based on clinical, light microscopic, immunohistochemical, and ultrastructural features. Semin Diagn Pathol 6:316–328, 1989.
4. Burger PC, Scheithauer BW, Vogel FS. Surgical Pathology of the Nervous System and Its Coverings. 3rd Ed. New York, Churchill Livingstone, 1991, pp 536–554.
5. Kepes JJ. Transitional cell tumor of the pituitary gland developing from a Rathke's cleft cyst. Cancer 41: 337–343, 1978.
6. McKeever PE, Blaivas M. Surgical pathology of the brain, spinal cord and meninges. In: Sternberg S, Antonioli D, Kempson R, Carter D, Eggleston J, Oberman H (eds). Diagnosis in Surgical Pathology. Vol 1. New York, Raven, 1989, pp 326–346.
7. Lana-Peixoto MA, Pittella JE, Arouca EM. Primary intracranial tumors: Analysis of a series of consecutive autopsies and biopsies. Arquivos de Neuroi-Psiquiatria 39:13–24, 1981.
8. Burger PC, Scheithauer BW, Vogel FS. Surgical Pathology of the Nervous System and Its Coverings. 3rd Ed. New York, Churchill Livingstone, 1991, pp 34–39.
9. Volpe R, Mazabraud A. A clinicopathologic review of 25 cases of chordoma. Am J Surg Pathol 7:161–170, 1983.
10. Austin MB, Mills SE. Neoplasms and neoplasm-like lesions involving the skull base. Ear, Nose Throat 65:25–52, 1986.
11. Perzin KH, Pushparaj N. Nonepithelial tumors of the nasal cavity, paranasal sinuses, and nasopharynx. Cancer 57:784–796, 1986.
12. Franquemont DW, Katsetos CD, Ross GW. Fatal acute pontocerebellar hemorrhage due to an unsuspected spheno-occipital chordoma. Arch Pathol Lab Med 113:1075–1078, 1989.
13. Kendall BE. Cranial chordomas. Br J Radiol 50:687–698, 1977.
14. Launay M, Fredy D, Merland JJ, Bories J. Narrowing and occlusion of arteries by intracranial tumors: Review of the literature and report of 25 cases. Neuroradiology 14:117–126, 1977.
15. Koga N, Kadota Y, Hatashita S, Hosaka Y, Sugamura J, Sakakibara T, Takagi S. A case of clivus chordoma showing hemorrhage in the posterior fossa. No Shinkei Geka 16:1417–1421, 1988.
16. Kontozoglou T, Qizilbash AH, Sianos J, Stead R. Chordoma: Cytologic and immunocytochemical study of four cases. Diagn Cytopathol 2:55–61, 1986.
17. Marigil MA, Pardo-Mindan FJ, Joly M. Diagnosis of chordoma by cytologic examination of cerebrospinal fluid. Am J Clin Pathol 80:402–403, 1983.
18. Apaja-Sarkkinen M, Vaananen K, Curran S, Siponen P, Autio-Harmainen H. Carcinomatous features of cervical chordoma in a fine needle aspirate. Acta Cytologica 31:769–773, 1987.
19. Finley JL, Silverman JF, Dabbs DJ, West RL, Dickens A, Felman PS, Frable WJ. Chordoma: Diagnosis by fine-needle aspiration biopsy with histologic, immunocytochemical, and ultrastructural confirmation. Diagn Cytopathol 2:330–337, 1986.
20. Nakajima T, Kameya T, Watanabe S, Hirota T, Sato Y, Shimosato Y. An immunoperoxidase study of S-100 protein distribution in normal and neoplastic tissues. Am J Surg Pathol 6:715–727, 1982.
21. Nakamura Y, Becker LE, Marks A. S-100 protein in human chordoma and human and rabbit notochord. Arch Pathol Lab Med 107:118–120, 1983.
22. Weiss SW, Langloss JM, Enzinger FM. Value of S-100 protein in the diagnosis of soft tissue tumors with particular reference to benign and malignant Schwann cell tumors. Lab Invest 3:299–308, 1983.
23. Miettinen M, Lehto V-P, Dahl D, Virtanen I. Differential diagnosis of chordoma, chondroid, and ependymal tumors as aided by anti-intermediate filament antibodies. Am J Pathol 112:160–169, 1983.
24. Seidman MD, Nichols RD, Raju UB, Mehta B, Levy HG. Extracranial skull base chondrosarcoma. Ear Nose Throat J 68:626–632, 1989.
25. Salisbury JR, Isaacson P. Demonstration of cytokeratins and an epithelial membrane antigen in chordomas and human fetal blood. Am J Surg Pathol 9:791–797, 1985.
26. Salisbury JR. Demonstration of cytokeratin: An epithelial membrane antigen in chondroid chordoma. J Pathol 153:37–40, 1987.
27. Rutherfoord GS, Davies AG. Chordomas—ultrastructure and immunohistochemistry: A report based on the examination of six cases. Histopathology 11:775–787, 1987.
28. Okajima K, Honda I, Kitagawa T. Immunohistochemical distribution of S-100 protein in tumors and tumor-like lesions of bone and cartilage. Cancer 61:792–779, 1988.
29. Meis JM, Giraldo AA. Chordoma: An immunohistochemical study of 20 cases. Arch Pathol Lab Med 112:553–556, 1988.
30. Schmitt FC, Bacchi CE. S-100 protein: Is it useful as a tumor marker in diagnostic immunocytochemistry? Histopathology 15:281–288, 1989.

31. Bouropoulou V, Bosse A, Roessner A, Vollmer E, Edel G, Wuisman P, Harle A. Immunohistochemical investigation of chordomas: Histogenetic and differential diagnostic aspects. Curr Top Pathol 80:183–203, 1989.

32. Coindre JM, Rivel J, Trojani M, DeMascarel I, DeMascarel A. Immunohistological study in chordomas. J Pathol 150:61–63, 1986.

33. Imrie SF, Sloane JP, Ormerod MG, Styles J, Dean CJ. Detailed investigation of the diagnostic value in tumour histopathology of ICR.2, a new monoclonal antibody to epithelial membrane antigen. Histopathology 16:573–581, 1990.

34. Burger PC, Makek M, Kleihues P. Tissue polypeptide antigen staining of the chordoma and notochordal remnants. Acta Neuropathol (Berl) 70:269–272, 1986.

35. Kay S, Schatzki PF. Ultrastructural observations of a chordoma arising in the clivus. Hum Pathol 3:403–413, 1972.

36. Pardo-Mindan FJ, Guillen FJ, Villas C, Vazquez JJ. A comparative ultrastructural study of chondrosarcoma, choroid sarcoma, and chordoma. Cancer 47:2611–2619, 1981.

37. Erlandson RA, Tandler B, Lieberman PH, Higinbotham NL. Ultrastructure of human chordoma. Cancer Res 28:2115–2125, 1968.

38. Ho KL. Ecchordosis physaliphora and chordoma: A comparative ultrastructural study. Clin Neuropathol 4:77–86, 1985.

39. Brooks JJ, LiVolsi VA, Trojanowski JQ. Does chondroid chordoma exist? Acta Neuropathol 72:229–235, 1987.

40. Mierau GW, Weeks DA. Chondroid chordoma. Ultrastruct Pathol 11:731–737, 1987.

41. Ohshima T, Sakamoto M, Takasugi S, Matsumoto K, Asano N, Kouyama Y. Three cases of intracranial chordoma. Typical chordoma and chondroid chordoma. No Shinkei Geka 12:591–598, 1984.

42. Hruban RH, Traganos F, Reuter VE, Huvos AG. Chordomas with malignant spindle cell components. A DNA flow cytometric and immunohistochemical study with histogenetic implications. Am J Pathol 137:436–447, 1990.

43. Cho KG, De Armond SJ, Barnwell S, Edwards MSB, Hoshino T. Proliferative characteristics of intracranial and spinal tumors of developmental origin. Cancer 62:740–748, 1988.

44. Sibley RK, Day DL, Dehner LP, Trueworthy RC. Metastasizing chordoma in early childhood: A pathological and immunohistochemical study with review of the literature. Pediatr Pathol 7:287–301, 1987.

45. Spaar F-W, Spaar U, Markakis E. DNA in chordomas of the clivus Blumenbachi. Neurosurg Rev 13:219–229, 1990.

46. Dutton J. Intracranial solitary chondroma: Case report. J Neurosurg 49:460–462, 1978.

47. Hoffman HJ. Craniopharyngiomas. Prog Exp Tumor Res 30:325–334, 1987.

48. Richmond I, Wilson CB. Parasellar tumors in children. I. Clinical presentation, preoperative assessment, and differential diagnosis. Child's Brain 7:73–84, 1980.

49. Petito CK, DeGirolami U, Earle KM. Craniopharyngiomas. Cancer 37:1944–1952, 1976.

50. Akimura T, Kameda H, Abiko S, Aoki H, Kido T. Intrasellar craniopharyngioma. Neuroradiology 31:180–183, 1989.

51. Byrne MW, Sessions DG. Nasopharyngeal craniopharyngioma. Case report and literature review. Ann Otol Rhinol Laryngol 99:633–639, 1990.

52. Neetens A, Selosse P. Oculomotor anomalies in sellar and parasellar pathology. Opthalmologica 175:80–104, 1977.

53. Hiramatsu K, Takahashi K, Ikeda A, Arimori S. A case of intrasellar craniopharyngioma. Tokai J Exp Clin Med 12:135–140, 1987.

54. Veyama Y, Kuratsuji T, Lee JY, Yamazaki T, Hata J, Tamaoki N. Congenital giant craniopharyngioma. Acta Pathol Jpn 35:1273–1277, 1985.

55. Freeman TB, Abati AD, Topsis J, Snyder JR, Beneck D, Lehman LB. Neonatal craniopharyngioma. NY State J Med Feb:81–83, 1988.

56. Lederman GS, Recht A, Loeffler JS, Dubusson D, Kleefield J, Schnitt SJ. Craniopharyngioma in an elderly patient. Cancer 60:1077–1080, 1987.

57. Young SC, Zimmerman RA, Nowell MA, Hackney DB, Grossman RI, Goldberg HI. Giant cystic craniopharyngiomas. Neuroradiology 29:468–473, 1987.

58. Kuwabara S, Seo H, Ishikawa S. Huge, dense, cystic craniopharyngioma with unusual extensions. Case report. Neurol Med Chir (Tokyo) 2737–41, 1987.

59. Hazen S, Friedberg SR, Thomas C, Wallman J, Clerkin EP, Lo TCM. Multiple distinct intracranial tumors: Association of pinealoma and craniopharyngioma. Surg Neurol 31:381–386, 1989.

60. Takahashi J, Makita Y, Nabeshima S, Tei T, Keyaki A, Miyamoto Y, Yagura T, Hamada S, Shoji K, Kitamura H, Hatabu H, Sano A, Kuroda Y. Craniopharyngioma associated with parathyroid adenoma, cerebral arteriovenous malformations, and persistent superior vena cava. Neurol Med Chir (Tokyo) 289:200–204, 1988.

61. Tsuji N, Kuriyama T, Iwamoto M, Shizuki K. Moya-moya disease associated with craniopharyngioma. Surg Neurol 21:588–592, 1984.

62. Ho KC, Meyer G, Cava J, Tieu TM, Prentiss A. Craniopharyngioma and "reactive" subependymoma of the third ventricle—a case report. Clin Neuropathol 6:12–15, 1987.

63. Strom EH, Tangsrud S-E. Craniopharyngioma in a body with centronuclear (myotubular) myopathy: Clinical and postmortem findings. Clin Neuropathol 5:84–87, 1986.

64. Patrick BS, Smith RR, Bailey TO. Aseptic meningitis due to spontaneous rupture of craniopharyngioma cyst. J Neurosurg 41:387–390, 1974.

65. Krueger DW, Larson EB. Recurrent fever of unknown origin, coma and meningismus due to a leaking craniopharyngioma. Am J Med 84:543–545, 1988.

66. Okamoto H, Harada K, Uozumi T, Goishi J. Spontaneous rupture of a craniopharyngioma cyst. Surg Neurol 24:507–510, 1985.

67. Burger PC, Vogel FS. Surgical Pathology of the Nervous System and its Coverings. 2nd Ed. New York, John Wiley & Sons, 1982, p 514.

68. Goodrich JT, Post KD, Duffy P. Ciliated craniopharyngioma. Surg Neurol 24:105–111, 1985.

69. Giangaspero F, Burger PC, Osborne DR, Stein RB. Suprasellar papillary squamous epithelioma ("papillary craniopharyngioma"). Am J Surg Pathol 8:57–64, 1984.

70. Crotty T, Scheithauer B, Young W, Davis D, Miller G, Burger P. Papillary craniopharyngiomas: Clinicopathologic features of 34 cases. Abstract. US

and Canada Academy of Pathology Annual Meeting, Chicago, March 17–22, 1991.

71. Sato K, Kubota T, Yamamoto S, Ishikura A. An ultrastructural study of mineralization in craniopharyngioma. J Neuropathol Exp Neurol 45:463–470, 1986.

72. Aza SL, Kovaks K, Bilbao JM, Penz G. Immunohistochemical localization of keratin in craniopharyngiomas and squamous cell nests of the human pituitary. Acta Neuropathol 54:257–260, 1981.

73. Cho KG, De Armond SJ, Barnwell S, Edwards MSB, Hoshino T. Proliferative characteristics of intracranial and spinal tumors of developmental origin. Cancer 62:740–748, 1988.

74. Franzini A, Ferraresi S, Giorgi C, Costa A, Alleganza A, Broggi G. Cell kinetic investigations in brain tumors studied by serial stereotactic biopsy. J Neuroncol 7:373–379, 1989.

75. Nelson GA, Bastian FO, Schlitt M, White RL. Malignant transformation in craniopharyngioma. Neurosurgery 22:427–429, 1988.

76. Barloon TY, Yuh WTC, Sato Y, Sickels WJ. Frontal lobe implantation of craniopharyngioma by repeated needle aspirations. AJNR 9:406–407, 1988.

77. Adamson TE, Wiestler OD, Kleihues P, Yasargil MG. Correlation of clinical and pathological features in surgically treated craniopharyngiomas. J Neurosurg 73:12–17, 1990.

78. Kahn EA, Gosch HH, Seeger JF, Hicks SP. Forty-five years experience with the craniopharyngiomas. Surg Neurol 1:5–12, 1973.

79. Szeifert GT, Julow J, Slowik F, Balint K, Lanyi F, Pasztor E. Pathological changes in cystic craniopharyngiomas following intracavital ^{90}Yttrium treatment. Acta Neurochir (Wien) 102:14–18, 1990.

80. Klonoff DC, Kahn DG, Rosenzweig W, Wilson CB. Hyperprolactinemia in a patient with a pituitary and an ovarian dermoid tumor: Case report. Neurosurgery 26:335–339, 1990.

81. Mortada A. Dermoid cysts of greater wing of sphenoid bone. Br J Ophthalmol 2:131–133, 1970.

82. Lippe BM, Edwards MSB, Braunstein GD, Halks-Miller M. A nonmalignant teratoma secreting HCG: Expanding the spectrum of ectopic hormone production. J Pediatr 105:765–768, 1984.

83. Hashimoto T, Kubota S, Shimizu T, Beppu T. A case of suprasellar tumor associated with so-called atypical angina pectoris. No Shinkei Geka (Neurol Surg) 4:979–984, 1976.

84. McKeever PE, Blaivas M. Surgical pathology of the brain, spinal cord and meninges. In: Sternberg S, Antonioli D, Kempson R, Carter D, Eggleston J, Oberman H (eds). Diagnosis in Surgical Pathology. Vol 1. New York, Raven, 1989, pp 345–346.

85. Okamoto S, Handa H, Yamashita J, Ishikawa M, Nagasawa S. Computed tomography of intra- and suprasellar epithelial cysts (symptomatic Rathke cleft cysts). Am J Neuroradiol 6:515–519, 1985.

86. Rubinstein LJ. Tumors of the Central Nervous System. Washington, DC, Armed Forces Institute of Pathology, 1972, pp 288–292.

87. McKeever PE, Blaivas M. Surgical pathology of the brain, spinal cord and meninges. In: Sternberg S, Antonioli D, Kempson R, Carter D, Eggleston J, Oberman H (eds). Diagnosis in Surgical Pathology. Vol 1. New York, Raven, 1989, pp 339–343.

88. Gyldensted C, Karle A. Computer tomography of intra- and juxtasellar lesions. Neuroradiology 14:5–14, 1977.

89. Tremblay R, Dussault J. Les tumeurs sellaires et suprasellaires. Laval Medical 38:639–646, 1967.

90. Lee BCP, Deck MDF. Sellar and juxtasellar lesions. Detection with MR. Radiology 157:143–147, 1985.

91. Mahoney W. Die Epidermoide des Zentralnervensystems. Gesamte Neurolog Psychiatr 155:416–472, 1936.

92. Sadeh M, Goldhammer Y, Schacked I, Tadmar R, Godel V. Basal encephalocele associated with suprasellar epidermoid cyst. Arch Neurol 39:250–252, 1983.

93. Tytus TS, Pennybacher J. Pearly tumours in relation to the central nervous system. J Neurol Nerosurg Psychiatry 19:241–259, 1958.

94. Salyer D, Carter D. Squamous carcinoma arising in the pituitary gland. Cancer 31:713–718, 1973.

95. Lewis AJ, Cooper PW, Kassel EE, Schwartz ML. Squamous cell carcinoma arising in suprasellar epidermoid cysts. J Neurosurg 59:538–541, 1983.

96. Russell DS, Rubinstein LJ. Pathology of Tumours of the Nervous System. Baltimore, Williams & Wilkins, 1988, pp 695–702.

97. Elkon D, Hightowser SI, Lim ML, et al. Esthesioneuroblastoma. Cancer 44:1087–1094, 1979.

98. Schochet SS Jr, Peters B, O'Neal J, McCormick WF. Intracranial esthesioneuroblastoma. A light and electron microscopic study. Acta Neuropath (Berl) 31:181–189, 1975.

99. Rosengren JE, Jing BS, Wallace S, Danziger J. Radiographic features of olfactory neuroblastoma. AJR 132:945–948, 1979.

100. Burke DP, Gabrielsen TO, Knake JE, Seeger JF, Oberman HA. Radiology of olfactory neuroblastoma. Radiology 137:367–372, 1980.

101. Takahashi H, Ohara S, Yamada M, Ikuta F, Tanimura K, Honda Y. Esthesioneuroepithelioma: A tumor of true olfactory epithelium origin. An ultrastructural and immunohistochemical study. Acta Neuropathol (Berl) 75:147–155, 1987.

102. Hg KH, Poon WS, Poon CYF, South JR. Intracranial olfactory neuroblastoma mimicking carcinoma: Report of two cases. Histopathology 12:393–403, 1988.

103. Durham JC: Olfactory neuroblastoma. Ear Nose Throat J 68:185–186, 1989.

104. Miyaguchi M, Kitaouku S, Sakai S, Uda H. Clinical and histopathological studies of olfactory neuroblastoma. Auris Nasus Larynx 16:157–163, 1989.

105. Levine PA, Paling MR, Black WC, Cantrell RW. MRI vs high resolution CT scanning: Evaluation of the anterior skull base. Otolaryngol Head Neck Surg 96:260–267, 1987.

106. Rodas RA, Erkman-Balis B, Cahill DW. Late intracranial metastasis form esthesioneuroblastoma: Case report and review of the literature. Neurosurgery 19:622–627, 1986.

107. Reznik M, Melon J, Lambricht M, Kaschten B, Beckers A. Neuroendocrine tumor of the nasal cavity (esthesioneuroblastoma). Apropos of a case with paraneoplastic Cushing's syndrome. Ann Pathol 7:137–142, 1987.

108. Mills SE, Frierson HF Jr. Olfactory neuroblastoma. A clinicopathologic study of 21 cases. Am J Surg Pathol 9:317–327, 1985.

109. Taxy JB, Bharani NK, Mills SE, Frierson HF Jr., Gould VE. The spectrum of olfactory neural tumors. A light-microscopic immunohistochemical and ultrastructural analysis. Am J Surg Pathol 10:687–695, 1986.

110. Ross GW, Mills SE, Frankfurter A, Collins VP,

Walker CC. Immunohistochemical characterization of human olfactory neuroblastomas with multiple markers. Abstract. J Neurol Exp Neurol *47*:349, 1988.

111. Perentes E, Rubinstein LJ. Immunohistochemical recognition of human neuroepithelial tumors by anti-Leu 7 (HNK-1) monoclonal antibody. Acta Neuropathol (Berl) *69*:227–233, 1986.

112. Takahashi H, Wakabayashi K, Ikuta F, Tanimura K. Esthesioneuroblastoma: A nasal catecholamine-producing tumor of neural crest origin. Demonstration of tyrosine hydroxylase-immunoreactive tumor cells. Acta Neuropathol (Berl) *76*:522–527, 1988.

113. Curtis JL, Rubinstein LJ. Pigmented olfactory neuroblastoma. A new example of melanotic neuroepithelial neoplasm. Cancer *49*:2136–2143, 1982.

114. Ferris CA, Schnadig VJ, Quinn FB, Des Jardins L. Olfactory neuroblastoma. Cytodiagnostic features in a case with ultrastructural and immunohistochemical correlation. Acta Cytol *32*:381–385, 1988.

115. Chaudhru AP, Haar JG, Koul A, Nickerson PA. Olfactory neuroblastoma (esthesioneuroblastoma): A light and ultrastructural study of two cases. Cancer *44*:554–579, 1979.

116. Spalke G, Mennel HD, Martin G. Histogenesis of olfactory neuroblastoma. I. Electron microscopy of typical human case. Pathol Res Pract *180*:516–520, 1985.

117. Kahn LB. Esthesioneuroblastoma: A light and electron microscopic study. Hum Pathol *5*:364–371, 1974.

118. Payne CM, Smith WL, Grogan TM, Nagle RB, Paplanus SH, Palmer T. Ultrastructural morphometry distinguishes Burkitt's-like lymphomas from neuroendocrine neoplasms: Useful criteria applied to the evaluation of a poorly differentiated neuroendocrine neoplasm of the nasal cavity masquerading as Burkitt's-like lymphoma. Mod Pathol *8*:35–45, 1989.

119. Albert RW. Esthesioneuroblastoma. Ear Nose Throat J *60*:522–526, 1981.

120. Fagan MF, Rone R. Esthesioneuroblastoma: Cytologic features with differential diagnostic considerations. Diagn Cytopathol *1*:322–326, 1985.

121. Frierson HF, Mills SE, Fechner RE, Taxy JB, Levine PA. Sinonasal undifferentiated carcinoma: An aggressive neoplasm derived from Schneiderian epithelium and distinct from olfactory neuroblastoma. Am J Surg Pathol *10*:771–779, 1986.

122. Levine PA, Frierson HF Jr, Stewart FM, Mills SE, Fechner RE, Cantrell RW. Sinonasal undifferentiated carcinoma: A distinctive and highly aggressive neoplasm. Laryngoscope *97*:905–908, 1987.

123. Palma L, Spagnoli LG, Yusuf MA. Intracerebral fibroma: Light and electron microscopic study. Acta Neurochirurg *77*:152–156, 1985.

124. Zulch KJ. Brain Tumors. Their Biology and Pathology. Berlin, Springer-Verlag, 1986, p 393.

125. Frank E, Derauz J-P, de Tribolet N. Chondromyxoid fibroma of the petrous-sphenoid junction. Surg Neurol *27*:182–186, 1987.

126. Gartman JJ Jr, Powers SK, Fortune M. Pseudotumor of the sellar and parasellar areas. Neurosurgery *24*:896–901, 1989.

127. Russell DS, Rubinstein LJ. Pathology of Tumours of the Nervous System. Baltimore, Williams & Wilkins, 1988, pp 289–306.

128. Oberc-Greenwood MA, McKeever PE, Kornblith

PL, Smith BH. A human ganglioglioma containing paired helical filaments. Hum Pathol *15*:834–838, 1984.

129. Zulch KJ. Biologie und Pathologie der Hirngeschwulste. In: Olivecrona H, Tonnis W (eds). Handbuch der Neurochirugie. Vol 3. Berlin, Springer-Verlag, 1956, p 381.

130. Sima AAF, Robertson DM. Subependymal giant cell astrocytoma. An ultrastructural case study. J Neurosurg *50*:240–245, 1979.

131. Nakamura Y, Becker LE. Subependymal giant-cell tumor: Astrocytic or neuronal? Acta Neuropathol *60*:271–277, 1983.

132. Bonnin JM, Rubinstein LJ, Papasozomenos SC, Marangos PJ. Subependymal giant cell astrocytoma. Significance and possible cytogenetic implications of an immunohistochemical study. Acta Neuropathol (Berl) *62*:185–193, 1984.

133. Burchield KJ, Shaw COM, Kelly WA. A mixed functional microadenoma and ganglioneuroma of the pituitary fossa. Case report. J Neurosurg *58*:416–420, 1983.

134. Kamel OW, Horoupian DS, Silverberg GD. Mixed gangliocytoma-adenoma. A distinct neuroendocrine tumor of the pituitary fossa. Hum Pathol *20*:1198–1203, 1983.

135. Bevan JS, Asa SL, Rossi ML, Esiri MM, Adams CBT, Burke CW. Intracellular gangliocytoma containing gastrin and growth hormone-releasing hormone associated with a growth hormone-secreting pituitary adenoma. Clin Endocrinol *30*:213–224, 1989.

136. Asa SL, Scheithauer BW, Bilbao JM, Horvath E, Ryan N, Kovacs K, Randall RV, Laws ER Jr, Suiger W, Ainfoot JA, Thorner MO, Vale W. A case of hypothalamic acromegaly: A clinicopathological study of six patients with hypothalamic gangliocytomas producing growth hormone-releasing factor. J Clin Endocrinol Metab *58*:796–803, 1984.

137. Burger PC, Scheithauer BW, Vogel FS. Surgical Pathology of the Nervous System and Its Coverings. 3rd Ed. New York, Churchill Livingstone, 1991, pp 388–398.

138. Jennings MT, Gelman R, Hochberg F. Intracranial germ-cell tumors: Natural history and pathogenesis. J Neurosurg *63*:155–167, 1985.

139. Inoue HK, Haganuma H, Ono N. Pathobiology of intracranial germ-cell tumors: Immunocytochemical, immunohistochemical, and electron microscopic investigations. J Neurooncol *5*:105–115, 1987.

140. Harms D, Janig U. Germ cell tumours of childhood. Report of 170 cases including 59 pure and partial yolk-sac tumours. Virchows Arch *409*:223–239, 1986.

141. Karnaze MG, Sartor K, Winthrop JD, Gado MH, Hodges FJ. Suprasellar lesions: Evaluation with MR imaging? Radiology *161*:77–82, 1986.

142. Fetell MR, Stein BM. Neuroendocrine aspects of pineal tumors. Neurol Clin *4*:877–905, 1986.

143. Ghatak NR, Hirano A, Zimmerman HM. Intrasellar germinomas: A form of ectopic pinealoma. J Neurosurg *31*:670, 1969.

144. Page RB, Plourde PV, Coldwell D, Heald JI, Weinstein J. Intrasellar mixed germ-cell tumor: Case report. J Neurosurg *58*:766, 1983.

145. Buchfelder M, Fahlbusch R, Walther M, Mann K. Endocrine disturbances in suprasellar germinomas. Acta Endocrinol (Copenh) *120*:337–342, 1989.

146. Legido A, Packer RJ, Sutton LN, D'Angio G, Rorke

LB, Bruce DA, Schut L. Suprasellar germinomas in childhood. Cancer *63*:340–344, 1989.

147. Konig R, Schonberger W, Grimm W. Mediastinal teratocarcinoma and hypophyseal stalk germinoma in a patient with Klinefelter syndrome. Klin Padiatr *202*:53–56, 1990.

148. Sugita K, Izumi T, Yamaguchi K, Fukuyama Y, Sato A, Kajita A. Cornelia de Lange syndrome associated with a suprasellar germinoma. Brain Dev *8*:541–546, 1986.

149. Shuangshoti S. Combined occurence of third ventricular germinoma and hypothalamic mixed glioma. J Surg Oncol *31*:148–152, 1986.

150. Karnaze MG, Sartor K, Winthrop JD, Gado MH, Hodges FJ. Suprasellar lesions: Evaluation with MR imaging. Radiology *161*:77–82, 1986.

151. Shen DY, Guay AT, Silverman ML, Hybels RL, Freidberg SR. Primary intrasellar germinoma in a woman presenting with secondary amenorrhea and hyperprolactemia. *15*:417–420, 1984.

152. Baskin DS, Wilson CB. Transsphenoidal surgery of intrasellar germinomas. Report of two cases. J Neurosurg *59*:1063–1066, 1983.

153. Kraichoke S, Cosgrove M, Chandrasoma PT. Granulomatous inflammation in pineal germinoma. A cause of diagnostic failure of stereotaxic brain biopsy. Am J Surg Pathol *12*:655–660, 1988.

154. Ono N, Inoue HK, Naganuma H, Kunimine H, Zama A, Tamura M. Diagnosis of germinal neoplasm in the thalamus and basal ganglia. Surg Neurol *26*:24–28, 1986.

155. Koide O, Iwai S, Kanno T, Kanda S. Isoenzymes of alkaline phosphatase in germinoma cells. Am J Clin Pathol *89*:611–616, 1988.

156. Wick MR, Swanson PE, Manivel JC. Placental-like alkaline phosphatase reactivity in human tumors: An immunohistochemical study of 520 cases. Hum Pathol *18*:946–954, 1987.

157. Saint-Andre JP, Alhenc-Gelas F, Rohmer V, Chretien MF, Bigorgne JC, Corvol P. Angiotensin-I-converting enzyme in germinomas. Hum Pathol *19*:208–213, 1988.

158. Rohmer V, Saint-Andre JP, Alhenc-Gelas F, Corval P, Vigorgne JC. Angiotensin I-converting enzyme in a suprasellar germinoma. Am J Clin Pathol *87*:281–284, 1987.

159. Yamagami T, Handa H, Yamashita J, Okumura T, Paine J, Haebara H, Furukawa F. An immunohistochemical study of intracranial germ cell tumours. Acta Neurochir *86*:33–41, 1987.

160. Scheithauer BW. Pathology of the pituitary and the sellar region: Exclusive of pituitary adenoma. In: Sommers SC, Rosen PP, Fechner RE (eds). Pathology. Norwalk, CT, Appleton-Century-Crofts, 1985, pp 67–155.

161. Nakagawa Y, Perentes E, Ross GW, Ross AN, Rubinstein LJ. Immunohistochemical differences between intracranial germinomas and their gonadal equivalents. An immunoperoxidase study of germ cell tumours with epithelial membrane antigen, cytokeratin, and vimentin. J Pathol *156*:67–72, 1988.

162. Vaquero J, Coca S, Magallon R, Ponton P, Martinez R. Immunohistochemical study of natural killer cells in tumor-infiltrating lymphocytes of primary intracranial germinomas. J Neurosurg *72*:616–618, 1990.

163. Sawamura Y, Hamou MF, Kuppner MC, de Tribolet N. Immunohistochemical and in vitro functional analysis of pineal-germinoma infiltrating lymphocytes: Report of a case. Neurosurgery *25*:454–457, 1989.

164. Saito T, Tanaka R, Kouno M, Washiyama K, Abe S, Kumanishi T. Tumor-infiltrating lymphocytes and histocompatibility antigens in primary intracranial germinomas. J Neurosurg *70*:81–85, 1989.

165. Paine JT, Handa H, Yamasaki T, Yamashita J. Suprasellar germinoma with shunt metastasis: Report of a case with an immunohistochemical characterization of the lymphocyte subpopulations. Surg Neurol *25*:55–61, 1986.

166. Ulbright TM, Roth LM, Brodhecker CA. Yolk sac differentiation in germ cell tumors. Am J Surg Pathol *10*:151–164, 1986.

167. Koide O, Iwai S, Matsumura H. Intranuclear membranous profiles in germinoma cells—a variant of nuclear pockets and intranuclear annulate lamellae. Acta Pathol Jpn *35*:605–619.

168. Hassoun J, Gambarelli D, Pellissier JF, Henin D, Toga M. Germinomas of the brain. Light and electron microscopic study. A report of seven cases. Acta Neuropathol (Suppl) (Berl) *7*:105–108, 1981.

169. Matsumura H, Setoguti T, Mori K, Ross ER, Koto A. Endothelial tubuloreticular structures in intracranial germinomas. Acta Pathol Jpn *34*:1–9, 1984.

170. Tabachi K, Yamada O, Nishimoto A. The ultrastructure of pinealomas. Acta Neuropathol (Berl) *24*:117, 1973.

171. Delahunt B. Suprasellar germinoma with probable extracranial metastases. Pathology *14*:215–218, 1982.

172. Ostertag CB, Volk B, Shibata T, Burger P, Kleihues P. The monoclonal antibody Ki-67 as a marker for proliferating cells in stereotactic biopsies of brain tumours. Acta Neurochir *89*:117–121, 1987.

173. Viale GL. Giant cell tumours of the sellar region. Acta Neurochir *38*:259–268, 1977.

174. Jacas R, and Bermejo A. Giant cell tumors of the sellar region. Acta Neurochirurgica (Suppl) *28*:416–417, 1979.

175. Wolfe JT, Scheithauer BW, Dahlin DC. Giant cell tumor of the sphenoid bone. Review of 10 cases. J Neurosurg *59*:322–327, 1983.

176. Martins AN, Dean DF. Giant cell tumor of sphenoid bone: Malignant transformation following radiotherapy. Surg Neurol *2*:105–107, 1974.

177. Wu KK, Ross PM, Mitchell DC, Sprague HH. Evolution of a case of multicentric giant cell tumor over a 23-year period. Clin Orthop Rel Res *213*:279–288, 1986.

178. Monda L, Wick MR. S-100 protein immunostaining in the differential diagnosis of chondroblastoma. Hum Pathol *16*:287–293, 1985.

179. Sara AS, Ayala AG, El-Naggar A, Ro JY, Raymond AK, Murray JA. Giant cell tumor of bone. A clinicopathologic and DNA flow cytometric analysis. Cancer *66*:2186–2190, 1990.

180. Huang CI, Chiou WH, Ho DM. Oligodendroglioma occurring after radiation therapy for pituitary adenoma. J Neurol Neurosurg Psychiatry *50*:1619–1624, 1987.

181. Kitanaka C, Shitara N, Nakagomi T, Nakamura H, Genka S, Nakagawa K, Akanuma A, Aoyama H, Takakura K. Postradiation astrocytoma: Report of two cases. J Neurosurg *70*:469–474, 1989.

182. Suda Y, Mineura K, Kowada M, Ohishi H. Malignant astrocytoma following radiotherapy in pitui-

tary adenoma: Case report. No Shinkei Geka 17:783–788, 1989.

183. Hufnagel TJ, Kim JH, Lesser R, Miller JM, Abrahams JJ, Piepmeier J, Manuelidis EE. Malignant glioma of the optic chiasm eight years after radiotherapy for prolactinoma. Arch Ophthalmol 106:1701–1705, 1988.

184. Zampieri P, Zorat PL, Mingrino S, Soattin GB. Radiation-associated cerebral gliomas. A report of two cases and review of the literature. J Neurosurg Sci 33:271–279, 1989.

185. Komaki S, Komaki R, Choi H, Correa-Paz F. Radiation and drug induced intracranial neoplasm with angiographic demonstration. Neurol Med Chir (Tokyo) 17:55–62, 1977.

186. Sogg RL, Donaldson SS, Yorke CH. Malignant astrocytoma following radiotherapy of a craniopharyngioma. J Neurosurg 48:622–627, 1978.

187. Gutjahr P, Dieterich E. Risiko zweiter manligne Neoplasien nach erfolgreicher Tumor behandlung im Kindersalter. Dtsch Med Wochenschr 104:969–972, 1979.

188. Piatt JH Jr, Blue JM, Schold SC Jr, Burger PC. Glioblastoma multiforme after radiotherapy for acromegaly. Neurosurgery 13:85–89, 1983.

189. Liwnicz BH, Berger TS, Liwnicz RG, Aron BS. Radiation-associated gliomas: A report of four cases and analysis of postradiation tumors of the central nervous system. Neurosurgery 17:436–445, 1985.

190. Maat-Schiemann MLC, Bots GTAM, Thomeer RTWM, Vielvoye GJ. Malignant astrocytoma following radiotherapy for craniopharyngioma. Br J Radiol 48:480–482, 1985.

191. Maruc G, Levin VC, Rutherfoord GS. Malignant glioma following radiotherapy for unrelated primary tumors. Cancer 58:886–894, 1986.

192. Ushio Y, Arita N, Yoshimine T, Nagatani M, Mogami H. Glioblastoma after radiotherapy for craniopharyngioma: Case report. Neurosurgery 21:33–38, 1987.

193. McKeever PE, Blaivas M. Surgical pathology of the brain, spinal cord and meninges. In: Sternberg S, Antonioli D, Kempson R, Carter D, Eggleston J, Oberman H (eds). Diagnosis in Surgical Pathology. Vol 1. New York, Raven, 1989, pp 317–318, 330, 346–348.

194. Masunaga S-I, Ono K, Abe M. A method for the selective measurement of the radiosensitivity of quiescent cells in solid tumors—combination of immunofluorescence staining of BrdU and Micronucleus Assay. Radiat Res 125:243–247, 1991.

195. Schmitt HP. Rapid anaplastic transformation in gliomas of adulthood. "Selection" in neuro-oncogenesis. Pathol Res Pract 176:313–318, 1983.

196. McKeever PE, Balentine JD. Histochemistry of the nervous system. In: Spicer SS (ed). Histochemistry in Pathologic Disease. Vol 22. In: Schwartz MK (ed). Clinical and Biochemical Analysis. New York, Marcel Dekker, 1987, pp 920–936.

197. Asa SL, Kovacs K, Horvath E, Ezrin C, Weiss MH. Sellar glomangioma. Ultrastruct Pathol 7:49–54, 1984.

198. Enzinger FM, Weiss SW. Soft Tissue Tumors. 2nd Ed. St Louis, CV Mosby, 1988, pp 581–959.

199. Kim YI, Kim JH, Suh JS, Ham EK, Suh KP. Glomus tumor of the trachea. Report of a case with ultrastructural observation. Cancer 64:881–886, 1989.

200. Rubinstein LJ. Tumors of the Nervous System. Washington, DC, Armed Forces Institute of Pathology, 1972, pp 314–315.

201. Mey vander AGL, Maaswinkel-Mooy PD, Cornelisse CJ, Schmidt PH, Kamp van de JJP. Genomic imprinting in hereditary glomus tumors: Evidence for new genetic theory. Lancet 8675:1292–1294, 1989.

202. Harvey JS, Walker F. Solid glomus tumor of the pterygoid fossa: A lesion mimicking an epithelial neoplasm of low-grade malignancy. Hum Pathol 18:965–966, 1987.

203. Gould EW, Manivel JC, Albores-Saavedra J, Monforte H. Locally infiltrative glomus tumors and glomangiosarcomas. Cancer 65:310–318, 1990.

204. Nuovo MA, Grimes MM, Knowles DM. Glomus tumors: A clinicopathologic and immunohistochemical analysis of forty cases. Surg Pathol 3:31–45, 1990.

205. Porter PL, Bigler SA, McNutt M, Gown AM. The immunophenotype of hemangiopericytomas and glomus tumors, with special reference to muscle protein expression: An immunohistochemical study and review of the literature. Mod Pathol 4:46–42, 1991.

206. Kovacs K, Horvath E. Tumors of the Pituitary Gland. Washington, DC, Armed Forces Institute of Pathology, 1986.

207. McCormick WF, Hamlmi BS. Absence of chromophobe adenomas from a large series of pituitary tumors. Arch Pathol 92:231–238, 1971.

208. Luse SA, Kernohan JW. Granular cell tumors of the stalk and posterior lobe of the pituitary gland. Cancer 8:616–622, 1955.

209. Enzinger FM, Weiss SW. Soft Tissue Tumors. 2nd Ed. St Louis, CV Mosby, 1988, pp 757–779.

210. Vaquero J, Leunda G, Gabezudo JM, Salazar AR, Miguel de J. Granular pituicytomas of the pituitary stalk. Acta Neurochir 59:209–215, 1981.

211. Becker DH, Wilson CB. Symptomatic parasellar granular cell tumor. Neurosurgery 8:173–180, 1981.

212. Russell DS, Rubinstein LJ. Pathology of Tumours of the Nervous System. 5th Ed. Baltimore, Williams & Wilkins, 1989, pp 378–573.

213. Lloyd RV, Warner TF. Immunohistochemistry of neuron-specific enolase. In: DeLellis RA (ed). Advances in Immunohistochemistry, Maison, 1984, pp 127–140.

214. Nathrath WBJ, Remberger K. Immunohistochemical study of granular cell tumors. Demonstration of neurone specific enolase, S100 protein, laminin and alpha-1-antichymotrypsin. Virchows Arch (Pathol Anat) 408:421–434, 1986.

215. Liwnicz BH, Liwnicz RG, Huff JS, McBride BH, Tew JM. Giant granular cell tumor of the suprasellar area: Immunohistochemical and electron microscopic studies. Neurosurgery 15:246–251, 1984.

216. Gambini C, Ruelle A, Palladino M, Boccardo M. Intracerebral granular cell tumor. Case report. Pathologica 82:83–88, 1990.

217. Dickson DW, Suzuki KI, Kanner R, Weitz S, Horoupian DS. Cerebral granular cell tumor: Immunohistochemical and electron microscopic study. J Neuropathol Exp Neurol 45:304–314, 1986.

218. Nakamura T, Hirato J, Hotchi M, Kyoshima K, Nakamura Y. Astrocytoma with granular cell tumor-like changes. Report of a case with histochem-

ical and ultrastructural characterization of granular cells. Acta Pathol Jpn *40*:206–211, 1990.

219. Thunold S, Von Eyben FE, Maehle B. Malignant granular cell tumor of the neck: Immunohistochemical and ultrastructural studies of a case. Histopathology *14*:655–662, 1989.

220. O'Donovan DG, Kell P. Malignant granular cell tumor with intraperitoneal dissemination. Histopathology *14*:417–428, 1989.

221. Rosenthal SA, Livolsi VA, Turrisi AT III. Adjuvant radiotherapy for recurrent granular cell tumor. Cancer *65*:897–900, 1990.

222. Russell D, Rubinstein LJ. Pathology of Tumours of the Nervous System. Baltimore, Williams & Wilkins, 1988, pp 711–717.

223. Schmidt E, Hallervorden J, Spatz J. Die Entstehung der Hamartome am Hypothalamus mit und ohne Pubertas praecox. Dtsch Z Nervenheilk *177*:235–262, 1957.

224. Wolman L, Balmforth GV. Precocious puberty due to a hypothalamic hamartoma in a patient surviving to late middle age. J Neurol Neurosurg Psychiatry *26*:275–280, 1963.

225. Asa SL, Bilbao JM, Kovacs K, Linfoot JA. Hypothalmic neuronal hamartoma associated with pituitary growth hormone cell adenoma and acromegaly. Acta Neuropathol *52*:231–234, 1980.

226. Scheithauer BW, Kovacs K, Randall RV, Horvath E, Okazaki H, Laws ER. Hypothalamic neuronal hamartoma and adenohypophyseal neuronal choristoma: Their association with growth hormone adenoma of the pituitary gland. J Neuropathol Exp Neurol *42*:633–648, 1983.

227. Slowik F, Fazekas I, Balint K, Gazso L, Pasztor E, Czirjak D, Lapis K. Intrasellar hamartoma associated with pituitary adenoma. Acta Neuropathol *80*:328–333, 1990.

228. Graber H, Kersting G. Pubertas praecox bei Hamartie des mediobasalen Hypothalamus mit heterotoper Retinaanlage. Dtsch Z Nervenheilk *173*:1–11, 1955.

229. Hall JG, Pallister PD, Clarren SK, Beckwith JB, Wiglesworth FW, Fraser FL, Cho S, Benke PJ, Reed SD. Congenital hypothalamic hamartoblastoma, hypopituitarism, imperforate anus, and postaxial polydactyly—a new syndrome? 1. Clinical, causal and pathogenic considerations. Am J Med Genet 7:47–74, 1980.

230. Nurbai MA, Tomlinson BE, Lorigan-Forsythe B. Infantile hypothalamic hamartoma with multiple congenital abnormalities. Neuropathol Appl Neurobiol *11*:61–70, 1985.

231. Rho YM. Von Hippel-Lindau's disease: A report of five cases. Can Med Assoc J *101*:135–142, 1969.

232. Dan NG, Smith DE. Pituitary hemangioblastoma in a patient with von Hippel-Lindau disease. Case report. J Neurosurg *42*:232–235, 1975.

233. Grisoli F, Gambarelli D, Raybaud C, Guibout M, Leclercq T. Suprasellar hemangioblastoma. Surg Neurol *22*:257–262, 1984.

234. Kupersmith MJ, Berenstein A. Visual disturbances in von Hippel-Lindau disease. Ann Ophthalmol *Feb*:195–197, 1981.

235. Kepes JJ, Rengachary SS, Lee SH. Astrocytes in hemangioblastomas of the central nervous system and their relationship to stromal cells. Acta Neuropathol (Berlin) *47*:99–104, 1979.

236. Deck JHN, Rubinstein LJ. Glial fibrillary acidic protein in stromal cells of some capillary heman-

gioblastomas: Significance and possible implications of an immunoperoxidase study. Acta Neuropathol (Berlin) *54*:173–181, 1981.

237. Tanimura A, Nakamura V, Hachisuka H, Tanimura Y, Fukumura A. Hemangioblastoma of the central nervous system: Nature of the stromal cells as studied by the immunoperoxidase technique. Hum Pathol *15*:866–869, 1984.

238. Kochi N, Tani E, Kaba K, Natsume S. Immunohistochemical study of fibronectin in hemangioblastomas and hemangiopericytomas. Acta Neuropathol (Berlin) *64*:229–233, 1984.

239. Kamitani H, Masauzawa H, Sato J, Kanazawa I. Capillary hemangioblastoma: Histogenesis of stromal cells. Acta Neuropathol (Berlin) *73*:370–378, 1987.

240. Feldenzer JA, McKeever PE. Selective localization of γ-enolase in stromal cells of cerebellar hemangioblastomas. Acta Neuropathol (Berlin) *72*:281–285, 1987.

241. Ironside JW, Stephenson TJ, Royds JA, Mills PM, Taylor CB, Rider CC, Timperley WR. Stromal cells in cerebellar haemangioblastomas: An immunohistochemical study. Histopathology *12*:29–40, 1988.

242. Grant JW, Gallagher PJ, Hedinger C. Hemangioblastoma. An immunohistochemical study of ten cases. Acta Neuropathol *76*:82–86, 1988.

243. Frank TS, Trojanowski JQ, Roberts SA, Brooks JJ. A detailed immunohistochemical analysis of cerebellar hemangioblastoma: An undifferentiated mesenchymal tumor. Mod Pathol *2*:638–651, 1989.

244. Ho K-L. Ultrastructure of cerebellar capillary hemangioblastoma. I. Weibel-Palade bodies and stromal cell histiogenesis. J Neuropathol Exp Neurol *43*:592–608, 1984.

245. Kawamura J, Garcia JH, Kamijyo Y. Cerebellar hemangiomas: Histogenesis of stromal cells. Cancer *31*:1528–1540.

246. Mills SE, Ross GW, Perentes E, Nakagawa Y, Scheithauer BW. Cerebellar hemangioblastoma: Immunohistochemical distinction from metastatic renal cell carcinoma. Surg Pathol *3*:121–132, 1990.

247. Clelland CA, Treips CS. Histological differentiation of metastatic renal carcinoma in the cerebellum from cerebellar hemangioblastoma in von Hippel-Lindau's disease. J Neurol Neurosurg Psychiatry *52*:162–166, 1989.

248. Bohling T, Haltia M, Rosenlof K, Fyhrquist F. Erythropoietin in capillary hemangioblastoma. An immunohistochemical study. Acta Neuropathol (Berlin) *74*:324–328, 1987.

249. Crocker J, Carey MP, Allcock R. Hemangioblastoma and renal clear cell carcinoma distinguished by means of the AgNOR method. Am J Clin Pathol *93*:555–557, 1990.

250. Chaudhry AP, Moutes M, Cohn GA. Ultrastructure of cerebellar hemangioblastoma. Cancer *42*:1834–1838, 1978.

251. Mann BS, Geddes JF. The nature of cytoplasmic inclusion in cerebellar hemangioblastomas. Acta Neuropathol (Berlin) *67*:174–176, 1985.

252. Voigt K, Yasargil MG. Cerebral cavernous hemangiomas or cavernomas. Neurochirurgia *19*:59–68, 1976.

253. Kawai K, Fukui M, Tanaka A, Kuramoto S, Kitamura K. Extracerebral cavernous hemangioma of the middle fossa. Surg Neurol *9*:19–25, 1978.

254. Shimabukuro H, Shinoda S, Yamada N, Iwasa H, Masuzawa T, Sato F. Parasellar cavernous heman-

gioma presenting with hyperprolactinemia. Case report. Neurol Med Chir (Tokyo) _24_:212–216, 1984.

255. Sansone ME, Liwnicz BH, Mandybur TI. Giant pituitary cavernous hemangioma. Case report. J Neurosurg _53_:124–126, 1980.

256. Moore T, Ganti SR, Mawad ME, Hilal SK. CT and angiography of primary extradural juxtasellar tumors. AJNR _145_:491–496, 1985.

257. Gray MH, Rosenberg AE, Dickersin GR, Bhan AK. Cytokeratin expression in epithelioid vascular neoplasms. Hum Pathol _21_:212–217, 1990.

258. Kumar PP, Good RR, Skultety FM, Masih AS, McComb RD. Spinal metastases from pituitary hemangiopericytic meningioma. Am J Clin Oncol _10_:428, 1987.

259. Austin MB, Mills SE. Neoplasms and neoplasm-like lesions involving the skull base. Ear Nose Throat J _65_:57–73, 1986.

260. Kumar PP, Good RR, Cox TA, Leibrock LG, Skultety FM. Reversal of visual impairment after interstitial irradiation of pituitary tumor. Neurosurgery. _18_:82–84, 1986.

261. Nikonov AA, Matsko DE. Pituitary hemangiopericytoma. Arkh Patol _47_:79–83, 1985.

262. Yokota M, Tani E, Maeda Y, Morimura T, Kakudo K, Uematsu K. Acromegaly associated with suprasellar and pulmonary hemangiopericytomas. Case report. J Neurosurg _62_:771, 1985.

263. Mangiardi JR, Flamm ES, Cravioto H, Fisher B. Hemangiopericytoma of the pituitary fossa: Case report. Neurosurgery _13_:58–62, 1983.

264. Orf G. "Angioretikulom" der Sella turcica. Acta Neurochir (Wien) _23_:63–78, 1970.

265. Eichhorn JH, Dickersin GR, Bhan AK, Goodman ML. Sinonasal hemangiopericytoma. A reassessment with electron microscopy, immunohistochemistry, and long-term follow-up. Am J Surg Pathol _14_:856–866, 1990.

266. D'Amore ES, Manivel JC, Sung JH. Soft-tissue and meningeal hemangiopericytomas: An immunohistochemial and ultrastructural study. Hum Pathol _21_:414–423, 1990.

267. Rice CD, Kersten RC, Mrak RE. An orbital hemangiopericytoma recurrent after 33 years. Arch Opthalmol _107_:552–556, 1989.

268. Winek RR, Scheithauer BW, Wick MR. Meningioma, meningeal hemangiopericytoma (angioblastic meningioma), peripheral hemangiopericytoma, and acoustic schwannoma. A comparative immunohistochemical study. Am J Surg Pathol _13_:251–261, 1989.

269. Davidson GS, Hope J. Meningeal tumors of childhood. Cancer _63_:1205–1210, 1989.

270. Iwaki T, Fukui M, Takeshita I, Tsuneyoshi M, Tateishi J. Hemangiopericytoma of the meninges: A clinicopathologic and immunohistochemical study. Clin Neuropathol _7_:93–99, 1988.

271. McKeever PE, Blaivas M. Surgical pathology of the brain, spinal cord and meninges. In: Sternberg S, Antonioli D, Kempson R, Carter D, Eggleston J, Oberman H (eds). Diagnosis in Surgical Pathology. Vol 1. New York, Raven Press, 1989, pp 357–359.

272. Burger PC, Scheithauer BW, Vogel FS. Surgical Pathology of the Nervous System and Its Coverings. 3rd Ed. New York, Churchill Livingstone, 1991, pp 107–112.

273. Kepes JJ. Meningiomas, Biology, Pathology and Differential Diagnosis. Chicago, Year Book Medical, 1982, pp 87–92.

274. Theunissen PH, Bebets TE, Baerts M, Blaauw G. Histogenesis of intracranial haemangiopericytoma and haemangioblastoma. An immunohistochemical study. Acta Neuropathol _80_:68–71, 1990.

275. Schurch W, Skalli O, Lagace R, Seemayer TA, Gabbiani G. Intermediate filament proteins and actin isoforms as markers for soft-tissue tumor differentiation and origin. III. Hemangiopericytomas and glomus tumors. Am J Pathol _136_:77–86, 1990.

276. Dardick I, Hammar SP, Scheithauer BW. Ultrastructural spectrum of hemangiopericytoma: A comparative study of fetal, adult, and neoplastic pericytes. Ultrastruct Pathol _15_:111–154, 1989.

277. Moss TH. Immunohistochemical characteristics of haemangiopericytic meningiomas: Comparison with typical meningiomas, haemangioblastomas and haemangiopericytomas from extracranial sites. Neuropathol Appl Neurobiol _13_:467–480, 1987.

278. Miettinen M. Antibody specific to muscle actins in the diagnosis and classification of soft tissue tumors. Am J Pathol _130_:205–215, 1988.

279. Nakamura M, Inoue HK, Ono N, Kunimine H, Tamada J. Analysis of hemangiopericytic meningiomas by immunohistochemistry, electron microscopy and cell culture. J Neuropathol Exp Neurol _46_:57–71, 1987.

280. Zulch KJ. Histological Typing of Tumours of the Central Nervous System. International Histological Classification of Tumours. No 21. Geneva, World Health Organization, 1979, pp 53–55.

281. Kumar PP, Good RR, Leibrock LG, Mawk JR, Yonkers AJ, Ogren FP. High activity iodine 125 endocurietherapy for recurrent skull base tumors. Cancer _61_:1518–1527, 1988.

282. Zulch KJ. Histological Typing of Tumours of the Central Nervous System. International Histological Classification of Tumours. No 21. Geneva, World Health Organization, 1979, pp 43–50.

283. Nelson JS, Tsukada Y, Schoenfeld D, Fulling K, Lamarche J, Peress N. Necrosis as a prognostic criterion in malignant supratentorial astrocytic gliomas. Cancer _52_:550–554, 1983.

284. Hou-Jensen K, Rawlinson DG, Hendrickson M. Proliferating histiocytic lesion (Histiocytosis-X?). Cancer _32_:809–821, 1973.

285. MacCumber MW, Hoffman PN, Wand GS, Epstein JI, Beschorner WE, Green R. Ophthalmic involvement in aggressive histiocytosis X. Ophthalmology _97_:22–27, 1990.

286. Rimoin DL. Hereditary forms of growth hormone deficiency and resistance. Birth Defects _12_:15–29, 1976.

287. Hirata Y, Sakamoto N, Yoshimoto Y, Kato Y, Matsukura S. Diabetes insipidus and galactorrhea caused by histiocytosis X. Endocrinol Jpn _22_:311–318, 1975.

288. Schneider J, Guthert H. Histiocytosis X of the hypothalamus. Zentralbl Allg Pathol _119_:49–55, 1975.

289. Gates RB, Friesen H, Samaan NA. Inappropriate lactation and amenorrhea: Pathological and diagnostic considerations. Acta Endocrinol _72_:101–114, 1973.

290. Lampert IA, Catovsky D, Bergier N. Malignant histiocytosis: A clinico-pathological study of 12 cases. Br J Haematol _40_:65–77, 1978.

291. Asai A, Matsutani M, Kohno T, Fujimaki T, Tanaka H, Kawaguchi K, Koike M, Takakura K. Leptomeningeal and orbital benign lymphophagocytic histiocytes. J Neurosurg 69:610–612, 1988.

292. Lopez P, Estes ML. Immunohistochemical characterization of the histiocytes in sinus histiocytosis with massive lymphadenopathy: Analysis of an extranodal case. Hum Pathol 20:711–715, 1989.

293. Mir R, Aftalion B, Kahn LB. Sinus histiocytosis with massive lymphadenopathy and unusual extranodal manifestations. Arch Pathol Lab Med 109:867–870, 1985.

294. Moscinski LC, Kleinschmidt-DeMasters BK. Primary eosinophlic granuloma of frontal lobe. Cancer 9:284–288, 1985.

295. Eriksen B, Janinis J, Variakojis D, Winter J, Russell E, Marder R, DelCanto MC. Primary histiocytosis X of the parieto-occipital lobe. Hum Pathol 19:611–614, 1988.

296. Knobler RM, Neumann RA, Gebhart W, Radaskiewicz TH, Ferenic P, Widhalm K. Xanthoma disseminatum with progressive involvement of the central nervous and hepatobiliary systems. J Am Acad Dermatol 23:341–346, 1990.

297. Carey MP, Case CP. Sinus histiocytosis with massive lymphadenopathy presenting as a meningioma. Neuropathol Appl Neurobiol 13:391–398, 1987.

298. Kahn HJ, Thorner PS. Monoclonal antibody MT1: A marker for Langerhans cell histiocytosis. Pediatr Pathol 10:375–384, 1990.

299. Ya-You JI, Yan-Fang L, Bo-Yun W, De-Yun Y. An immunocytochemical study on the distribution of ferritin and other markers in 36 cases of malignant histiocytosis. Cancer 64:1281–1289, 1989.

300. Salisbury JR, Hall PA, Williams HC, Mangi MH, Mufti GJ. Multicentric reticulohistiocytosis. Detailed immunophenotyping confirms macrophage origin. Am J Surg Pathol 14:687–693, 1990.

301. Sacchi S, Artusi T, Selleri L, Temperani P, Zucchini P, Vecchi A, Emilia G, Torelli U. Sinus histiocytosis with massive lymphadenopathy: Immunological, cytogenetic and molecular studies. Blut 60:339–344, 1990.

302. Rabkin MS, Kjeldsberg CR, Wittwer CT, Marty J. A comparison study of two methods of peanut agglutinin staining with S-100 immunostaining in 29 cases of histiocytosis X (Langerhans' cell histiocytosis). Arch Pathol Lab Med 114:511–515, 1990.

303. Ornvold K, Ralfkiaer E, Carstensen H. Immunohistochemical study of the abnormal cells in Langerhans cell histiocytosis (histiocytosis X). Virchows Arch 416:403–410, 1990.

304. Eisen RN, Buckley PJ, Rosai J. Immunophenotypic characterization of sinus histiocytosis with massive lymphadenopathy. Semin Diagn Pathol 7:74–82, 1990.

305. Nemes Z, Thomazy V. Diagnostic significance of histiocyte-related markers in malignant histiocytosis and histiocytic lymphoma. Cancer 62:1970–1980, 1988.

306. Andreesen R, Brugger W, Sohr GW, Kross KJ. Human macrophages can express the Hodgkin's cell-associated antigen Ki-1 (CD30). Am J Pathol 134:187–192, 1989.

307. Burger PC, Scheithauer BW, Vogel FS. Surgical Pathology of the Nervous System and Its Coverings. 3rd Ed. New York, Churchill Livingstone, 1991, pp 6–13.

308. McLelland J, Newton J, Malone M, Camplejohn RS, Chu AC. A flow cytometric study of Langerhans cell histiocytosis. Br J Dermatol 120:485–491, 1989.

309. Russell DS, Rubinstein LJ. Pathology of Tumours of the Nervous System. Baltimore, Williams & Wilkins, 1988, pp 377, 378.

310. Scothorne CM. Glioma of the posterior lobe of the pituitary gland. J Pathol Bacteriol 69:109–112, 1955.

311. Liss L, Kahn EA. Pituicytoma. Tumor of the sella turcica. A clinicopathologic study. J Neurosurg 15:481–488, 1958.

312. Roggli VL, Suzuki M, Armstrong D, McGavran M. Pituitary microadenoma and primary lymphoma of brain associated with hypothalamic invasion. Am J Clin Pathol 71:724–727, 1979.

313. Patrick AW, Campbell IW, Ashworth B, Gordon A. Primary cerebral lymphoma presenting with cranial diabetes insipidus. Postgrad Med J 65:771–772, 1989.

314. Hirata K, Izaki A, Tsutsumi K, Kaminogo M, Baba H, Shibata S, Mori K, Shimada O, Tsuda N. A case of primary hypothalamic malignant lymphoma with diabetes insipidus. No Shinkei Geka 17:461–466, 1989.

315. Peters Ft, Keuning JJ, deRooy HA. Primary cerebral malignant lymphoma with endocrine defect. Case report and review of the literature. Neth J Med 29:406–410, 1986.

316. Ashworth B. Cerebral histiocytic lymphoma presenting with loss of weight. Neurology 32:894–896, 1982.

317. Case records of the Massachusetts General Hospital. Weekly clinicopathological exercises. Case 31–1982. A 50-year-old woman with an acute neurologic disorder and changing CT-scan findings. N Engl J Med 307:359–368, 1982.

318. Hadfield MG, Vennart GP, Rosenblum WI. Hypoglycemia: Invasion of the hypothalamus by lymphosarcoma. Metastasis to blood glucose regulating centers. Arch Pathol 94:317–321, 1972.

319. McKeever PE, Blaivas M. Surgical pathology of the brain, spinal cord and meninges. In: Sternberg S, Antonioli D, Kempson R, Carter D, Eggleston J, Oberman H (eds). Diagnosis in Surgical Pathology. Vol 1. New York, Raven Press, 1989, pp 351–352.

320. Garvin AJ, Spicer SS, McKeever PE. The cytochemical demonstration of intracellular immunoglobulin. II. In neoplasms of lymphoreticular tissue. Am J Pathol 82:457–478, 1976.

321. Nakhleh RE, Manivel Carlos, Hurd D, Sung JH. Central nervous system lymphomas: Immunohistochemical and clinicopathologic study of 26 autopsy cases. Arch Pathol Lab Med 113:1050–1056, 1989.

322. Murphy JK, O'Brien CJ, Ironside JW. Morphologic and immunophenotypic characterization of primary brain lymphomas using paraffin-embedded tissue. Histopathology 15:449–460, 1989.

323. Sano T, Kovacs K, Scheithauer BW, Rosenblum MK, Petito CK, Greco CM. Pituitary pathology in acquired immunodeficiency syndrome. Arch Pathol Lab Med 113:1066–1070.

324. Amendola BE, McClatchey KD, Amendola MA, Gebarski SS. Primary large-cell lymphoma of the central nervous system. Am J Clin Oncol 9:204–208, 1986.

325. Davey FR, Elghetany MT, Kurec AS. Immunophenotyping of hematologic neoplasms in paraffin-

embedded tissue sections. Am J Clin Pathol (Suppl)93:S17–S26, 1990.

326. Feiden W, Bise K, Steude U. Diagnosis of primary cerebral lymphoma with particular reference to CT-guided stereotactic biopsy. Virchows Arch *417*:21–28, 1990.

327. Hitchcock E, Morris CS. Immunocytochemical techniques in stereotactic biopsy. Stereotact Funct Neurosurg 53:21–28, 1989.

328. Nakamine H, Yokote H, Itakura T, Hayashi S, Komai N, Takano Y, Saito K, Moriwaki H, Nishino E, Takenaka T, Maeda J, Matsumori T. Non-Hodgkin's lymphoma involving the brain. Diagnostic usefulness of stereotactic needle biopsy in combination with paraffin-section immunohistochemstry. Acta Neuropathol (Berl) *78*:462, 1989.

329. Namiki TS, Nichols P, Young T, Martin SE, Chandrasoma P. Stereotaxic biopsy diagnosis of central nervous system lymphoma. Am J Clin Pathol *90*:40–45, 1988.

330. Bayliss KM, Kueck BD, Hanson CA, Matthaeus WG, Almagro UA. Richter's syndrome presenting as primary central nervous system lymphoma. Transformation of an identical clone. Am J Clin Pathol 93:117–123, 1988.

331. Handt S, Hofstadter F. What's new in the application of Southern blot analysis of malignant lymphomas? Path Res Pract *184*:455–463, 1989.

332. Burger PC, Scheithauer BW, Vogel FS. Surgical Pathology of the Nervous System and Its Coverings. 3rd Ed. New York, Churchill Livingstone, 1991, pp 359–369.

333. Hanson CA, Ross CW. The molecular genetics of the immunoglobulin and T-cell receptors: Applications in diagnostic hematopathology. Adv Pathol *3*:33–74, 1990.

334. Aozasa K, Ohsawa M, Yamabe H, Shima N, Kirimoto K, Yamane T, Tsujimoto M, Kobayashi Y, Kurata A, Osada H, Konishi F, Nagashima K. Malignant lymphoma of the central nervous system in Japan: Histologic and immunohistologic studies. Int J Cancer *45*:632–636, 1990.

335. Nishiyama A, Saito T, Abe S, Kumanishi T. An immunohistochemical analysis of T cells in primary B cell malignant lymphoma of the brain. Acta Neuropathol (Berl) *79*:27–29, 1989.

336. Shibata S. Sites of origin of primary intracerebral malignant lymphoma. Neurosurgery *25*:14–19, 1989.

337. Egerter DA, Beckstead JH. Malignant lymphomas in the acquired immunodeficiency syndrome. Additional evidence for a B-cell origin. Arch Pathol Lab Med *112*:602–606, 1988.

338. Garson JA, Bourne SP, Allan PM, Leather C, Brownell DB, Coakham HB. Immunohistological diagnosis of primary brain lymphoma using monoclonal antibodies: Confirmation of B-cell origin. Neuropathol Appl Neurobiol *14*:19–37, 1988.

339. Warnke RA, Gatter KC, Fallini B, Hildreth P, Woolston RE, Pulford K, Cordell JL, Cohen B, De Wolf-Peeters C, Mason DY. Diagnosis of human lymphoma with monoclonal antileukocyte antibodies. N Engl J Med *309*:1275–1281, 1983.

340. Kurtin PJ, Pinkus GS. Leukocyte common antigen—diagnostic discriminant between hematopoietic and nonhematopoietic neoplasms in paraffin sections using monoclonal antibodies: Correlation with immunologic studies and ultrastructural localization. Hum Pathol *16*:353–365, 1985.

341. Slowik F, Jellinger K. Membranous changes in primary malignant CNS lymphomas. Acta Neuropathol 79:86–93, 1989.

342. Johnson PC. Ultrastructural study of two central nervous system lymphomas. Acta Neuropathol (Suppl) (Berl) *6*:155–160, 1975.

343. Scholtz CL, Siu K. Melanoma of pituitary. Case report. J Neurosurg 1976:45:101–103.

344. Roos B. Isolated melanoma of the pituitary. Fortschr Hals Nasen Ohrenheilkd *12*:193–198, 1965.

345. Neilson J McE, Moffat AD. Hypopituitarism caused by a melanoma of the pituitary gland. J Clin Pathol *16*:144–149, 1963.

346. Kasumova Siu, Inauri GA. Melanotic tumor of the hypophysis. Vopr-Onkol *26*:64–66, 1980.

347. Shinbor T, Vyama E, Eto K, Kohrogi H, Araki S. An autopsy cases of malignant melanoma possibly originating in the sphenoid sinus. Rinsho-Shinkeigaku *28*:636–642, 1988.

348. Moseley RP, Davies AG, Bourne SP, Popham C, Carrel S, Monro P, Coakham HB. Neoplastic meningitis in malignant melanoma: Diagnosis with monoclonal antibodies. J Neurol Neurosurg Psychiatry *52*:881–886, 1989.

349. Wick MR, Stanley SJ, Swanson PE. Immunohistochemical diagnosis of sinonasal melanoma, carcinoma, and neuroblastoma with monoclonal antibodies HMB-45 and anti-synaptophysin. Arch Pathol Lab Med *112*:616–620, 1988.

350. Christensen E. Two cases of primary intracranial melanomata. Acta Chir Scand *85*:90–98, 1941.

351. Gibson JB, Burrows D, Weir WP. Primary melanoma of the meninges. J Pathol Bacteriol *74*:419–438, 1957.

352. Duray PH, Ernstoff MS, Titus-Ernsoff L. Immunohistochemical phenotyping of malignant melanoma: A procedure whose time has come in pathologic practice. Pathol Annu *25*(pt 2):351–377, 1990.

353. McKeever PE, Balentine JD. Histochemistry of the nervous system. In: Spicer SS (ed). Histochemistry in Pathologic Disease. Vol 22. In: Schwartz MK (ed). Clinical and Biochemical Analysis. New York, Marcel Dekker, 1987, pp 941–942.

354. Shoup SA, Johnston WW, Siegler HF, Tello JW, Schlom J, Bigner DD, Bigner SH. A panel of antibodies useful in the cytologic diagnosis of metastatic melanoma. Acta Cytol *34*:385–392, 1990.

355. McKeever PE, Blaivas M. Surgical pathology of the brain, spinal cord and meninges. In: Sternberg S, Antonioli D, Kempson R, Carter D, Eggleston J, Oberman H (eds). Diagnosis in Surgical Pathology. Vol 1. New York, Raven Press, 1989, p 355.

356. Heitz PU. Neuroendocrine tumor markers. Curr Pathol *77*:279–306, 1987.

357. Erlandson RA. Diagnostic transmission electron microscopy of human tumors: The interpretation of submicroscopic structures in human neoplastic cells. New York, Masson, 1983, pp 71–79.

358. Banna M, Baker HL Jr, House OW. Pituitary and parapituitary tumours on computed tomography. Br J Radiol *53*:1123–1143, 1980.

359. Ugrumov VM, Ignatyeva GE, Olushin VE, Tigliev GS, Polenov AL. Parasellar meningiomas: diagnosis and possibility of surgical treatment according to the place of original growth. Acta Neurochirurgica (Suppl)*28*:373–374, 1979.

360. Bonnal J, Brotchi J, Boru J. Meningiomas of the lateral portion of the sella turcica. Acta Neurochirurgica (Suppl)*28*:385–386, 1979.

361. Solero CL, Giombini S, Morello G. Suprasellar and olfactory meningiomas. Report on a series of 153 personal cases. Acta Neurochirurgica 67:181–194, 1983.

362. Cushing H, Eisenhardt L. Meningiomas: Their Classification, Regional Behavior, Life History and Surgical End Result. New York, Hafner, 1962, pp 224–297.

363. Olivercrona H. The surgical treatment of intracranial tumours. In: Olivercrona H, Tönnis W (eds). Handbuch der Neurochirurgie. Vol IV/4. Berlin, Springer-Verlag, 1967, pp 23–111.

364. Synom L. Olfactory groove and suprasellar meningiomas. In: Krayenbühl H (ed). Advances and Technical Standards in Neurosurgery. Vol 4. New York, Springer-Verlag, 1977, pp 67–91.

365. Ehlers N, Malmros R. The suprasellar meningioma. A review of the literature and presentation of a series of 31 cases. Acta Ophthalmol (Suppl)121:1–73, 1973.

366. Ley A, Gabas E. Meningiomas of the tuberculum sellae. Acta Neurochirurgica (Suppl)28:402–404, 1979.

367. Krenkel W, Frowein RA. Suprasellar meningiomas. Acta Neurochirurgica 31:280, 1974.

368. Russell D, Rubinstein LJ. Pathology of Tumours of the Nervous System. London, Arnold, 1971, pp 48–64, 454.

369. Busch E, Mahneke A. A case of meningioma from the diaphragm of the sella turcica. Zentralbl Neurochir 14:25–28, 1954.

370. Demailly PW, Guiat G. Meningiomes du diaphragme sellaire. Bull Soc D'Ophthalmol 2:191–193, 1970.

371. Guiat G, Montrieul B, Goutelle A. Comoy J, Langie S. Meningiomes suprasellaires retro-chiasmatiques. Neurochirurgie 16:273–285, 1970.

372. Papo I, Villani R, Giovanelli M, Scarpelli M, Salvolini V, Pasquini U, Tomei G. Angioblastic parasellar extradural tumours. Acta Neurochirururgica (Suppl)28:438–444, 1979.

373. Grisoli F, Vincentelli F, Raybaud C, Harter M, Guibout M, Baldini M. Intrasellar meningioma. Surg Neurol 20:36–41, 1983.

374. Hardy J, Roberst F. Un meningiome de la sella turcique variete sous diaphragmatique (exerese par voie transphenoidale) Neurochirurgie 15:535–544, 1969.

375. Shah RP, Leavens ME, Samaan NA. Galactorrhea, amenorrhea, and hyperprolactinemia as manifestations of parasellar meningioma. Arch Intern Med 140:1608–1612, 1980.

376. Kepes JJ. Meningiomas. Biology, Pathology and Differential Diagnosis. New York, Masson, 1982, pp 64–149.

377. Sutherland G, Sima AAF. Incidence and clinicopathological features of meningioma. In: Schmidek H (ed). Meningiomas and Their Surgical Management. Philadelphia, WB Saunders, 1991, pp 10–21.

378. Memoli VA, Brown EF, Gould VE. Glial fibrillary acidic protein (GFAP) immunoreactivity in peripheral nerve sheath tumors. Ultrastruct Pathol 7:269–275, 1984.

379. Yamada K, Hatayama T, Ohta M, Sakoda K, Uozumi T. Coincidental pituitary adenoma and parasellar meningioma. Case report. Neurosurgery 19:267–270, 1986.

380. O'Connell JEA. Intracranial meningiomata associated with other tumors involving the central nervous system. Br J Surg 48:373–383, 1961.

381. Kitamura K, Nakamura N, Terao H, Hayakawa I, Kamano S, Ishijima T, Sano K. Primary brain tumors. Brain Nerve 17:109–117, 1965.

382. Probst VA. Kombination eines Cushing-Syndromes, Hypophysenadenoms und suprasellaren Meningeoms—Fallbericht. Zentralbl Neurochir 32:75–82, 1971.

383. Bunick EM, Mills LC, Rose LI. Association of acromegaly and meningiomas. JAMA 240:1267–1268, 1978.

384. Hyoda A, Nose T, Maki Y, Enomoto T. Pituitary adenoma and meningioma in the same product. Neurochirurgia (Stuttg) 25:66–67, 1982.

385. Brennan TG, Jr, Rao CVGK, Robinson W, Itani A. Case Report: Tandem lesions. Chromophobe adenoma and meningioma. J Comput Assist Tomogr 1:517–520, 1977.

386. Friede RL, Yasargil MG. Suprasellar neoplasm with a granular cell component. J Neuropathol Exp Neurol 36:769–782, 1977.

387. Mitsumori K, Maronpot RR, Boorman GA. Spontaneous tumors of the meninges in rats. Vet Pathol 24:50–58, 1987.

388. Meis JM, Ordonez NG, Bruner JM. Meningiomas: An immunohistochemical study of 50 cases. Arch Pathol Lab Med 110:934–937, 1986.

389. Meyrignae C, N'Guyen JP, Blatrix C, Degos JDD. Meningiome post radique. Complication tardive de l'irradiation de la sella turcique. La Nouv Presse Med 10:3246–3247, 1981.

390. Nagatoni M, Mori M, Takomoto N, Arita N, Ushio Y, Hayakawa T, Gen M, Uozumi T, Mogami H. Primary myxoma in the pituitary fossa: Case report. Neurosurgery 20:329–331, 1987.

391. Branch CL Jr, Laster DW, Kelly DL Jr. Left atrial myxoma with cerebral emboli. Neurosurgery 16:675–680, 1985.

392. Enzinger FM, Weiss SW. Soft Tissue Tumors. 2nd Ed. St Louis, CV Mosby, 1988, pp 912–928.

393. Pulitzer DR, Reed JR. Nerve-sheath myxoma (perineural myxoma). Am J Dermatopathol 7:409–421, 1985.

394. Stout AP. The tumor of primitive mesenchyme. Ann Surg 127:706–719, 1948.

395. Ghosh BC, Huvos AG, Gerold FP, Miller TR. Myxoma of the jaw bones. Cancer 31:237–240, 1973.

396. Shanmugaratham K, Chan SH, De-The G, Goj JE, Khor TH, Simons MJ. Histopathology of nasopharyngeal carcinoma. Correlations with epidemiology, survival rates and other biological characteristics. Cancer 44:1029–1044, 1979.

397. Million RR. The myth regarding bone and cartilage involvement by cancer and the likelihood of cure by radiotherapy. Head Neck 11:30–40, 1989.

398. Miura T, Hirabuki N, Hishiyama K, Hashimoto T, Kawai R, Yoshida J, Sasaki R, Matsunaga T, Kozuka T. Computed tomographic findings of nasopharyngeal carcinoma with skull base and intracranial involvement. Cancer 65:29–37, 1990.

399. Hsu YC, Chen CL, Hsu MM, Lynn TC, Tu SM, Huang SC. Pathology of nasopharyngeal carcinoma. Proposal of a new histologic classification correlated with prognosis. Cancer 59:945–951, 1987.

400. Taxy JB, Hidvegi DF, Battifora H. Nasopharyngeal carcinoma: Antikeratin immunohistochemistry and electron microscopy. Am J Clin Pathol 83:320–325, 1985.

401. Ward PH, Thompson R, Calcaterra T, Kadin MR. Juvenile angiofibroma: A more rational therapeu-

tic approach based upon clinical and experimental evidence. Laryngoscope *84*:2181–2194, 1974.

402. Franquemont DW, Fechner RE, Mills SE. Histologic classification of sinonasal intestinal-type adenocarcinoma. Am J Surg Pathol *15*:368–375, 1991.

403. Matson D. Neurosurgery of Infancy and Childhood. Springfield, IL, Charles C Thomas, 1969, pp 523–536.

404. Reese AB. Tumors of the eye and adnexa. In: Atlas of Tumor Pathology. Fascicle 38. Washington, DC, Armed Forces Institute of Pathology, 1956, pp 31–42.

405. Russell DS, Rubinstein LJ. Pathology of Tumours of the Nervous System. Baltimore, Williams & Wilkins, 1988, pp 370–376.

406. Borit A, Richardson EP Jr. The biological and clinical behaviour of pilocytic astrocytoma of the optic pathway. Brain *105*:161–187, 1982.

407. Horwich A, Bloom HJG. Optic gliomas: Radiation therapy and prognosis. Int J Radiol Oncol Biol Phys *11*:1067–1079, 1985.

408. Alvord EC Jr, Lofton S. Gliomas of the optic nerve or chiasm. Outcome by patients age, tumor site, and treatment. J. Neurosurg *68*:85–98, 1988.

409. Verhoeff FH. Tumors of the optic nerve. In: Penfield W (ed). Cytology and Cellular Pathology of the Nervous System. Vol 3. New York, Hoeber, 1932, p. 1027.

410. Rubinstein LJ. Tumeurs et hamartomes dans la neurofibromatose central. In: Michaux L, Feld M (eds). Les Phakomatoses Cerebrales. Paris, SPEI Editeurs, 1963, p 427.

411. Hoyt WF, Mechel LG, Lessell S, Schatz NJ, Suckling RD. Malignant optic glioma of adulthood. Brian *96*:121–132, 1973.

412. Spoor TL, Kernnerdell JS, Martinez AJ, Zorub D. Malignant gliomas of the optic nerve pathways. Am J Ophthalmol *89*:284–292, 1980.

413. Davis FA. Primary tumors of the optic nerve (a phenomenon of Recklinghausen's disease): A clinical and pathological study with a report of five cases and review of the literature. Arch Ophthalmol *23*:735–821, 1940.

414. Huvos AG. Pathology of osteogenic sarcoma. In: Rosen G (ed). Pharmanual. A Comprehensive Guide to the Therapeutic Use of Methotrexate in Osteogenic Sarcoma. Pharmalibri, 1984, pp 1–16.

415. Dahlin DL, Uuni KK. Bone Tumors. 4th Ed. Springfield, IL, Charles C Thomas, 1986, p 271.

416. Kleinsasser O, Albrecht H. Zur Kenntnis der Osteosarcome des Stirn-und Keilbeines. Arch Ohren Heilk *170*:595–603, 1957.

417. Reichenthal E, Cohen ML, Manor R, Marshak G, Matz S, Shalit MN. Primary osteogenic sarcoma of the sellar region. Case report. J Neurosurg *55*:299–302, 1981.

418. Lee YY, Van Tassel P, Raymond AK, Edeiken J. Craniofacial osteosarcomas: Plain film, CT, and MR findings in 46 cases. AJR *150*:1397–1402, 1988.

419. Tanaka S, Nishio S, Morioka T, Fukui M, Kitamura K, Hikita K. Radiation-induced osteosarcoma of the sphenoid bone. Neurosurgery *25*:640–643, 1989.

420. Swanson PE, Wick MR. HLA-DR (Ia-like) reactivity in tumors of bone and soft tissue: An immunohistochemical comparison of monoclonal antibodies LN3 and LK8D3 in routinely processed specimens. Mod Pathol *3*:113–118, 1990.

421. Roessner A, Mellin W, Hiddenmann W, Voss B, Vollmer E, Grundmann E. New cytomorphologic methods in the diagnosis of bone tumors: Possibilities and limitations. Semin Diagn Pathol *1*:199–214, 1984.

422. Bilbao JM, Horvath E, Kovacs K, Singer W, Hudson AT. Intrasellar paraganglioma associated with hypopituitarism. Arch Path Lab Med *102*:95–98, 1978.

423. Lloyd V, Sisson JC, Shapiro B, Verhofstad AAJ. Immunohistochemical localization of epinephrine, norepinephrine, catecholamine-synthesizing enzymes, and chromogranin in neuroendocrine cells and tumors. Am J Path *125*:45–54, 1986.

424. Tapia FJ, Barbosa AJA, Marangos PJ, Polak JM, Bloom SR, Dermody C, Pearse AGE. Neuron-specific enolase is produced by neuroendocrine tumors. Lancet *1*:808–811, 1981.

425. Scheithauer BW. Pathology of the pituitary and the sellar region: Exclusive of pituitary adenoma. In: Sommers SC, Rosen PP, Fechner RE (eds). Pathology. Norwalk, CT, Appleton-Century-Crofts, 1985, pp 99–105.

426. Silverstein AM, Quint DJ, McKeever PE. Intradural paraganglioma of the thoracic spine. Am J Neuroradiol *11*:614–616, 1990.

427. Fu Y-S, Perzin KH. Nonepithelial tumors of the nasal cavity, paranasal sinuses and nasopharynx. A clinicopathologic study. IX. Plasmacytomas. Cancer *42*:2399–2406, 1978.

428. Poon M-C, Prchal JT, Murad TM, Galbraith JG. Multiple myeloma masquerading as chromophobe adenoma. Cancer *43*:1513–1516, 1979.

429. Bitterman P, Ariza A, Black RA, Allen WE, Lee SH. Multiple myeloma mimicking pituitary adenoma. Comput Radiol *10*:201–205, 1986.

430. Urbanski SF, Bilbao JM, Horvath E, Kovacs K, So W, Ward JV. Intrasellar solitary plasmacytoma terminating in multiple myeloma: A report of a case including electron microscopical study. Surg Neurol *14*:233–236, 1980.

431. Calvo A, Purriel JA, Bastarrica E, Haberbeck MA. Tumors of the sellar region and the cavernous sinus. Evaluation of diagnostic procedures and therapeutic orientation. Acta Neurol Latinoam *26*:111–122, 1980.

432. Estopinan V, Riobo P, Fernandez G, Varela C. Intrasellar plasmacytoma simulating a pituitary adenoma. Letter. Med Clin (Barc) *89*:128, 1987.

433. Pinkus GS, Kurtin PJ. Epithelial membrane antigen—diagnostic discriminant in surgical pathology: Immunohistochemical profile in epithelial, mesenchymal, and hematopoietic neoplasms using paraffin sections and monoclonal antibodies. Hum Pathol *16*:929–940, 1985.

434. Kurabayashi H, Kubota K, Murakami H, Tamura J, Sawamura M, Nogiwa E, Shinonome S, Miyawaki S, Sato S, Omine M, Naruse T, Shirakura T, Tsuchiya J. Ultrastructure of myeloma cells in patients with common acute lymphoblastic leukemia antigen (CALLA)-positive myeloma. Cancer Res *48*:6234–6237, 1988.

435. Van Camp B, Durie BGM, Spier C, De Waele M, Van Riet I, Vela E, Frutiger Y, Richter L, Grogan TM. Plasma cells in multiple myeloma express a natural killer cell-associated antigen: CD56 (NKH-1; Leu-19). Blood *76*:377–382, 1990.

436. Dehou MF, Schots R, Lacor P, Arras N, Verhavert P, Kloppel G, Van Camp B. Diagnostic and prog-

nostic value of the MB2 monoclonal antibody in paraffin-embedded bone marrow sections of patients with multiple myeloma and monoclonal gammopathy of undetermined significance. Am J Clin Pathol *94*:287–291, 1990.

437. Boccadoro M, Gavarotti P, Fossati G, Pileri A, Marmont F, Neretto G, Gallamini A, Olta C, Tribalto M, Testa MC, Amadori S, Mandelli F, Durie BGM. Low plasma cell ³(H) thymidine incorporation in monoclonal gammopathy of undetermined significance (MGUS), smouldering myeloma and remission phase myeloma: A reliable indicator of patients not requiring therapy. Br J Haematol *58*:689–696, 1984.

438. Campana D, Coustan-Smith E, Janossy G. Double and triple staining methods for studying the proliferative activity of human B and T lymphoid cells. J Immunol *107*:79–88, 1988.

439. Cordell J, Falini B, Erber WN, Ghosh AK, Abdulaziz Z, Macdonald S, Polford K, Stein H, Mason DY. Immunoenzymatic labelling of monoclonal antibodies using immune complexes of alkaline phosphatase and monoclonal anti-alkaline phosphatase (APAAP complexes). J Histochem Cytochem *31*:219–229, 1984.

440. Dolbeare F, Beisker W, Pallavicini MG, Vanderlaan M, Gray JW. Cytochemistry of bromodeoxyuridine/DNA analysis: Stoichiometry and sensitivity. Cytometry *6*:521–530, 1985.

441. Durie BGM, Salmon SE, Moon TE. Pretreatment to tumor mass, cell kinetics, and prognosis in multiple myeloma. Blood *55*:363–372, 1980.

442. Gratzner HG. Monoclonal antibody to 5-bromo and 5-iododeoxyuridine: A new reagent for detection of DNA replication. Science *218*:474–475, 1982.

443. Greipp PR, Witzig TE, Gonchoroff NJ, Habermann TM, Katzmann JA, O'Fallon WM, Kyle RA. Immunofluorescene labeling indices in myeloma and related monoclonal gammopathies. Mayo Clin Proc *62*:969–977, 1987.

444. Houck DW, Loken MR. Simultaneous analysis of cell surface antigens, bromodeoxyuridine incorporation and DNA content. Cytometry *6*:531–538, 1985.

445. Latreille J, Barlogie B, Johnston D, Drewinko B, Alexanian R. Ploidy and proliferative characteristics in monoclonal gammopathies. Blood *59*:43–51, 1982.

446. Kucharczyk W, Peck WW, Kelly WM, Norman D, Newton TH. Rathke cleft cysts: CT, MR imaging, and pathologic features. Radiology *165*:491–495, 1987.

447. Matsushima T, Fukui M, Fujii K, Kinoshita K, Yamakawa Y. Epithelial cells in symptomatic Rathke's cleft cysts. A light- and electron-microscopic study. Surg Neurol *30*:197–203, 1988.

448. Yoshida J, Kobayashi T, Kageyama N, Kanzaki M. Symptomatic Rathke's cleft cyst. Morphological study with light and electron microscopy and tissue culture. J Neurosurg *47*:451–458, 1977.

449. Seidel FG, Towbin R, Kaufman RA. Normal pituitary stalk size in children: CT study. Am J Roentgenol *145*:1297–1302, 1985.

450. Barrow DL, Spector RH, Takei Y, Tindall GT. Symptomatic Rathke's cleft cysts located entirely in the suprasellar region: Review of diagnosis, management, and pathogenesis. Neurosurgery *16*:766–772, 1985.

451. Hirano A, Hirano M. Benign cystic lesions in the central nervous system. Light and electron microscopic observations of cyst walls. Childs Nerv Syst *4*:325–333, 1988.

452. Marin F, Boya J, Lopez-Caronell AL, Borregon A. Immunohistochemical localization of intermediate filament and S-100 proteins in several non-endocrine cells of the human pituitary gland. Arch Histol Cytol *52*:241–248, 1989.

453. Kasper M, Karsten U. Coexpression of cytokeratin and vimentin in Rathke's cysts of the human pituitary gland. Cell Tissue Res *253*:419–424, 1988.

454. Inoue T, Matsushima T, Fukui M, Iwaki T, Takeshita I, Kuromatsu C. Immunohistochemical study of intracranial cysts. Neurosurgery *23*:576–581, 1988.

455. Ikeda H, Yoshimoto T, Suzuki J. Immunohistochemical study of Rathke's cleft cyst. Acta Neuropathol *77*:33–38, 1988.

456. Pearl GS, Seyama S, Takei N, Tindall GT, Kurisaka M. Cyst prolactinoma: A variant of "transitional cell tumor" of the pituitary. Am J Surg Pathol *5*:85–91, 1981.

457. Cinti S, Sbarbati A, Balercia G, Cigolini M. An ultrastructural study on muciparous microcysts of the human adenohypophysis. Acta Anat *121*:94–98, 1985.

458. Nishio S, Mizuno J, Barrow DL, Takei Y, Tindall GT. Pituitary tumors composed of adenohypophysial adenoma and Rathke's cleft cyst elements: A clinicopathological study. Neurosurgery *21*:371–377, 1987.

459. Verkijk A, Bots GT. An intrasellar cyst with both Rathke's cleft and epidermoid characteristics. Acta Neurochir *51*:203–207, 1980.

460. Schaeffer BT, Som PM, Sacher M, Lanzieri CF, Solodnik P, Lawson W, Biller HF. Coexistence of a nasal mucoepidermoid carcinoma and sphenoid mucoceles: CT diagnosis and treatment implications. J Comput Assist Tomogr *9*:803–805, 1985.

461. Alleva MD, Werber JL, Kimmelman CP. Pathologic quiz case 2. Fibromyxoma of the ethmoidal sinus with secondary sphenoidal sinus mucocele. Arch Otolaryngol Head Neck Surg *115*:878–879, 1989.

462. Terry RD, Hyams VJ, Davidoff LM. Combined non-metastasizing fibrosarcoma and chromophobe tumor of the pituitary. Cancer *12*:791–798, 1959.

463. Walzp TA, Brownell B. Sarcoma: A possible late result of effective radiation therapy for pituitary adenoma. Report on two cases. J Neurosurg *24*:901–907, 1966.

464. Shi T, Farrell MA, Kaufman JCE. Fibrosarcoma complicating irradiated pituitary adenoma. Surg Neurol *22*:277–283, 1984.

465. Powell HC, Marshall LF, Ignelzi RJ. Post-irradiation pituitary sarcoma. Acta Neuropathol (Berl) *39*:165–167, 1977.

466. Amendola BE, Amendola MA, McClatchey KD, Miller CH Jr. Radiation associated sarcoma; A review of 23 patients with postradiation sarcoma over a 50-year period. Am J Clin Oncol *12*:411–415, 1989.

467. Amine ARC, Sugar O. Suprasellar osteogenic sarcoma following radiation for pituitary adenoma J Neurosurg *44*:88–91, 1976.

468. Gerlach J, Janisch W. Intrakranielles Sarkom nach Bestrahlung eines Hypophysen-adenoms. Zentralbl Neurochir *40*:136–141, 1976.

469. Pieterse S, Dinning TAR, Blumbergs PC. Postir-

radiation sarcomatous transformation of a pituitary adenoma: A combined pituitary tumor. J Neurosurg 56:283–286, 1982.

470. Willis RA. Pathological study of tumors of the pituitary region. Med J Aust 1:281–291, 1938.

471. Anderson WR, Cameron JD, Tsai SH. Primary intracranial leiomyosarcoma. Case report with ultrastructural study. J Neurosurg 53:401–405, 1980.

472. Urich H. Pathology of tumors of cranial nerves, spinal nerve roots, and peripheral nerves. In: Dyck PJ, Thomas PK, Lamber EH, Bunge R (eds). Peripheral Neuropathy. Vol 2. Philadelphia, WB Saunders, 1984, pp 2253–2299.

473. Ho K-L. Schwannoma of the trochlear nerve. J Neurosurg 55:132–134, 1981.

474. Lennda G, Vaquero J, Cabezudo J, Garcia-Uria J, Bravo G. Schwannoma of the oculomotor nerve. Report of four cases. J Neurosurg 57:563–565, 1982.

475. Wilberger JE Jr. Primary intrasellar schwannoma. Case report. Surg Neurol 32:156–158, 1989.

476. Perone TP, Robinson B, Holmes SM. Intrasellar schwannoma: Case report. Neurosurgery 14:71–73, 1984.

477. Goebel HH, Shimokawa K, Schaake TH, Kremp A. Schwannoma of the sellar region. Acta Neurochirurg 48:191–197, 1979.

478. Chadduk WN. Unusual lesions involving the sella turcica. South Med J 66:948–955, 1973.

479. Russell DS, Rubinstein LJ. Pathology of Tumours of the Nervous System. Baltimore, Williams & Wilkens, 1988, p 538.

480. Tekeuchi J, Morik, Moritake K, Tani F, Waga S, Handa H. Teratomas in the suprasellar region:

Report of five cases. Surg Neurol 3:247–255, 1975.

481. Page RB, Plourde PV, Coldwell D, Heald JI, Weinstein J. Intrasellar mixed germ-cell tumor. Case report. J Neurosurg 58:766–770, 1983.

482. Merchut MP, Biller J, Ghobrial M, Fine M. Adult intrasellar teratoid tumor. J Clin Neuro-ophthalmol 6:175–180, 1986.

483. Wilson JW, Gehweiler JA. Teratoma of the face associated with a patent canal extending into the cranial cavity (Rathke's pouch) in a three-week-old child. J Pediatr Surg 5:349–359.

484. Senae MO, Segall HD. CT diagnosis of an atypical nasopharyngeal teratoma in a newborn. AJNR 8:710–712, 1987.

485. Russell DS, Rubinstein LJ. Pathology of Tumours of the Nervous System. 5th Ed. Baltimore, Williams & Wilkins, 1989.

486. Jennings MT, Gelman R, Hochberg F. Intracranial germ-cell tumors: Natural history and pathogenesis. J Neurosurg 63:155–167, 1985.

487. McKeever PE, Blaivas M. Surgical pathology of the brain, spinal cord and meninges. In: Sternberg S, Antonioli D, Kempson R, Carter D, Eggleston J, Oberman H (eds). Diagnosis in Surgical Pathology. Vol 1. New York, Raven Press, 1989, pp 361–365.

488. Perentes E, Rubinstein LJ. Recent applications of immunoperoxidase histochemistry in human neuro-oncology. An update. Arch Pathol Lab Med 111:796–812, 1987.

489. McKeever PE, Blaivas M. Surgical pathology of the brain, spinal cord and meninges. In: Sternberg S, Antonioli D, Kempson R, Carter D, Eggleston J, Oberman H (eds). Diagnosis in Surgical Pathology. Vol 1. New York, Raven Press, 1989, pp 340–342.

14

MEDICAL TREATMENT OF PITUITARY ADENOMAS

JAMIE DANANBERG and ALAN C. DALKIN

PROLACTIN-SECRETING ADENOMAS

Physiology of Prolactin Secretion

Prolactin is secreted by the pituitary lactotroph in both a constitutive and a pulsatile fashion (1, 2). Hypothalamic regulation of prolactin occurs via the inhibitory action of dopamine. A decline in hypothalamic dopaminergic activity results in an increase in pituitary prolactin, which in turn stimulates dopamine synthesis and secretion, forming a negative feedback–loop type of regulation (3, 4). Other hormones such as thyrotropin releasing hormone (TRH) (5), vasoactive intestinal peptide (6), serotonin (7), and the gonadotropin releasing hormone (GnRH)–associated peptide (GAP) (8) may alter prolactin release, but their role in normal physiology remain uncertain.

Serum prolactin concentrations are generally less than 25 ng/ml in a man or a non-pregnant, non-lactating woman. The etiologies of hyperprolactinemia are numerous (9–13), and different mechanisms may result in elevated prolactin levels. Physiological increases of prolactin usually range from 25 to 40 ng/ml and may occur following stress or during sleep; hence mild increases may be observed in the early morning hours. Several determinations of serum prolactin may be needed at later times of the day to distinguish between pathologic and physiological hyperprolactinemia. Numerous medications have been shown to reduce dopamine synthesis, alter dopamine secretion or block dopamine receptors at the lactotroph, resulting in an elevated serum prolactin. This point deserves particular emphasis, as a careful medication history should be part of any evaluation of hyperprolactinemia. Estrogens may increase prolactin (14, 15), though their role in the formation of prolactinomas is controversial (16, 17). Up to 25% of patients with polycystic ovarian syndrome have mild hyperprolactinemia, which may be secondary to elevated levels of estrone (18). Patients with severe or protracted primary hypothyroidism may have increased prolactin levels that normalize with thyroid hormone replacement (19). Other reasons for hyperprolactinemia include chronic renal failure (20), breast feeding (21) and direct nipple or chest wall stimulation.

Non-pathologic causes of hyperprolactinemia are rarely associated with prolactin levels of greater than 100 to 150 ng/ml. Nonfunctioning pituitary tumors or metastatic disease to the hypothalamus or pituitary can disrupt dopamine delivery and elevate prolactin levels to a modest degree. However, prolactin-producing pituitary tumors are associated with the greatest degree of hyperprolactinemia, and values greater than 200 ng/ml are virtually diagnostic of prolactinomas. Additionally, the highest prolactin levels are associated with large adenomas. Hence, if careful medication history and physical examination fail to elucidate an etiology, a prolactinoma should be suspected.

Clinical Presentation and Evaluation

In general, the clinical presentation of patients with prolactinomas relates either to the hormonal consequences of hyperprolactinemia or to the mass effect of the tumor itself. Prolactinomas are the most common pituitary tumor in either sex, though significant differences exist between women and men. Hyperprolactinemia is found more often in women (22), and menstrual dysfunction or infertility are the most common symptoms (23). Elevated prolactin reduces GnRH pulse frequency (24) and thereby alters normal ovarian function. The incidence of galactorrhea is highly variable (25, 26). This may be related to different degrees of hypoestrogenemia, as estrogen is needed for galactorrhea. Additionally, reduced estrogen secretion can result in diminished libido and dyspareunia (13, 25). Headache occurs in up to 50% of women with prolactinomas, though this complaint does not correlate with tumor size (27). Perhaps because of the relative sensitivity of the menstrual cycle to hormonal dysregulation, which brings patients to medical attention, women tend to present with microadenomas (<10 mm) rather than macroadenomas (> 10 mm), so visual field defects are uncommon.

Hyperprolactinemia may present in a more subtle fashion in men than in women. Hypogonadism secondary to hyperprolactinemia appears to be less prevalent in men than in women. The mean age of diagnosis is approximately 10 years greater in men (22), and men present with a higher proportion of macroadenomas. Concomitant with the large tumors, visual field defects and hypopituitarism are more common. While 15% to 20% of women with secondary amenorrhea have increased prolactin (28, 29), less than 10% of men with infertility have hyperprolactinemia (30, 31). These differences in symptom complex and tumor characteristics often dictate differences in therapeutic approach for men and women with prolactinomas.

Therapeutic Approach

The finding that hypothalamic secretion of dopamine acts to inhibit prolactin secretion forms the basis for the medical management of prolactinomas. Dopamine agonists, in particular bromocriptine (Parlodel), which have longer half lives than dopamine, have proved safe and effective in the treatment of prolactinomas.

Bromocriptine

Bromocriptine is an ergot-alkaloid derivative that has significant dopaminergic properties. Acting via the dopamine receptor on lactotrophs (32), bromocriptine has been shown to reduce both prolactin synthesis and prolactin secretion. The effect of bromocriptine is rapid, and peak plasma concentrations occur within 2 to 3 hours, coinciding with maximum reductions of prolactin secretion. The action of bromocriptine persists for 8 to 12 hours and hence can be given orally on a b.i.d./t.i.d. basis. Bromocriptine may be preferentially concentrated by prolactinomas (33), and tumor size reduction may be observed over days to weeks (34–39). Following therapy with bromocriptine, prolactinomas have reduced amounts of rough endoplasmic reticulum and Golgi apparatus (40–43) as well as diminished prolactin mRNA and DNA synthesis rates (44, 45).

The usual dose of bromocriptine necessary to suppress prolactin to normal limits is 2.5 mg po t.i.d., though doses of up to 30 mg per day have been required in some patients. Though the majority of prolactinomas respond to bromocriptine (42), a number of case reports have documented resistance to bromocriptine based on probable receptor or post-receptor defects in the tumors (46, 47). Additionally, spontaneous tumor enlargement while on therapy has been documented (48). The major side effects of bromocriptine include dizziness, lightheadedness, headache, nausea, nasal congestion and orthostatic hypotension. These symptoms are more prevalent early in therapy or when the medication is taken on an empty stomach. In cases where bromocriptine is poorly tolerated, administration of small doses at bedtime with gradual increments in dosage may be indicated.

Bromocriptine in Microadenomas. The indications for initiation of bromocriptine therapy in prolactinomas remain somewhat controversial and depend on tumor size, clinical presentation, therapeutic goal and patient preference. The available therapies for microprolactinomas include observation, bromocriptine or transsphenoidal resection. Studies detailing longitudinal changes in microadenomas without therapy have been conflicting. Some case reports document tumor progression (49, 50), while others have shown little, if any, change in tumor size over 4 to 5 years of follow-up (51–53). Therefore, no medical intervention may be an acceptable approach in patients with microadenomas, mild or absent galactorrhea and normal gonadal function. Conversely, in those patients with significant symptoms (e.g., headaches, galactorrhea, hypogonadism) bromocriptine has shown to be effective. Between 70% and 100% of patients with microprolactinomas respond to bromocriptine in terms of reduced serum prolactin, diminished galactorrhea, tumor shrinkage and resumption of menses within 1 to 2 months of initiation of therapy (53–56). Additionally, bromocriptine appears to be safe for long-term treatment. The majority of patients note recurrence of their initial symptoms following the discontinuation of therapy (57, 58), although approximately 15% may continue to have normal prolactin levels without reinstitution of therapy (59). Patients with smaller tumors or initial prolactin levels less than 100 ng/ml are more likely to be "cured" by bromocriptine, and hence therapy should be discontinued for 2 to 3 weeks annually to identify those patients no longer requiring therapy.

Bromocriptine in Macroadenomas. In contrast to smaller pituitary tumors, macroprolactinomas are rarely cured with surgical resection alone, and hence bromocriptine is the cornerstone for management for these neoplasms. At least two thirds of patients with macroprolactinomas have a diminution in serum prolactin and tumor size in response to bromocriptine (34, 40, 42, 54, 55, 60–63). Visual field defects improve in approximately 85% of patients, with improvement noted in days to weeks (64). Despite the excellent response of macroprolactinomas to bromocriptine, most patients require long-term therapy, and few cases of "cure" have been reported (65). Generally, larger tumors show less response to bromocriptine (48, 66). Hence bromocriptine may produce rapid and beneficial responses in macroprolactinomas, but additional modes of therapy, including surgical resection, are often necessary to effect satisfactory long-term treatment and allow discontinuation of bromocriptine.

Surgical resection of macroprolactinomas can improve hyperprolactinemia and anatomic complications but is rarely curative.

Short courses of bromocriptine given preoperatively have resulted in marked reduction in tumor size, visual defect improvement and diminished hyperprolactinemia without affecting surgical outcome (67, 68). However, bromocriptine has been felt by some neurosurgeons to induce fibrotic changes in these tumors, which may make surgical resection more difficult (69). Prospective studies have concluded that these fibrotic changes may relate to the duration of therapy (70). We often employ bromocriptine for up to 6 weeks prior to surgery if indicated. Bromocriptine therapy may also play a role in postoperative management of macroprolactinomas and may diminish the recurrence rate (71).

Other Agents With Dopamine Agonist Properties

As bromocriptine often requires multiple doses per day, long-acting preparations of bromocriptine mesylate have been developed. Parlodel L.A. is an injectable, long-acting form of bromocriptine that lowers prolactin within hours, has fewer side effects and a duration of action that is apparently greater than 21 days. It is effective in rapidly shrinking macroadenomas (72, 73) and is equal to the standard form of bromocriptine in overall tumor responsiveness (74, 75). Bromocriptine mesylate may be given via vaginal suppository to further reduce side effects (76). Pergolide is a synthetic derivative of bromocriptine that can be given orally once daily and may be of equal (77) or slightly greater (78, 79) efficacy than bromocriptine itself.

A variety of other agents have been assessed in the therapy of hyperprolactinemia. Carbergoline is a synthetic, long-acting ergoline derivative that can reduce prolactin secretion for up to 7 days following a single oral dose (80). Two studies have documented that 80% to 100% of patients with macroadenomas responded to this medication while encountering few side effects (81, 82). Lisuride, and its derivative terguride, are synthetic ergolines that can lower prolactin levels and reduce tumor size, although their advantages over bromocriptine remain uncertain (83–85). Somatostatin analogues, useful in the therapy of other pituitary neoplasms, have not been shown to be effective in the treatment of prolactinomas (86).

In summary, the mainstay of medical management of prolactinoma is bromocriptine. This medication is safe and effective and can be used in conjunction with other therapeutic modalities. Bromocriptine analogues are currently being developed that may improve compliance and decrease side effects.

GROWTH HORMONE–SECRETING ADENOMAS

Physiology of Growth Hormone Secretion

Growth hormone (GH) secretion, like secretion of pituitary glycoprotein hormones, occurs in a pulsatile fashion (87). Though proof in humans is lacking, this intermittent GH signal appears necessary for target tissue sensitivity (88). Regulation of GH release is primarily via hypothalamic growth hormone releasing hormone (GHRH) and somatostatin, which act via specific pituitary receptors (89, 90). GHRH secretion is the primary stimulus for GH release, and the pulsatile pattern of GH reflects pulsatile GHRH (91, 92). GHRH induces GH synthesis and has a mitogenic effect on the somatotroph (93). Additionally, pulsatile exogenous GHRH is more effective than continuous administration in promoting GH release and rat somatic growth (94). Hypothalamic somatostatin exerts an inhibitory effect on GH release. Somatostatin does not act in a pulsatile fashion, but rather "tonically" regulates interpulse GH secretion, although it may also influence pulsatile GH, as portal levels may decline prior to release of GHRH (90). Somatostatin may further act to diminish the GH response to GHRH and oppose the mitogenic effect of GHRH (93).

Tissue responses to GH include metabolic changes (gluconeogenesis and glycolysis) as well as hepatic secretion of insulin-like growth factor I (IGF I) (95, 96). In turn, increased IGF I exerts negative feedback on GH secretion via increased somatostatin and diminished responsiveness to GHRH (95). Thus, a complex pattern of stimulatory and inhibitory signals serve to regulate normal GH secretion.

Physiological GH secretion follows a diurnal pattern that is characterized by GH surges occurring predominantly between midnight and 8:00 A.M. (97) and periods of basal secretion during the day. Hence, single GH values of 20 to 40 µg/L can be seen in normal individuals in the early morning (98). However, the majority of random samples will be less than 5 µg/L in men and 10 µg/L in women. Therefore, single estimates of GH are insufficient on which to document either GH excess or deficiency. Further, as GH increases in response to hypoglycemia and is at least partially excreted in the urine, poorly controlled diabetes mellitus or significant declines in creatinine clearance may result in elevated GH levels.

Clinical Presentation and Evaluation

Excess GH secretion results in a constellation of signs and symptoms. The review by Nabarrow (99) of 256 acromegalics extensively details the complications of this disorder. Cardiac dysfunction may be observed in up to one third of patients with acromegaly (99–102). Predominantly these patients experience cardiac hypertrophy, normal or increased cardiac output, normal or diminished total peripheral resistance and congestive heart failure that may be refractory to standard therapy (110, 103–105). Although hypertension is also common in acromegaly (99), acromegalic cardiomyopathy can occur in the absence of an elevated blood pressure level and is thought to be a direct effect of GH on the heart (104). Concomitant with this cardiomyopathy is a high mortality secondary to arrhythmia (106), and overall heart disease is felt to be the leading cause of death in acromegaly (107).

Another cause of morbidity and mortality in acromegaly is respiratory tract disease (108). Nasal polyps, laryngeal changes with deepening of the voice and sinus reshaping with frontal bossing are common. Glossal and epiglottic hypertrophy may narrow airways (99). Mandibular enlargement results in worsening dentition. Vertebral deformities, in particular kyphosis, may significantly inhibit respiratory function. Total lung capacity may be increased (109), perhaps secondary to chronic obstructive lung disease, and bronchitis and emphysema have been reported.

The dermatological manifestations of acromegaly include hyperhidrosis (110), deepening of the skin furrows and soft tissue enlargement resulting in growth of hands and feet. Pigmented skin tags are present in up to 50% of patients (99). Acanthosis nigricans that improves with treatment has been reported (111, 112).

Patients with acromegaly appear to have an increased risk of abnormal carbohydrate metabolism. Impaired glucose tolerance may be seen in up to 60%, but overt diabetes mellitus is noted in only 15% to 25% (88, 89, 104, 113). In general, those patients with more severe hyperglycemia tend to have the greatest degree of GH excess (99). Treatment of diabetes in acromegalic patients can usually be managed by diet therapy with or without oral hypoglycemic agents, although some patients do require insulin. Neuropathic and vascular complications of diabetes appear infrequently in acromegaly (99, 115). Treatment of GH excess may restore euglycemia in a significant portion of the patients.

Amenorrhea has been noted in approximately 45% of women with acromegaly (99). Half of these may be secondary to coexisting hyperprolactinemia, either as a result of mass effect of the tumor or co-secretion of prolactin by the adenoma. Hirsutism is somewhat common, with an incidence of approximately 25% (99), and the majority of cases are associated with amenorrhea. Galactorrhea is found in 10% of women with acromegaly and is also associated with hyperprolactinemia (99, 116). A significant proportion of men with acromegaly experience impotence with hypogonadotropic hypogonadism. Again, this may be a result of hyperprolactinemia or secondary to tumorous compression of the pituitary. Despite a large tumor burden, most acromegalics do not have coexisting pertubation of the hypothalamic-pituitary-adrenal axis.

Though the signs and symptoms will be similar, abnormal secretion of GHRH, GH, or IGF I can result in acromegaly. Pituitary adenomas secreting GH represent the majority (greater than 99% of cases). These tumors are usually benign and slow growing; however, a subset may be invasive (117) and, rarely, malignant. Mixed tumors with cells secreting either GH or prolactin are seen in 15% of cases, and pluri-hormonal adenomas, in which a single cell type secretes multiple hormones (GH, prolactin, adrenocorticotropic hormone [ACTH], thyroid-stimulating hormone [TSH] and α subunit), are seen in 5% of cases. Eighty percent of GH-producing tumors are macroadenomas at the time of diagnosis, and approximately half of those are locally invasive (118). Ectopic pituitary glands do occur, and case reports have documented acromegaly as a result of adenomas outside of the sella (119, 120). Ectopic GH secretion from tumors other than pituitary are quite rare but may arise from gastrointestinal, pulmonary, breast or pancreatic islet tissue (121).

Dysregulation of GHRH may result in acromegaly. Hypothalamic tumors have been described that secrete excess GHRH (122). Altered GHRH pulse frequency has been proposed as a mechanism by which pituitary adenomas may arise (97). Ectopic GHRH production by malignant neoplasms has been reported in such tumors as bronchial or intestinal carcinoid, pancreatic islet cell and pheochromocytomas (123–125).

As previously mentioned, multiple factors can increase GH levels, and hence random GH values are of little benefit in the diagnosis of acromegaly. The majority of patients with acromegaly have GH levels between 3 and 10 μg/L, although values up to 100 μg/L have been observed (98). While these latter "extreme" values are virtually diagnostic of acromegaly, other indirect assessments of GH secretion are often needed to definitively diagnose acromegaly.

IGF I, synthesized and secreted from the liver, has a half-life of hours. An excellent correlation between serum IGF I levels and mean 24-hour GH secretion has been established (97, 126–128). A single elevated IGF I is nearly 100% accurate in terms of both sensitivity and specificity and can reliably establish the diagnosis of acromegaly (129). Adjunctive studies such as glucose tolerance testing, glucagon suppression and TRH stimulation are generally reserved for research protocols.

Radiographic detection of pituitary tumors in patients with acromegaly is not difficult, as most have tumors greater than 10 mm at the time of diagnosis. Both computed tomography (CT) and magnetic resonance imaging (MRI) are effective. As with prolactinomas, CT scans better define bony involvement, and MRI scans better delineate tumor involvement with surrounding soft tissue structures.

Therapeutic Approach

Somatostatin

Although somatostatin can significantly reduce excessive GH secretion, it is of limited pharmacological use, as its half-life is on the order of 2 to 3 minutes. In 1980, a somatostatin analogue, octreotide acetate (Sandostatin), was synthesized. Octreotide is a synthetic octapeptide that shares a 4–amino acid sequence with native somatostatin (f130). Because of incomplete oral absorption, administration has been chiefly via subcutaneous and intravenous routes. Octreotide is rapidly absorbed subcutaneously, has a peak serum concentration in 30 minutes (131) and circulates in the blood, with approximately 65% of the drug bound to protein. Octreotide is at least 100 times more potent than somatostatin in suppressing GH secretion (132) and, with a half-life of 120 minutes after subcutaneous injection, can be given on a t.i.d. basis. GH levels should reach a nadir approximately 20 to 30 minutes after a single subcutaneous injection of octreotide (133).

In addition to its GH-suppressing properties, octreotide has effects on other endocrine and non-endocrine systems. In healthy subjects it will inhibit the TSH response to TRH (133, 134), although clinical hypothyroidism is not observed. Octreotide can delay gastrointestinal transit and thereby promote reabsorption of fluids and electrolytes (135). Fecal fat excretion may increase, however, and loose, malodorous stools may be present at the onset of therapy (136). This may be accompanied by abdominal discomfort, cramping, nausea and even vomiting, which should be self-limited. The use of pancreatic enzyme replacements may be of some benefit (133). Cholelithiasis and occasionally cholecystitis have been reported in up to 60% of acromegalics receiving octreotide (137–139). Octreotide appears to inhibit post-prandial contraction of the gallbladder (140) and diminish secretion of cholecystokinin (140, 141). Hence, some clinicians have cautioned that the high incidence of cholecystitis should be considered before initiating therapy with octreotide (142). Octreotide can inhibit insulin secretion and, to a lesser extent, glucagon secretion. Although post-prandial hyperglycemia has been noted, octreotide does not appear to significantly alter the level of glycemic control in patients with non–insulin-dependent diabetes mellitus (143). Most acromegalics receiving octreotide experience no change (144) or improved glycemic control (50–59), though some individuals may worsen (133, 146).

The recommended starting dose of octreotide is 50 to 100 μg subcutaneously given every 8 hours (147, 148). Furthermore, studies employing a constant total daily dose of octreotide have shown that smaller doses (333 μg) given t.i.d. may be more effective than larger doses (500 μg) given b.i.d. (146) Wang *et al.* (149) reported that treatment with octreotide every 2 hours may be more effective than treatment given every 8 hours in diminishing GH levels, though both regimens reduced IGF I levels to a similar degree.

Approximately 75% of the patients have a significant decline in GH levels with this regimen (50 to 100 μg subcutaneously/t.i.d.) (127, 144, 146, 150–155). However, only 35% have complete normalization of GH and IGF I levels (156). As this lack of responsiveness may correlate with tumor somatostatin receptor number (157), further studies using higher doses of octreotide have been undertaken. Although not all studies have employed maximal doses of octreotide, doses of up to 1500 μg per day have been used, and the overall response rate is approximately 80%, with nearly 50% having normal GH profiles and IGF I levels (158–159). Hence, incremental alterations in octreotide dose may be necessary for maximum responsiveness in some acromegalics.

The clinical response to octreotide is often rapid and dramatic. Most patients experience reduction in soft tissue mass, weight loss of 2 to 5 kg, diminished hand volume and improved facial appearance within 1 to 4 weeks of initiating therapy (98, 145, 149), and clinical improvement may be greater than would be predicted by GH and IGF I response (165). Reduction in tumor size is variable and appears to be evident in 30% to 75% of patients in most series (136, 149, 156, 159, 161, 166, 169). However, these series often include patients receiving prior therapy for their acromegaly (low-dose octreotide, radiation therapy and surgery), and hence, response rates in previously untreated acromegalics with octreotide may be higher (149, 170). Though the degree of tumor shrinkage is usually less than 50%, preoperative therapy with octreotide may improve surgical resectibility and thereby overall cure rates (98).

Dopamine Agonists

As previously mentioned, bromocriptine (Parlodel) is a synthetic dopamine agonist that can be orally administered on a b.i.d./t.i.d. basis. Its GH-lowering effect has been documented since 1972 (171), and many subsequent studies have reported its effectiveness at doses of up to 30 mg per day in patients with acromegaly. These results have been previously summarized (98). Whereas greater than 50% of patients given bromocriptine have a decrease in GH levels, only 20% "normalize" their GH profiles, and less than 10% have normal IGF I levels. Another objective criteria used to assess the response to bromocriptine is improvement in glucose intolerance. This has been noted in up to 80% of patients (171, 172), 65% of whom may experience normalization (173). As with octreotide, the rate of symptomatic improvement may exceed that of biochemical improvement, as response rates of greater than 90% have been reported (174, 175). Bromocriptine is less effective than octreotide in reducing tumor size (176), and hence is no longer considered a suitable initial therapy for acromegaly. It can be used in combination with other modalities (surgery and radiation therapy) and has been shown to rarely increase the effectiveness of octreotide (177).

Other dopamine agonists have been employed in the therapy of acromegaly and are generally equal to or of less efficacy than bromocriptine itself. However, two compounds merit notation. Carbergoline can be given on a once-per-week basis and can reduce GH and IGF I levels (178). Though terguride may not acutely lower GH secretion, chronic administration may normalize GH levels and significantly reduce IGF I concentrations in some patients (179, 180).

In summary, octreotide is the most effective medical therapy for GH-secreting pituitary tumors. Though other modalities need to be employed to affect a cure, octreotide is of benefit in both acute and chronic therapeutic schemes. Bromocriptine may be a useful adjunct in tumors that show a poor response to octreotide.

ACTH-SECRETING ADENOMAS: CUSHING'S DISEASE

Physiology of ACTH Secretion

ACTH is a 39–amino acid peptide secreted by corticotroph cells in the anterior pituitary. The peptide is but one of several derived from a larger precursor molecule, pro-opiomelanocortin (POMC) (181). Post-translational processing varies in different tissues so that different species of POMC products are found in anterior or posterior pituitary and brain. Other peptides derived from POMC include α-melanocyte stimulating hormone (MSH), β-lipotropic hormone (LPH), and β-endorphin (182, 183). ACTH is secreted in a pulsatile manner superimposed on a cyclic diurnal variation that is related to the sleep-wake cycle (184).

The secretion of ACTH is positively regulated by a variety of neurotransmitters and is negatively controlled by glucocorticoids. Corticotropin-releasing factor (CRF) is a hypothalamic factor felt to be the most important positive physiological regulator of ACTH release (185–187). The neurotransmitters acetylcholine (188), serotonin (189) and opioids (190) have also been shown to affect ACTH secretion. Cortisol regulation of ACTH occurs both at the level of the hypothalamus by affecting CRF gene transcription (191) and directly on the pituitary by altering POMC mRNA (191) and ACTH secretion (192). Other humoral mediators of ACTH release include vasopressin (192, 193), epinephrine and norepinephrine (192), vasoactive intestinal polypeptide (194), and angiotensin II (195), although the physiological importance of these substances has not been fully determined.

Clinical Presentation and Evaluation

The excess secretion of ACTH from a pituitary adenoma (Cushing's disease) causes hypercortisolemia, with the eventual development of the hallmark features of Cushing's syndrome. The specific features of Cushing's syndrome have been well characterized over the years and include centripetal obesity, lanugal hirsutism, tinea versicolor, violaceous striae, and hyperpigmentation (196). These are in contrast to less specific findings that may be present in patients with obesity without hypercortisolism, such as glucose intolerance, acne, male-pattern hirsutism and hypertension. The male-to-female ratio of Cushing's disease is 10:1 (196, 197), in contrast to syndromes of ectopic ACTH production, which are twofold more common in men (196). Because of the profound symptoms associated with Cushing's disease, this diagnosis tends to be made earlier, so that large tumors causing visual field changes and headache are less common.

In the patient presenting with hypercortisolism, the differential diagnosis includes a pathologic primary increase in adrenal cortisol production versus an ACTH-stimulated event. In the latter case, it is important to distinguish between pituitary and non-pituitary sources of ACTH. Patients with Cushing's disease make up approximately 80% of patients found to have endogenous hypercortisolemia (183).

The presence of an elevated 24-hour urinary-free cortisol level is perhaps the simplest screening test to evaluate the potential of Cushing's syndrome. Elevated urinary cortisol excretion and an increased ACTH level exclude primary adrenal pathology. The overproduction of cortisol is confirmed by administering 1 mg of dexamethasone p.o. at 11 P.M. and measuring a plasma cortisol the following morning at 8 A.M. Cortisol levels greater than 5 µg/dl confirm the diagnosis of Cushing's syndrome. Distinguishing pituitary from non-pituitary ACTH-dependent forms of Cushing's syndrome may require a series of additional investigations. A 2-day, high-dose dexamethasone suppression test (2 mg p.o. every 6 hours for 2 days) has been shown to lower plasma cortisol in patients with pituitary-dependent forms of hypercortisolism (198). An overnight test (8 mg p.o. at 11 P.M.) has been shown to be more reliable and easier to perform (199, 200). In the latter test, patients with Cushing's disease have a decline in plasma cortisol by more than 50% of the baseline level (200). Despite the success of these suppression tests, there are a considerable number of false-positive and false-negative results (201). A corticotropin releasing hormone (CRH) stimulation test has been devised in which there is an exaggerated response of ACTH of greater than 50% and of plasma cortisol of greater than 20% in patients with pituitary-dependent Cushing's syndrome (202). Ectopic sources of ACTH may occasionally respond in this manner (203). When results of CRH stimulation and dexamethasone suppression testing are integrated, the accuracy of the combined testing increases to 98% (204).

Tumors that are greater than 1 cm at the time of presentation can almost always be imaged with a high-resolution CT scan; however, only 35% of those less than 1 cm can be detected by this means (196). Because 70% of corticotroph adenomas are microadenomas (201), additional imaging techniques are frequently warranted. MRI with gadolinium contrast increases detection sensitivity considerably (205). In difficult cases, the use of simultaneous bilateral inferior petrosal sinus sampling has gained favor. This study confirms the pituitary origin of excess ACTH secretion (206) by revealing at least a twofold increase in ACTH levels versus peripheral samples. False-positives may occur rarely in the case of ectopic production of CRF. In some cases, this study may also help lateralize the location of the adenoma in the pituitary; however, this is not highly accurate (206–208). Petrosal sinus sampling should be undertaken in those individuals in whom biochemical tests suggest the presence of a pituitary adenoma, but radiologic imaging studies are unable to conclusively detect the tumor.

Therapeutic Approach

The primary management of Cushing's disease is transsphenoidal exploration in an attempt at selective adenomectomy. When treated in this way at a center with physicians experienced in performing this procedure, the cure rate has been reported to be approximately 90% (196, 209). These rates fall significantly if no adenoma is found at pituitary microsurgery or if primary corticotropic cell hyperplasia exists. Friedman et al. reported that in those patients in whom Cushing's syndrome recurred despite transsphenoidal surgery, remission was achieved in 24 of 33 patients who underwent repeat pituitary exploration (210). The best evidence of successful surgery is post-operative hypocortisolism (196, 211). Medical therapy for those individuals with continued evidence of recurrent disease following transsphenoid adenomectomy or hypophysectomy is discussed below.

Medical Therapy for Cushing's Disease

The study of the chemotherapy of Cushing's disease has centered around the use of three drugs: octreotide (a somatostatin analogue), bromocriptine (a dopamine receptor agonist) and cyproheptadine (a serotonin antagonist). These agents have proved useful in other types of secretory pituitary adenomas. In addition, there are a variety of agents that can be used to control the peripheral manifestations of Cushing's syndrome by blocking the adrenal production of cortisol.

Bromocriptine, an agent highly successful in the treatment of prolactinomas, has been shown to be partially effective in the treatment of Cushing's disease (212, 213), though response is not universal (214). Bromocriptine has also been shown to be helpful in some cases of Nelson's syndrome (215, 216). Cyproheptadine is another agent that was shown to be partially effective in some patients with Cushing's disease (217). However, the effects of both of these drugs are present only as long as they are continued, and over time, medication failures occur. Although octreotide was shown to inhibit CRF-stimulated ACTH release from pituitary adenoma cells in culture (218) and in patients with Nelson's syndrome (219–221) or ectopic ACTH–producing tumors (222, 223), this agent does not appear to have an effect on ACTH or cortisol levels in patients with Cushing's disease (219).

The mainstay of therapy in failed resection or inoperable disease is anti-adrenal agents. Metapyrone, an inhibitor of 11β-hydroxylase, and aminoglutethamide, which blocks conversion of cholesterol to 20α-hydroxycholesterol in its metabolic conversion to pregnenolone, may be useful in remitting the clinical effects of hypercortisolism. However, these agents have significant gastrointestinal, skin, and central nervous system side effects. Mitotane, an adrenolytic agent, inhibits cortisol production and causes adrenal cortical destruction with some preservation of zona glomerulosa and mineralocorticoid production (224). Ketoconazole, developed as an anti-fungal agent, blocks adrenal and gonadal steroidogenesis. This agent is very useful in lowering cortisol levels (225). It is generally well tolerated, and its gastrointestinal adverse effects are often not severe; hepatitis is its most serious side effect. At this time, ketoconazole should be considered the agent of choice in patients with Cushing's disease who require medical therapy.

Like chemotherapy, radiation therapy has been relegated to a second-line therapy in the treatment of ACTH-secreting adenomas. Although this modality of therapy has been used a great deal in the past, its effects are not apparent for 6 to 18 months (226). Furthermore, results with radiation therapy have not been as good as those with transsphenoidal surgery, ranging from 50% to 80% (226, 227). A significant proportion of patients treated by radiation develop panhypopituitarism (226), although this appears to occur more often in cases of acromegaly than Cushing's disease.

TSH-SECRETING ADENOMAS

Physiology of TSH Secretion

TSH is a glycoprotein hormone secreted by the thyrotroph cells of the anterior pituitary. The protein shares a common α subunit with follicle-stimulating hormone (FSH), luteinizing hormone (LH) and chorionic gonadotropin (CG) and has a distinct β subunit that confers biological activity. Secretion of TSH appears to be pusatile (228) and is superimposed on a circadian rhythm, with peak TSH levels near midnight (229). TSH undergoes a series of post-translational modifications involving the addition of sulfated and sialated oligosaccharide moieties to the protein structure that are felt to alter TSH bioactivity (230, 231). In many cases of thyrotropic adenomas, the TSH secreted is atypical in structure.

Regulation of the secretory pattern of this peptide involves a number of positive and negative factors from neuroendocrine and humoral origins. Among the neural regulators of TSH secretion are thyrotropin releasing hormone (TRH) (232), dopamine (233, 234), somatostatin (234, 235, 236), norepinephrine and serotonin (237). Thyroid hormone is the best studied and the most important humoral factor that regulates TSH secretion. Both thyroxine (T_4) and triiodothyronine (T_3) have been shown to decrease TSH α and β subunit mRNA concentration (238, 239). Furthermore, these substances inhibit basal and TRH-stimulated TSH secretion. Although there is evidence to suggest that gonadal steroids may alter TSH subunit gene expression (240–242), these data are contradictory in terms of the direction of change in steady-state mRNA levels and do not support a major role for these substances in the regulation of TSH secretion.

Clinical Presentation and Evaluation

By all accounts, TSH-secreting pituitary adenomas are rare and are probably the least common of the secretory tumors, with fewer than 100 case reports in the literature since 1970. Hamilton and co-workers described the first case of secondary hyperthyroidism due to a pituitary adenoma since the advent of sensitive assays for TSH (243). A number of in-depth reviews have been published analyzing these cases (244–247). Depending on the source, the incidence among cases of pituitary adenomas may vary from 2 to 15 cases per 1000 (248–251), and the male-to-female ratio is approximately 3:4. Goiter is present in over 90% of the cases in which a thyroid examination is performed, and roughly one half of patients have defects on formal visual field examinations (245). In virtually all patients, clinical hyperthyroidism is present. The presence of hyperthyroidism combined with the rarity of these tumors has led to many patients with TSH-secreting adenomas initially being treated with anti-thyroid medications for a time, leading to a delay in diagnosis and treatment (252). Perhaps for this reason, these tumors tend to be macroadenomas at the time of diagnosis. As such, these tumors often cause compressive symptoms such as headache and optic chiasmal impingement with visual field defects.

The range of hyperthyroid symptoms varies considerably, and there is poor correlation between measured TSH and thyroxine levels or degree of hyperthyroidism. Some of this variability may be explained by the secretion of thyrotropin molecules with altered biological activity or a failure to couple α and TSH β subunits. Tumor cells isolated in culture have been shown to secrete free α subunit (253–256). In one study, the evaluation of immunoreactive TSH in a patient with a TSH-secreting adenoma was found to have a number of sub-fractions by electrofocusing with different bioactivities (257). The expression of TSH β subunit mRNA does not appear to vary between normal and adenomatous pituitary tissues, implying altered translation in the neoplasms (258). These findings are consistent with the hypothesis that TSH bioactivity can be modified post-translationally by differential glycosylation (230).

The diagnosis of TSH-secreting pituitary adenomas requires the presence of an elevated serum thyroxine and usually with clinical evidence of hyperthyroidism and an inappropriately high TSH. This criteria necessitates the use of an ultrasensitive immunometric assay for TSH to be able to distinguish between fully suppressed and low-normal levels. Once these features have been verified, several investigations may help establish the diagnosis and distinguish this condition from the rare case of thyroid hormone resistance, which may have similar biochemical features. Because these tumors secrete increased amounts of free α subunit, a measured molar ratio of α subunit to intact TSH greater than 1.0 strongly suggests the presence of a pituitary adenoma (245). It should be remembered that α subunit is present in the other glycoprotein hormones, so that conditions that elevate LH, FSH, or human chorionic gonadotropin (hCG), such as pregnancy or gonadal failure, can reduce the specificity of this assessment.

The use of provocative testing in the diagnosis of TSH-secreting adenomas is of interest but not generally necessary. TRH stimulation testing was previously thought to help in the diagnosis of adenomas, in that these patients frequently had no TSH response to TRH. Although the test is fairly specific, the false-negative rate can be high so that the predictive value of the test is limited (245).

In summary, the diagnosis of TSH-secreting adenoma should be entertained in patients with clinical hyperthyroidism in whom hyperthyroxinemia is present and TSH is detectable in an ultrasensitive assay. Included in the differential diagnosis in these patients is a condition known as "non-tumoral inappropriate secretion of TSH," which occurs in an otherwise normal pituitary. The cause of this condition is unknown, but it is postulated that the basis of the disorder is thyroid hormone resistance occurring primarily at the level of the pituitary and therefore leading to clinical hyperthyroidism (259). In contrast to patients with adenomas, these patients have a dramatic increase in TSH during TRH stimulation testing and will have a normal α subunit–to-TSH molar ratio (259). These tests may be indicated in individuals with biochemical features of TSH-secreting adenomas in whom radiographic procedures fail to demonstrate the presence of a tumor.

Secretion of other pituitary hormones in addition to TSH is well documented. These include GH (260, 261), prolactin (262, 263) and the gonadotropins (264). No cases of simultaneous TSH and ACTH secretion have been reported. In patients with co-existing GH secretion, acromegalic features are invariably present (261). Hyperprolactinemia is often but not exclusively associated with amenorrhea/galactorrhea (245). The secretion of prolactin in some cases may not be directly from the tumor but instead may be related to a mass effect of the macroadenoma, thereby mimicking hypophyseal stalk transection and resulting in loss of dopaminergic suppression of prolactin release.

Radiologic assessment of patients suspected of having TSH-secreting adenomas is essential. For reasons previously discussed, these tumors tend to be macroadenomas at diagnosis and as such are well visualized by CT. In the future, as ultrasensitive TSH assays become more widespread, the diagnosis of secondary hyperthyroidism with detectable levels of TSH may be made sooner, and a greater percentage of smaller tumors will be evident. If a microadenoma is suspected, the use of MRI may be employed. As in the evaluation of all patients with sellar masses, in particular with tumors larger than 10 mm, formal visual field testing should be employed.

Therapeutic Approach

The primary management of TSH-secreting adenomas is the surgical excision of the tumor. Although several medical therapies appear promising, these tumors are usually large and frequently are found to be invasive at the time of diagnosis; hence, results with these therapies have been less than ideal (265). Therefore, interest in the medical therapy of these tumors is aimed at improving surgical outcomes by reducing tumor mass pre-operatively or by post-operative management of residual tumor. Because of the rarity of TSH-secreting tumors, the role of pre-operative medical treatment of these adenomas has not been well evaluated. The remainder of this section will focus on the post-surgical management of TSH-secreting tumors. Among the treatments that have been studied are somatostatin analogue therapy, dopamine agonists therapy, radiotherapy, and anti-thyroid therapies.

Somatostatin

As previously noted, somatostatin has been shown to inhibit the release of TSH from the anterior pituitary. The short half-life of so-matostatin made it difficult to assess its potential role as a therapeutic agent. Early studies suggested that somatostatin could cause a mild diminution of TSH secretion from a pituitary adenoma (266). Since the introduction of a longer acting somatostatin analogue, octreotide (Sandostatin [SMS 201–995]), additional work has been done in this area. In a study of five patients with thyrotropic adenomas, three of whom had previously undergone pituitary surgery, octreotide significantly reduced serum TSH levels in four of the patients, including the two who received octreotide pre-operatively individuals. In one patient treated for 16 months, follow-up CT and MRI showed that the size of the tumor did not change (267). In another study reported by Beck-Peccoz et al. (268) of four patients with thyrotropin adenomas, all four showed a return to normal the TSH levels and marked reduction in the α subunit in all patients. Furthermore, in the three patients in whom biochemical hyperthyroidism was present prior to treatment, the free T_3 also returned to normal values. All four patients had previously undergone transsphenoidal surgery. The effectiveness of octreotide continued in one patient followed for 30 days. Other case reports have found similar improvements (269–271). In these cases, the dose of somatostatin analogue ranged from 50 to 150 μg/day in three divided doses.

At this time, current data support the use of somatostatin analogue in cases of active residual tumor after hypophysectomy or in cases in which the tumor is felt to be unresectable.

Bromocriptine

Dopaminergic agonists like bromocriptine have been highly effective in the treatment of prolactin-secreting tumors (272). This agent markedly reduces prolactin secretion and tumor size. Its efficacy in TSH-secreting tumors is limited, however. Dopamine agonists have been shown in some cases to partially suppress TSH secretion in patients with adenomas (240, 273). The length and degree of response is limited. Others have reported either no effect of bromocriptine on TSH secretion (274) or a paradoxical increase of TSH following L-dopa administration (275).

Other treatment modalities

In addition to the treatment of the tumor itself, therapy aimed at hyperthyroidism is also mandated if cure cannot be obtained. These patients should be treated in a fashion similar to cases of primary hyperthyroidism with consideration of β-blockers to reduce the systemic effects of hyperthyroxinemia as well as anti-thyroid agents like propylthiouracil. The use of radioiodine for thyroid ablation may be required if TSH cannot be modulated by other means. Because prolonged hypothyroidism may itself cause pituitary enlargement, it is possible that inducing hypothyroidism in a patient may increase tumor growth.

External pituitary radiation beam therapy has been used by itself and as an adjunct with surgery. Previous reviews have found that irradiation alone is associated with poor results; however, when coupled with surgery, there is some improvement in outcome (245).

GONADOTROPIC ADENOMAS

Physiology of Gonadotropin Secretion

GnRH is a decapeptide synthesized by and secreted from neurons in the hypothalamus into the hypophyseal portal venous system. To date, only a single hypothalamic factor, GnRH, has been identified that stimulates pituitary secretion of the gonadotropins LH and FSH. These hormones in turn regulate gonadal steroid production and gametogenesis. Because LH and FSH are secreted from a common gonadotrope cell and levels of the gonadotropins may vary in either parallel or divergent patterns, much research has been aimed at delineating the mechanisms allowing differential regulation. Modulation of the GnRH pulse pattern in addition to both inhibitory and stimulatory effects of gonadal steroids (testosterone, estrogen and progesterone) and peptides (inhibin) serves to induce the dynamic changes observed in the hypothalamic-pituitary-gonadal axis.

It has long been known that LH, and by inference GnRH, is released in a pulsatile manner (276). Work by Clarke and Cummins (277) further documented this relationship between GnRH and LH pulsatile release. The correlation between GnRH and FSH is more complex, as this glycoprotein hormone has a longer half-life than LH, making pulse detection more difficult. However, work by Urban *et al.* (278) has provided a scheme to detect pulsatile FSH release and may allow

for better comparison with LH and GnRH secretion. The pulsatile pattern of GnRH secretion is essential for normal gonadotrope function, as continuous infusion of exogenous GnRH will not increase gonadotropin secretion (279). Conversely, pulsatile GnRH increases LH and FSH in GnRH-deficient subjects (280), can induce pubertal maturation (281) and restores normal menstrual function and fertility (282–284).

One mechanism whereby differential secretion of the gonadotropins may be accomplished is via alterations in GnRH pulse amplitude and frequency. Faster pulse frequencies and lower pulse amplitudes favor LH, while slower pulse frequencies and higher pulse amplitudes increase FSH (279, 280, 285). Though GnRH-producing neurons may have an inherent rhythmicity (286), higher CNS input can alter the GnRH signal. Catecholamines can increase LH secretion (287), whereas endogenous opioids inhibit GnRH and slow LH pulse frequency (288). Progesterone, in the presence of estradiol, may act via the opioid pathway to slow GnRH pulse frequency during the luteal phase of the menstrual cycle (289, 290). Additionally, prolactin may increase opioid tone and diminish GnRH release, with resulting amenorrhea (291).

Modulation of the action of GnRH directly at the pituitary may also result in altered gonadotrope responsiveness. Estradiol may augment LH release at the time of the midcycle LH surge (292), an effect that may be prolonged by progesterone (293). Conversely, estradiol exerts a predominantly inhibitory action on FSH synthesis and secretion (294). Finally, gonadal peptides such as inhibin and activin have been shown *in vitro* to selectively regulate FSH synthesis and secretion (295), and passive immunoneutralization of inhibin can increase the ovulation rate in the rat (296). It is presumed that the loss of inhibin, in addition to gonadal steroids, accounts for the greater increase in FSH than LH commonly observed in postmenopausal women. However, the role of inhibin and activin in human physiology remains uncertain.

Clinical Presentation and Diagnosis

At one point, it was felt that gonadotropin-secreting adenomas were very rare tumors occurring in older men. However, more recent work has provided compelling evidence that gonadotropin-secreting adenomas affect a broader group. Part of the difficulty in tracking the incidence and characteristics of this disorder is that clinical syndromes related to excessive gonadotropin secretion, specifically FSH, generally do not occur. As such, patients with these tumors usually present with headaches, visual field defects and radiologic evidence of large pituitary masses with extra-sellar involvement (297, 298). Rarely, men may present with bilateral testicular enlargement due to FSH effect on the seminiferous tubules (299) or with elevated testosterone levels when the tumor hypersecretes LH (300, 301).

Case reviews of patients over the past few decades have shown that patients found to have gonadotropin-secreting adenomas tend to be men above 40 years of age (297). Snyder reviewed the experience with these tumors at the University of Pennsylvania (297). Of 31 men with FSH or α subunit excess, virtually all of them gave histories of normal pubertal development, and most had fathered children. In this study, 17% of men with pituitary tumors were of gonadotropic origin. Beckers *et al.* demonstrated similar findings (302). Establishing the diagnosis of a gonadotropin-secreting adenomas in older women is difficult in that the population of women likely to have such a tumor are postmenopausal and would normally have high levels of circulating gonadotropins. That these tumors are not exclusively found in men has been reported by Daneshdoost *et al.*. This group showed that in 11 of 16 women with apparently nonsecreting pituitary adenomas, provocative testing of the LH-β and intact LH and FSH responses to TRH revealed that these tumors were of gonadotropic origin (303). Furthermore, FSH-β and LH-β mRNAs have been identified within these tissues (304).

Patients with these tumor types are most commonly found to have elevated levels of intact FSH (297); however, secretion of LH (300, 301, 305, 306), LHβ (303), FSHβ (307) and α subunits (307, 308–310), as well as TSH (311), from these adenomas has also been recognized. To some extent, this distinguishes patients with adenomas from those with primary hypogonadism. The latter group will have elevated intact FSH and LH levels but lower circulating levels of the subunit species (247, 303, 307).

Therapeutic Approach

The primary modality of therapy is transsphenoidal resection. As previously discussed, these patients frequently present with headaches and evidence of optic nerve compression. Surgical decompression performed in a timely fashion can ameliorate these complications. The role of ancillary medical therapy in the treatment of gonadotropin-secreting tumors has not been well evaluated. An examination of non-secretory adenomas showed that a portion of these had somatostatin receptors (312). Because many nonsecreting tumors are probably of gonadotropic origin, investigators have tested the effectiveness of octreotide in gonadotropin-secreting adenomas. Vos *et al.* studied a patient with an LH-secreting tumor and increased testosterone levels in whom octreotide was effective in lowering circulating LH levels (313). Sassolas *et al.* also showed an effect of octreotide on α-subunit secretion in a patient with an adenoma secreting only that peptide. However there was no effect in two women with FSH and α-subunit–secreting adenomas (314). Bromocriptine lowers gonadotropin secretion in normal subjects and has also been tested in patients with glycoprotein-secreting adenomas. In the few patients examined, bromocriptine was able to reduce FSH, LH, and α-subunit levels (315–317). No study has documented a significant decrease in tumor size with medical therapy alone, but more studies in the use of these compounds need to be completed before recommendations regarding their use can be made.

Additional studies have been carried out using GnRH agonists and antagonists. In normal subjects, chronic infusion of GnRH agonist down-regulates receptor-mediated events, thereby decreasing gonadotropin secretion. When GnRH was administered to patients with adenomas, no such effect was found by two groups (318, 319), but lowering of LH or FSH levels was achieved in one other study (320). The use of GnRH antagonist appears to be more promising. When this agent was administered in repetitive injections, Daneshdoost *et al.* were able to show a lowering of FSH levels to normal in four of five patients studied (321). These findings raise the question of whether development of gonadotropin-secreting tumors is a GnRH-dependent process, a question that remains unanswered. Changes in tumor size were not evaluated.

The use of radiation therapy is directed at those patients who have undergone transsphenoidal resection and in whom significant residual tumor remains or rapid regrowth occurs. This modality of therapy is also useful in patients in whom little residual tumor remains but rapid tumor growth is demonstrated at a later date. Recurrence without rapid expansion may be treated by repeat surgery (322).

At present, surgical decompression with or without radiation therapy is the standard therapy for gonadotropin-secreting pituitary adenomas. The use of GnRH antagonist may provide some improvement in biochemical changes, but whether this will turn out to be an effective long-term modality of therapy has not been determined.

REFERENCES

1. Leighton PC, McNeilly AS, Chad T. Short-term variations in blood levels of prolactin in women. J Endocrinol 68:177–178, 1976.
2. Saunders A, Terry LC, Audet L, Brazeau P, Martin JD. Dynamic studies of growth hormone and prolactin secretion in the female rat. Neuroendocrinology 21:193–203, 1976.
3. Demarest KT, Moore KE. Accumulation of L-dopa in the median eminence: An index of tuberinfundibular dopaminergic activity. Endocrinology 106:463–468, 1980.
4. Gudelsky GA, Simpkins J, Mueller GP, Meites J, Moore KE. Selective actions of prolactin on catecholamine turnover in the hypothalamus and on serum LH and FSH. Neuroendocrinol 22:206–215, 1976.
5. Tashjian AH, Barowski NJ, Jensen DK. Thyrotropin-releasing hormone: Direct evidence for stimulation of prolactin production by pituitary cells in culture. Biochem Biophys Res Commun 43:516–523, 1971.
6. Frawley LS, Neill JD. Stimulation of prolactin secretion in rhesus monkeys by vasoactive intestinal peptide. Neuroendocrinology 33:79–83, 1981.
7. Wehrenberg WB, McNicol D, Frantz AG, Ferin M. The effects of serotonin on prolactin and growth hormone concentrations in normal pituitary stalk sectioned monkeys. Endocrinology 107:1747–1750, 1980.
8. Seeburg PH, Mason AJ, Stewart TA, Nikolics K. The mammalian GnRH gene and its pivotal role in reproduction. Recent Prog Horm Res 43:69–98, 1987.
9. Dalkin A, Marshall JC. The medical therapy of hyperprolactinemia. Endocrinol Metab Clin North Am 18:259–268, 1989.
10. Jordan R, Kohler PO. Recent advances in diagnosis and treatment of pituitary tumors. Adv Intern Med 32:299–323, 1987.
11. Molitch ME. Management of prolactinomas. Ann Rev Med 40:225–232, 1989.
12. Vance ML, Thorner MO. Prolactinomas. Endocrinol Metab Clin North Am 16:731–753, 1987.
13. Jacobs H, Franks S, Murray MAF, Hull MGR, Steele SJ, Nabarro JDN. Clinical and endocrine features of hyperprolactinemic amenorrhea. Clin Endocrinol 5:439–454, 1976.
14. Franks S. Regulation of pituitary secretion by estrogens: Physiological and pathological significance. Clin Sci 65:457–462, 1983.
15. Nakao H, Koga M, Arao M, Nakao M, Sato B, Kishimoto S, Saitoh Y, Arita N, Mori S. Enzyme-immunoassay for estrogen receptors in human pituitary adenomas. Acta Endocrinol 120:233–238, 1989.
16. Veldhuis JD. The estrogen-prolactinoma nexus in humans—fact or fable. Mayo Clin Proc 64:1190–1192, 1989.
17. Bevan JS, Sussman J, Roberts A, Hourihan M, Peters JR. Development of an invasive macroprolactinoma: A possible consequence of prolonged estrogen replacement. Case report. Br J Obstet Gynecol 96:1440–1444, 1989.
18. Falaschi P, del Pozo E, Rocco A, Toscano V, Petrangeli E, Pompei P, Frajese G. Prolactin release in polycystic ovarian syndrome. Obstet Gynecol 55:579–582, 1980.
19. Edwards CRW, Forsyth IA, Besser GM. Amenorrhea, galactorrhea and primary hypothyroidism with high circulating levels of prolactin. Br Med J 3:462–464, 1971.
20. Weizman R, Weizman A, Levi J, Guva V, Zevin D, Maoz B, Wijsenbneck H, Ben-David M. Sexual dysfunction associated with hyperprolactinemia in males and females undergoing hemodialysis. Psychosom Med 42:259–269, 1983.
21. Molitch ME. Pregnancy and the hyperprolactinemic woman. N Engl J Med 312:3164–3170, 1985.
22. Franks S, Jacobs HS. Hyperprolactinemia. Clin Endocrinol 3:641–668, 1983.
23. Koppelman MC, Jaffe MJ, Rieth KG, Caruso RC, Loriaux DL. Hyperprolactinemia, amenorrhea and galactorrhea. Ann Intern Med 100:115–121, 1984.
24. Sauder SE, Frager M, Case GD, Kelch RP, Marshall JC. Abnormal patterns of pulsatile luteinizing hormone secretion in women with hyperprolactinemia and amenorrhea: Responses to bromocriptine. J Clin Endocrinol Metab 59:941–948, 1984.
25. Nabarro JDN. Pituitary prolactinomas. Clin Endocrinol 17:129–155, 1982.
26. Thorner MO, McNeilly AS, Hagan C, Besser GM. Long-term treatment of galactorrhea and hypogonadism with bromocriptine. Br Med J 2:419–422, 1974.
27. Kemmann E, Jones JR. Hyperprolactinemia and headaches. Am J Obstet Gynecol 145:668–671, 1983.
28. Bohnet GH, Dabler GH, Wutke W, Schneider HPG. Hyperprolactinemic anovulatory syndrome. J Clin Endocrinol Metab 42:132–143, 1975.
29. Boyar RM, Kapen S, Finkelstein JW, Perlow M, Sassin JF, Fukushima DK, Weitzman ED, Hellman L. Hypothalamic-pituitary function in diverse hyperprolactinemic states. J Clin Invest 53:1588–1598, 1974.
30. Segal S, Polishuk W, Ben-David M. Hyperprolactinemic male infertility. Fertil Steril 27:1425–1427, 1976.
31. Wong T, Jones T. Hyperprolactinemia and male infertility. Arch Pathol Lab Med 108:35–39, 1985.
32. Corrodi H, Fuxe K, Hokfelt T, Lidbrink P, Ungerstedt U. Effect of ergot drugs on cerebral cat-

echolamine neurons: Evidence for a stimulation of central dopamine neurons. J Pharm Pharmacol 25:409–412, 1973.

33. Muhr C, Lundberg PO, Antoni G, Hartvig P, Lunquist H, Langstrom B, Stalnacke CG. 11C-bromocriptine uptake and pituitary adenomas. In: Macleod RM, Thorner MO, Scapagnini U (eds): Prolactin. Basic and Clinical Correlates. New York, Springer-Verlag, 1985, pp 729–737.

34. Spark RF, Baker R, Bienfang DC, Bergland R. Bromocriptine reduces pituitary tumor size and hypersecretion. JAMA 247:311–316, 1982.

35. Landolt AM, Mindler H, Osterwalter V, Caudolt T. Bromocriptine reduces the size of cells in pro-lactin secreting pituitary adenomas. Experientia 39:625–626, 1983.

36. Molitch ME, Elton RL, Blackwell RE, Caldwell B, Change J, Jaffe R, Joplan G, Robbins RJ, Tyson J, Thorner MO. Bromocriptine as primary therapy for prolactin-secreting adenomas: Results of a multi-center trial. J Clin Endocrinol Metab 60:698–705, 1985.

37. Thorner MO, Martin WH, Rogol AD, Morris JL, Perryman RL, Conway BP, Howards SS, Wolfman MG, MacLeod RM. Rapid regression of pituitary prolactinomas during bromocriptine therapy. J Clin Endocrinol Metab 51:438–445, 1980.

38. Fahlbus F, Buchfelder M, Schnell U. Short-term preoperative therapy of macroprolactinomas by dopamine agonists. J Neurosurg 67:807–815, 1987.

39. Bassetti M, Spada A, Pezzo G, Giannattasio G. Bromocriptine treatment reduced the cell size in human macroprolactinomas: A morphometric study. J Clin Endocrinol Metab 58:268–273, 1984.

40. Horvath E, Kovacs K. Pathology of prolactin cell adenomas of the human pituitary. Semin Diagn Pathol 3:4–17, 1986.

41. Nissim M, Ambrosi B, Berasconi V, Giannattasio G, Giovanelli MA, Bassetti M, Vaccari U, Moriondo P, Spada A, Travaglini P, Faglier G. Bromocriptine treatment of macroprolactinomas: studies on the time course of tumor shrinkage and morphology. J Endocrinol Invest 5:409–415, 1982.

42. McComb DJ, Kovacs K, Horvath E, Singer W, Kilinger DW, Symth HS, Ezrin L, Weiss ML. Cor-relative ultrastructural morphometry of human prolactin-producing adenomas. Acta Neurochir 53:217–225, 1980.

43. Tindall JT, Kovacs K, Horvath E, Thorner MO. Human prolactin-producing adenomas and bro-mocriptine: A histological, immunohistochemical, ultrastructural and morphometric study. J Clin Endocrinol Metab 55:1178–1183. 1982.

44. Lloyd HM, Jacobi JM, Meares JD. DNA synthesis and depletion of prolactin in the pituitary gland of the male rat. J Endocrinol 77:129–136, 1978.

45. Maurer RA. Transcriptional regulation of the pro-lactin gene by ergocryptine and cyclic AMP. Nature 294:94–97, 1981.

46. Pellegrini I, Costa R, Grisoli F, Jaquet P. Abnormal dopamine sensitivity in some human prolactino-mas. Hor Res 31:19–23, 1989.

47. Pellegrini I, Gunz G, Bertran P, Delivet S, Jedynak CP, Kordon C, Peillon F, Jaquet P, Enjalbert A. Resistance to bromocriptine in prolactinomas. J Clin Endocrinol Metab 69:500–509, 1989.

48. Dallabonzana D, Spelta B, Oppizzi G, Tonon C, Luccarelli G, Chiodini PG, Liuzzi L. Reenlarge-

ment of macroprolactinomas during bromocriptine therapy: Report of two cases. J Endocrinol Invest 6:47–50, 1983.

49. March CM, Kletzky DA, Davajan V, Teal J, Weiss M, Apuzzo MLJ, Marus RP, Mishell DR. Longitu-dinal evaluation of patients with untreated prolac-tin-secreting pituitary adenomas. Am J Obstet Gy-necol 139:835–844, 1981.

50. Pontiroli AE, Falsetti L. Development of pituitary adenomas in women with hyperprolactinemia: Clinical, endocrine and radiologic characteristics. Br Med J 288:515–518, 1984.

51. Malarkey WB, Martin TL, Kim M. Patients with idiopathic hyperprolactinemia infrequently de-velop pituitary tumors. In: MacLeod RM, Thorner MO, Scapagnini U (eds). Prolactin. Basic and Clin-ical Correlates. New York, Springer-Verlag, 1981, pp 705–708.

52. Sisam DA, Sheehan JP, Sheeler LR. The natural history of untreated microprolactinomas. Fertil Steril 48:67–71, 1987.

53. Johnston DG, Prescot R, Kendall-Taylor P, Hall K, Crombie A, Hall R, McGregor A, Watson MJ, Cook DB. Hyperprolactinemia. Long-term effects of bromocriptine. Am J Med 75:868–874, 1983.

54. Corenblum B, Taylor PJ. Long-term follow-up of hyperprolactinemic women treated with bromo-criptine. Fertil Steril 40: 596–599, 1983.

55. Winfield A, Finkel DM, Schatz NJ, Salino PJ, Snyder PJ. Bromocriptine treatment of prolactin-secreting pituitary adenomas may restore pituitary function. Ann Intern Med 101:783–785, 1984.

56. Jordan RM, Kohler PO. Recent advances in diag-nosis and treatment of pituitary tumors. Adv In-tern Med 32:299–323, 1987.

57. Zarate A, Canales ES, Cano L, Pilonieta CJ. Follow-up of patients with prolactinomas after discontin-uation of long-term therapy with bromocriptine. Acta Endocrinol 104:139–142, 1983.

58. Thorner MO, Perryman RL, Rogol AD, Conway BP, MacLeod RM, Lopi TS, Morris JL. Rapid changes of prolactinoma volume after withdrawal and reinstitution of bromocriptine. J Clin Endo-crinol Metab 53:480–483, 1981.

59. Winkelman W, Allolio B, Deuss U, Heesen D, Karlen D. Persisting normo-prolactinemia after withdrawal of bromocriptine long-term therapy in patients with prolactinomas. In: MacLeod RM, Thorner MO, Scapagnini U (eds). Prolactin. Basic and Clinical Correlates. New York, Springer-Ver-lag, 1985, pp 817–822.

60. Barrow DL, Tindall G, Kovacs K, Thorner MO, Horvath E, Hoffman JC. Clinical and pathological effects of bromocriptine on prolactin-secreting and other pituitary tumors. J Neurosurg 60:1–7, 1984.

61. Vance ML, Evans WS, Thorner MO. Bromocrip-tine. Ann Intern Med 100:78–91, 1984.

62. Wass JA, Williams J, Charlesworth M, Kingsley DP, Halliday AM, Donaich I, Rees LH, MacDonald WI, Besser GM. Bromocriptine in management of large pituitary tumors. Br Med J 284:1908–1911, 1982.

63. van't Verlaat JW, Croughs RJM, Hendriks MJ, Bosma MJ. Results of primary therapy with bro-mocriptine of prolactinomas with extracellular ex-tension. Can J Neurol Sci 17:71–73, 1990.

64. Lesser RL, Zheutlin GD, Bogher D, O'Dell JG, Robbins RJ. Visual function improvement in pa-tients with macroprolactinomas treated with bro-mocriptine. Am J Ophthalmol 109:535–543, 1990.

65. Arita K, Uozumi T, Ohta M. A case of large prolactinoma supposed to be cured by bromocriptine therapy. Endocrinol Jpn 35:503–509, 1988.

66. Breidahl DH, Topliss DJ, Pike JW. Failure of bromocriptine to maintain reduction in the size of macroprolactinoma. Br Med J 287:451–452, 1983.

67. Hubbard JL, Scheithauser BW, Abboud CF, Laws ER. Prolactin-secreting adenomas: The preoperative response to bromocriptine therapy and surgical outcome. J Neurosurg 67:816–821, 1987.

68. Fahlbusch R, Buchfelder M, Schrell U. Short-term preoperative therapy of macroprolactinomas by dopamine agonists. J Neurosurg 67:807–815, 1987.

69. Landolt AM, Osterwalder V. Perivascular fibrosis and prolactinomas: Is it increased with bromocriptine. J Clin Endocrinol Metab 58:1179–1183, 1984.

70. Bevan JS, Adams CBT, Burke CW, Morton KE, Moore RA, Esiri MM. Factors in the outcome of transsphenoidal surgery for prolactinoma and nonfunctioning pituitary tumors, including preoperative bromocriptine therapy. Clin Endocrinol 26:541–556, 1987.

71. Candrina R, Galli G, Bollati A, Pizzocolo G, Orlandini A, Giustina G. Results of combined surgery and medical therapy in patients with prolactin-secreting pituitary macroadenomas. Neurosurgery 21:894–897, 1987.

72. Bronstein MD, Cardim CS, Marino R. Short-term management of macroprolactinomas with a new injectable form of bromocriptine. Surg Neurol 28:31–37, 1987.

73. Zarate A, Moran C, Miranda R, Lloyd DM, Modine M, Fonseca ME. Long-acting bromocriptine for the acute treatment of large macroprolactinomas. Endocrinol Invest 10:233–236, 1987.

74. Kocijancic K, Prezel J, Urbovec I, Lan Cranjan I. Parlodel LAR in the therapy of macroprolactinomas. Acta Endocrinol 122:272–276, 1990.

75. van't Verlaat JW, Lancranjan I, Hendricks MJ, Croughs RJM. Primary treatment of microprolactinomas with Parlodel LAR. Acta Endocrinol 119:51–55, 1988.

76. Katz E, Schran HF, Adashi EY. Successful treatment of prolactin-producing pituitary macroadenomas with intravaginal bromocriptine mesylate: A novel approach to intolerance of oral therapy. Obstet Gynecol 73:517–520, 1989.

77. Kletzky DA, Borenstein R, Milekowsky GN. Pergolide and bromocriptine for the therapy of patients with hyperprolactinemia. Am J Obstet Gynecol 154:431–435, 1986.

78. Mattox JH, Bernstein J, Buckman MT. Control of hyperprolactinemia with pergolide. Int J Fertil 30:39–43, 1986.

79. Ahmed SR, Shalet SM. Discordent responses of prolactinoma to two different dopamine agonists. Clin Endocrinol 24:421–426, 1986.

80. Ferrari C, Barbieri C, Caldara R, Mucci M, Codecasa F, Paracchi A, Romano C, Boghen M, Dubini A. Long-acting prolactin-lowering effect of carbergoline, a new dopamine agonist in hyperprolactinemia patients. J Clin Endocrinol Metab 63:941–945, 1986.

81. Ferrari C, Mattei A, Melis GV, Peracchi A, Muratoni M, Faglia G, Sghedoni D, Crosignani PG. Carbergoline: Long-acting oral therapy of hyperprolactinemic disorders. J Clin Endocrinol Metab 68:1201–1206, 1989.

82. Mullis GB, Mais V, Gambacchiani M, Sghedoni D, Paoletti AM, Fioretti P. Reduction in the size of prolactin-producing pituitary tumors after carbergoline administration. Fertil Steril 52:412–415, 1989.

83. Crosignani PG. Therapy of hyperprolactinemic stage with different drugs: A study of bromocriptine, metergoline and lisuride. Fertil Steril 37:61–67, 1982.

84. Verde G. Effectiveness of the dopamine agonist lisuride and the therapy of acromegaly and pathological hyperprolactinemic stage. J Endocrinol Invest 4:405–414, 1980.

85. Dallabonzana D, Liuzzi A, Oppizzi G, Verde G, Chiodini PG, Dorow R, Horowski R. Effect of the new ergot derivative terguride on plasma prolactin and growth hormone levels in patients with pathological hyperprolactinemia or acromegaly. J Endocrinol Invest 8:147–151, 1985.

86. Lamberts SWJ, Zweens M, Klinn JG, van Vroonhoven CC, Stefanko SJ, Del Pozo E. The sensitivity of growth hormone and prolactin secretion to the somatostatin analogue SMS 102–995 in patients with prolactinomas and acromegaly. Clin Endocrinol 25:201–212, 1986.

87. Tannenbaum GS, Martin JB. Evidence for an endogenous ultradian rhythm governing growth hormone secretion in the rat. Endocrinology 98:562–570, 1976.

88. Maiter D, Underwood LE, Maes M, Davenport ML, Ketelslegers JM. Different effects of intermittent and continuous growth hormone (GH) administration on serum somatomedin-C/insulin-like growth factor I and liver GH receptors in hypophysectomized rats. Endocrinology 123(2):1053–1059, 1988.

89. Ikuyama, H, Natori S, Nawata H, Kato K, Ibayashi H, Kariya T, Sakai T, Rivier J. Characterization of growth hormone-releasing hormone receptors in pituitary adenomas from patients with acromegaly. J Clin Endocrinol Metab 66(6):1265–1271, 1988.

90. Moyse E, Le Dafniet M, Epelbaum J, Pagesy P, Peillon F, Kordon C, Enjalbert A. Somatostatin receptors in human growth hormone and prolactin-secreting pituitary adenomas. J Clin Endocrinol Metab 61(1):988–103, 1985.

91. Plotsky PM, Vale W. Patterns of growth hormone-releasing factor and somatostatin secretion into the hypophyseal-portal circulation of the rat. Science 230:461–463, 1985.

92. Wehrenberg WB, Brazeau P, Luben R, Bohlen P, Guillemin R. Inhibition of the pulsatile secretion of growth hormone by monoclonal antibodies to the hypothalamic growth hormone releasing factor (GRF). Endocrinology 111(6):2147–2148, 1982.

93. Billestrup N, Swanson LW, Vale W. Growth hormone-releasing factor stimulates proliferation of somatotrophs in vitro. Proc Natl Acad Sci USA 83:6854–6857, 1986.

94. Clark RG, Robinson ICA. Growth induced by pulsatile infusion of an amidated fragment of human growth hormone releasing factor in normal and GHRF-deficient rats. Nature 314:281–283, 1985.

95. Berelowitz M, Szabo M, Frohman LA, Firestone S, Chu L. Somatomedin-C mediates growth hormone negative feedback by effects on both the hypothalamus and the pituitary. Science 212:1279–1281, 1981.

96. Barkan AL, Beitins IZ, Kelch RP. Plasma insulin-

like growth factor-I/somatomedin-C in acromegaly: Correlation with the degree of growth hormone hypersecretion. J Clin Endocrinol Metab 67(1):69–73, 1988.

97. Barkan AL, Stred SE, Reno K, Markovs M, Hopwood NJ, Kelch RP, Beitins IE. Increased growth hormone pulse frequency in acromegaly. J Clin Endocrinol Metab 69(6):1225–1233, 1989.

98. Barkan AL. Acromegaly. Diagnosis and treatment. Endocrinol Metab Clin North Am 18(2):277–310, 1989.

99. Nabarro JND. Acromegaly. Clin Endocrinol 26:481–512, 1987.

100. Martins JB, Kerber RE, Sherman BM, Marcus ML, Ehrhardt JC. Cardiac size and function in acromegaly. Circulation 56:(5):863–869, 1977.

101. Silinkova-Malkova E, Kolbel F. Relationship between symptoms of acromegaly and its complications, principally cardiovascular, in 86 patients. Acta Univ Carol Med 16(5/6):553–569, 1970.

102. McGuffin WL Jr, Sherman BM, Roth J, Gorden P, Kahn CR, Roberts WC, Frommer PL. Acromegaly and cardiovascular disorders. Ann Intern Med 81(1):11–18, 1974.

103. Mather HM, Boyd MJ, Jenkins JS. Heart size and function in acromegaly. Br Heart J 41:697–701, 1979.

104. Smallridge RC, Rajfer S, Davia J, Schaaf M. Acromegaly and the heart. Am J Med 66:22–27, 1979.

105. Savage DD, Henry WL, Eastman RC, Borer JS, Gorden P. Echocardiographic assessment of cardiac anatomy and function in acromegalic patients. Am J Med 67:823–829, 1979.

106. Rossi L, Thiene, G, Caregaro L, Giordano R, Lauro S. Dysrhythmias and sudden death in acromegalic heart disease. Chest 72:495–498, 1977.

107. Randall R. Acromegaly and gigantism. In: DeGroot LJ, Cahill Jr GF, Martini L, Nelson DH, Winegrod AI, Odell WD, Potts Jr JT, Steinberger E (eds). Textbook of Endocrinology. Philadelphia, WB Saunders, 1989, pp 330–350.

108. Wright AD, Hill DM, Lowy C, Fraser TR. Mortality of acromegaly. Q J Med 39:1–16, 1970.

109. Harrison DW, Millhouse KA, Harrington M, Nabarro JDM. Lung function in acromegaly. Q J Med 188:517–532, 1978.

110. Jadresic A, Banks LM, Child DF, Diamant L, Doyle FH, Fraser TG, Joplin GF. The acromegaly syndrome. Q J Med 202:189–204, 1982.

111. Hofeldt F, Levin S, Schneider V, Becker N, Forsham P. Clinical features of acromegaly and response to cryohypophysectomy. Rocky Mtn Med J 70:21–24, 1973.

112. Brown J, Winkelmann RK, Randall RV. Acanthosis nigricans and pituitary tumors. JAMA 198(6):151–155, 1966.

113. Kanis JA, Gillingham FJ, Harris P, Horn DB, Hunter WM, Redpath AT, Strong JA. Clinical and labaoratory study of acromegaly: Assessment before and one year after treatment. Q J Med 171:409–431, 1974.

114. Wass JAH, Cudworth AG, Bottazzo GF, Woodrow JC, Besser GM. An assessment of glucose intolerance in acromegaly and its response to medical treatment. Clin Endocrinol 12:53–59, 1980.

115. Ballintine EJ, Foxman S, Gorden P, Roth J. Rarity of diabetic retinopathy in patients with acromegaly. Arch Intern Med 141:1625–1627, 1981.

116. Tindall G, Tindall S. Transsphenoidal surgery for acromegaly: Long-term results in 50 patients. In: Black P, Zervas NT, Ridgway EC, Martin JB (eds). Secretory Tumor of the Pituitary Gland. New York, Raven Press, 1984, pp 175–178.

117. Melmed S, Braunstein GD, Horvath E, Ezrin C, Kovacs K. Pathophysiology of acromegaly. Endocr Rev 4(3):271–290, 1983.

118. Scheithauer BW, Kovacs K, Randall RV, Horvath E, Laws ER Jr. Pathology of excessive production of growth hormone. Clin Endocrinol Metab 15(3):655–681, 1986.

119. Corenblum B, LeBlanc FE, Watanabe M. Acromegaly with an adenomatous pharyngeal pituitary. JAMA 243(14):1456–1457, 1980.

120. Warner BA, Santen RJ, Page RB. Growth hormone and prolactin secretion by a tumor of the pharyngeal pituitary. Arch Intern Med 96:56–68, 1982.

121. Melmed S, Ezrin C, Kovacs K, Goodman RS. Frohman LA. Acromegaly due to secretion of growth hormone by an ectopic pancreatic islet-cell tumor. New Engl J Med 312(1):9–17, 1985.

122. Asa SL, Scheithauer BW, Bilbao JM, Horvath E, Ryan N, Kovacs K, Randall RV, Laws ER Jr, Singer W, Linfoot JA, Thorner MO, Vale W. A case for hypothalamic acromegaly: A clinicopathological study of six patients with hypothalamic gangliocytomas producing growth hormone-releasing factor. J Clin Endocrinol Metab 58(5):796–803, 1984.

123. Sano T, Asa SL, Kovacs K. GHRH-producing tumors: Clinical, biochemical and morphological manifestations. Endocr Rev 9:357–373, 1988.

124. Thorner MO, Perryman RL, Cronin MJ, Rogol AD, Draznin M, Johanson A, Vale W, Horvath E, Kovacs K. Somatotroph hyperplasia. J Clin Invest 70:965–977, 1982.

125. Barkan AL, Shenker Y, Grekin RJ, Vale WW, Lloyd RV, Beals TF. Acromegaly due to ectopic growth hormone (GH)-releasing hormone (GHRH) production: Dynamic studies of GH and ectopic GHRH secretion. J Clin Endocrinol Metab 63:(5):1057–1064, 1986.

126. Gianello-Neto D, Wajchenberg B, Mendonca B. Criteria for the cure of acromegaly: Comparison between basal growth hormone and SmC concentrations in active and nonactive acromegalic patients. J Endocrinol Invest 11:57–60, 1988.

127. Lamberts SWJ, Uitterlinden P, Schuijff PC, Klijn JGM. Therapy of acromegaly with sandostatin: The predictive value of an acute test, the value of serum somatomedin-C measurements in dose adjustment and the definition of a biochemical "cure." Clin Endocrinol 29:411–420, 1988.

128. Roefsema F, Frolich M, Van Dulken H. Somatomedin-C levels in treated and untreated patients with acromegaly. Clin Endocrinol 26:137–144, 1987.

129. Clemmons DR, Van Wyk JJ, Ridgway EC, Kliman B, Kjellberg RN, Underwood LE. Evaluation of acromegaly by radioimmunoassay of somatomedin-C. N Engl J Med 301:1138–1142, 1979.

130. Pless J, Bauer W, Briner U. Chemistry and pharmacology of SMS 201–995, a long-acting octapeptide analogue of somatostatin. Scand J Gastroenterol 21:54–64, 1986.

131. Kutz K, Nuesch E, Rosenthaler J. Pharmacokinetics of SMS 201–995 in healthy subjects. Scand J. Gastroenterol 2165–72, 1986.

132. Bauer W, Briner U, Doepfner W, Haller R, Hyu-

guenin R, Marbach P, Petcher TJ, Pless J. SMS 201–995: A very potent and selective octapeptide analogue of somatostatin with prolonged action. Life Sci *31*:1133–1140, 1982.

133. Barkan AL, Kelch RP, Hopwood NJ, Beitins IZ. Treatment of acromegaly with the long-acting somatostatin analog SMS 201–995. J Clin Endocrinol Metab *66*(1):16–23, 1988.

134. Del Pozo E, Kutz K. SMS 201–995, a new somatostatin analogue: Pharmacology profile. Neuroendocrinol Lett *7*:111–113, 1985.

135. Dueno M, Pai J, Santangelo W, Kregs G. Effect of somatostatin analog on water and electrolyte transport and transit time in human small bowel. Dig Dis Sci *32*:1092–1096, 1987.

136. Stevenaert A, Beckers A, Kovacs K, Bastings E, de Longueville M, Henner G. Experience with sandostatin in various groups of acromegalic patients. In: Lamberts SWJ (ed). Sandostatin in the Treatment of Acromegaly. New York, Springer, 1988, pp 95–101.

137. Plockinger U, Dienemann D, Quabbe H. Gastrointestinal side-effects of octreotide during long term treatment of acromegaly. J Clin Endocrinol Metab *71*(6):1658–1662, 1990.

138. Comi R. Somatostatin and somatostatin analog (SMS 201–995) in treatment of hormone-secreting tumors of the pituitary and gastrointestinal tract and non-neoplastic diseases of the gut. Ann Intern Med *110*:35–50, 1989.

139. Wass J, Anderson JV, Besser GM, Dowling RH. Gall stones and treatment with octreotide for acromegaly. Letter. Br Med J *299*:1162–1163, 1989.

140. Van Liessum PA, Hopman WPM, Pieters GFF, Jansen JBM, Smals AGH, Rosenbusch G, Kloppenborg PWC, Lamers CBH. Postprandial gallbladder motility during long term treatment with the long-acting somatostatin analog SMS 201–995 in acromegaly. J Clin Endocrinol Metab *69*(3):557–562, 1989.

141. Lembcke B, Creutzfeldt W, Schlesser S, Ebert R, Shaw C, Koop I. Effect of the somatostatin analogue sandostatin (SMS 201–995) on gastrointestinal, pancreatic and biliary function and hormone release in normal men. Digestion *36*:108–124, 1987.

142. Daughaday WH. Octreotide is effective in acromegaly but often results in cholelithiasis. Ann Intern Med *112*(3):159–160, 1990.

143. Williams G, Fuessl H, Kranenzlin M. Postprandial effects of SM 201–995 on gut hormones and glucose tolerance. Scand J Gastroenterol *21*(suppl 119):73–93, 1986.

144. Plewe G, Schrezenmeir J, Nolken G, Krause U, Beyer J, Kasper H, del Pozo E. Long-term therapy of acromegaly with the somatostatin analogue SMS 201–995 over 6 months. Lkin Wochenschr *64*:389–392, 1986.

145. Ho KY, Weissberger AJ, Marbach P, Lazarus L. Therapeutic efficacy of the somatostatin analog SMS 201–995 (Octreotide) in acromegaly. Ann Intern Med *112*:173–191, 1990.

146. Sandler LM, Burrin JM, Williams G, Joplin GF, Carr DH, Bloom SR. Effective long-term treatment of acromegaly with a long-acting somatostatin analogue (SMS 201–995). Clin Endocrinol *26*:85–95, 1987.

147. Plewe G, Krause U, Beyer J, Neufeld M, del Pozo E. Long-acting and selective suppression of growth hormone secretion by somatostatin analogue SMS 201–995 in acromegaly. Lancet *2*:782–784, 1984.

148. Lamberts SWJ, Oosterom R, Neufeld M, del Pozo E. The somatostatin analog SMS 201–995 induces long-acting inhibition of growth hormone secretion without rebound hypersecretion in acromegalic patients. J Clin Endocrinol Metab *60*(6):1161–1165, 1985.

149. Wang C, Lam KSL, Arceo E, Chan FL. Comparison of the effectiveness of 2-hourly *versus* 8-hourly subcutaneous injections of a somatostatin analog (SMS 201–995) in the treatment of acromegaly. J Clin Endocrinol Metab *69*(3):670–677, 1989.

150. Comi RJ, Gorden P. The response of serum GH levels to the long-acting somatostatin analog SMS 201–995 in acromegaly. J Clin Endocrinol Metab *64*:37–42, 1987.

151. Ch'ng LJ, Sandler LM, Kraenzlin ME, Burrin JM, Joplin GF, Bloom SR. Long-term treatment of acromegaly with a long-acting analogue of somatostatin. Br Med J *1*:284–285, 1985.

152. Timsit J, Chanson P. Larger E, Duet M, Mosse A, Guillausseau PJ, Harris AG, Moulonguet M, Warnet A, Lubetzki J. The effect of subcutaneous infusion versus subcutaneous injections of a somatostatin analogue (SMS 201–995) on the diurnal GH profile in acromegaly. Acta Endocrinologica (Copenh) *116*:108–112, 1987.

153. Spinas GA, Zapf J, Landolt AM, Stuckmann G, Froesch ER. Pre-operative treatment of 5 acromegalics with a somatostatin analogue: Endocrine and clinical observations. Acta Endocrinologica (Copenh) *114*:249–256, 1987.

154. Pieters GF, Smals AEM, Smals AGH, von Gennep JA, Kloppenborg PW. The effect of minisomatostatin and anomalous GH responses in acromegaly. Acta Endocrinol *114*:537–542, 1987.

155. Fredstorp L, Harris A, Haas G, Werner S. Short term treatment of acromegaly with the somatostatin analog octreotide: The first double-blind randomized placebo-controlled study on its effects. J Clin Endocrinol Metab *71*(5):1189–1194, 1990.

156. Harris AG, Prestele H, Herold K, Boerlin V. Long-term efficacy of sandostatin (SMS 201–995, Octreotide) in 178 acromegalic patients. Results from the International Multicenter Acromegaly Study Group. In: Lamberts SWJ (ed). Sandostatin in the Treatment of Acromegaly. New York, Springer, 1988, pp 117–125.

157. Reubi JC, Landolt AM. The growth hormone responses to octreotide in acromegaly correlate with adenoma somatostatin receptor status. J Clin Endocrinol Mehab *68*:844–850, 1989.

158. Barkan A, Lloyd RV, Chandler WF, Hatfield MK, Gebarski SS, Kelch RP, Beitins IZ. Treatment of acromegaly with SMS 201–995 (Sandostatin): Clinical, biochemical and morphologic study. In: Lamberts SWJ (ed). Sandostatin in the Treatment of Acromegaly. New York, Springer, 1988, pp 103–108.

159. Liuzzi A, Chiodini PG, Cozzi R, Dallabonzana D, Oppizzi G, Petroncini MM. Dopaminergic agonists and long-term somatostatin. In: Lamberts SWJ (ed). Sandostatin in the Treatment of Acromegaly. New York, Springer, 1988, pp 75–79.

160. Sassolas G, Fossati P, Chanson P, Costa R, Estour B, Deidier A, Harris AG. Effects of long-term administration of Sandostatin (SMS 201–905) at increasing doses in 40 acromegalic patients. Results

from the French Sandostatin Acromegaly Study Group. In: Lamberts SWJ (ed). Sandostatin in the Treatment of Acromegaly. New York, Springer, 1988, pp 89–94.

161. Jackson IMD, Barnard L, Cobb W, Hein M, Perez R. Long-term treatment of resistant acromegaly with a somatostatin analog (SMS 102–995, Sandostatin). In: Lamberts SWJ (ed). Sandostatin in the Treatment of Acromegaly. New York, Springer, 1988, pp 133–139.

162. Vance ML, Kaiser DK, Thorner MO. Sandostatin (SMS 201–995) in the treatment of acromegaly. In: Lamberts SWJ (ed). Sandostatin in the Treatment of Acromegaly. New York, Springer, 1988, pp 149–150.

163. Wass JAH, Davidson K, Medbak S, Besser GM. Somatostatin octapeptide (SMS 201–995, Sandostatin) in the medical treatment of acromegaly. In: Lamberts SWJ (ed). Sandostatin in the Treatment of Acromegaly. New York, Springer, 1988, pp 151–152.

164. Schophol J, Muller OA, von Werder K. SMS 201–995 (Sandostatin) treatment of therapy resistant acromegaly. In: Lamberts SWJ (ed). Sandostatin in the Treatment of Acromegaly. New York, Springer, 1988, pp 153–156.

165. Tauber JP, Babin T, Tauber MT, Vigoni F, Bonafe A, Ducasse M, Harris AG, Bayard F. Long term effects of continuous subcutaneous infusion of the somatostatin analog octreotide in the treatment of acromegaly. J Clin Endocrinol Metab 68(5):917–924, 1989.

166. Shi YF, Harris AG, Zhu XF, Deng JY. Clinical and biochemical effects of incremental doses of the long-acting somatostatin analogue SMS 201–995 in ten acromegalic patients. Clin Endocrinol 32:695–705, 1990.

167. Salmela PI, Juustila H, Pyhtinen J, Jokinen K, Alavaikko M, Ruokonen A. Effective clinical response to long term octreotide treatment, with reduced serum concentrations of growth hormone, insulin-like growth factor-1, and the aminoterminal propeptide of type III procollagen in acromegaly. J Clin Endocrinol Metab 70(4):1193–1201, 1990.

168. Quabbe H, Plockinger U. Dose-response study and long term effect of the somatostatin analog octreotide in patients with therapy-resistant acromegaly. J Clin Endocrinol Metab 68(5):873–881, 1989.

169. Sassolas G, Harris AG, James-Deidier A. The French SMS 201–995 Acromegaly Study Group. Long term effect of incremental doses of the somatostatin analog SMS 201–995 in 58 acromegalic patients. J Clin Endocrinol Metab 71(2):391–397, 1990.

170. Barkan A, Lloyd RV, Chandler WF, Hatfield MK, Gebarski SS, Kelch RP, Beitins IZ. Preoperative treatment of acromegaly with long-acting somatostatin analog SMS 201–995: Shrinkage of invasive pituitary macroadenomas and improved surgical cure rate. J Clin Endocrinol Metab 67:1040–1048, 1988.

171. Chiba T, Chihara K, Minamitani N, Goto B, Kadowaki S, Taminato T, Matsukura S, Fujita T. Effect of long term bromocriptine treatment of glucose intolerance in acromegaly. Horm Metab Res 14:57–61, 1982.

172. Feek CM, McLelland J, Seth J, Toft AD, Irvine WJ, Padfield PL, Edwards CR. How effective is external pituitary irradiation for GH-secreting pituitary tumors? Clin Endocrinol 20:401–408, 1984.

173. Wass JA, Thorner MO, Morris DV, Rees LH, Mason AS, Jones AE, Besser GM. Long-term treatment of acromegaly with bromocriptine. Br Med J 1:875–878, 1977.

174. Besser GM, Wass JAH, Thorner MO. Bromocriptine in the medical management of acromegaly. In: Goldstein M, et al (eds). Advances in Biochemical Psychopharmacology. New York, Raven, 1980, pp 191–198.

175. Carlson HE, Levin SR, Braunstein GD, Spencer EM, Wilson SE, Hershman JM. Effect of bromocriptine on serum hormones in acromegaly. Horm Res 19:142–152, 1984.

176. Oppizzi G, Liuzzi A, Chiodini P, Dallabonzana D, Speita B, Silvestrini F, Borghi G, Tonon C. Dopaminergic treatment of acromegaly. Different effects on hormone secretion and tumor size. J Clin Endocrinol Metab 58:988–992, 1984.

177. Chiodini PG, Cozzi R, Dallabonzana D, Oppizzi G, Verde G, Petroncini M, Liuzzi A, del Pozo E. Medical treatment of acromegaly with SMS 201–995, a somatostatin analog: A comparison with bromocriptine. J Clin Endocrinol Metab 64:447–453, 1987.

178. Ferrari C, Paracchi A, Romano C, Gerevini G, Boghen M, Barreca A, Fortini P, Dubini A. Long-lasting lowering of serum GH and prolactin levels by single and repetitive cabergoline administration in dopamine-responsive acromegalic patients. Clin Endocrinol 29:467–476, 1988.

179. Dallabonzana D, Luizzi A, Oppizzi G, Verde G, Chiodini PG, Dorow R, Horowski R. Effect of the new ergot derivative terguride on plasma PRL and GH levels in patients with pathological hyperprolactinemia or acromegaly. J Endocrinol Invest 8:147–151, 1985.

180. Dallabonzana D, Liuzzi A, Oppizzi G, Cozzi R, Verde G, Chiodini P, Rainer E, Dorow R, Harowski R. Chronic treatment of pathological hyperprolactinemia and acromegaly with the new ergot derivative terguride. J Clin Endocrinol Metab 63:1002–1007, 1986.

181. Mains RE, Eipper BA. Biosynthesis of adrenocorticotropic hormone in mouse pituitary tumor cells. J Biol Chem 251:1313:4115–4120, 1976.

182. Imura H. ACTH and related peptides: Molecular biology, biochemistry and regulation of secretion. Clin Endocrinol Metab 14(4):845–866, 1985.

183. Frohman LA. Disease of the anterior pituitary. In: Felig P, Baxter JD, Broadus AE, Frohman LA (eds). Endocrinology and Metabolism. New York, McGraw-Hill, 1987, pp 247–337.

184. Desir D, Van Cauter E, Fang VS, Martino E, Jadot C, Spire JP, Noel P, Refetoff S, Copinschi G, Golstein J. Effects of "jet lag" on hormonal patterns. I. Procedures, variations in total plasma proteins, and disruption of adrenocorticotropin-cortisol periodicity. J Clin Endocrinol Metab 52(44):628–641, 1981.

185. Vale W, Spiess J, Rivier C, Rivier J. Characterization of a 41-residue ovine hypothalamic peptide that stimulates secretion of corticotrophin and β-endorphin. Science 213:1394–1987, 1981.

186. Gibbs DM, Vale W. Effect of serotonin reuptake inhibitor fluoxetine on corticotropin-releasing factor and vasopressin secretion into hypophyseal portal blood. Brain Res 250:176–179, 1983.

187. Plotzky PM, Vale W. Hemorrhage-induced secretion of corticotropin-releasing factor-like immunoreactivity into the rat hypophyseal portal circu-

lation and its inhibition by glucocorticoids. Endocrinology 114:164–169, 1984.

188. Risch SC, Kalin NH, Janowsky DS, Cohen RM, Pickar D, Murphy DL. Co-release of ACTH and beta-endorphin immunoreactivity in human subjects in response to central cholinergic stimulation. Science 222(4619):77, 1983.

189. Imura H, Nakai Y, Yoshimi T. Effect of 5-hydroxytryptophan (5-HTP) on growth hormone and ACTH release in man. J Clin Endocrinol Metab 36:204–207, 1973.

190. Stubbs WA, Delitala G, Jones A, Jeffocoate WJ, Edwards CR, Ratter SJ, Besser GM, Bloom SR, Alberti KG. Hormonal and metabolic responses to an enkephalin analogue in normal man. Lancet 2(8102):1225–1227, 1978.

191. Jingami H, Matsukura, S, Numa S, Imura H. Effects of adrenalectomy and dexamethasone administration on the level of prepro-CRF mRNA in the hypothalamus and ACTH/β-LPH precursor mRNA in the pituitary in rats. Endocrinology 117:1314–1320, 1985.

192. Vale W, Vaughan J, Smith M, Yamamoto G, Rivier J, Rivier C. Effects of synthetic ovine corticotropin-releasing factor, glucocorticoids, catecholamines, neurohypophysial peptides, and other substances on cultured corticotropic cells. Endocrinology 113(33):1121–1131, 1983.

193. Gillies G, Lowry P. Corticotrophin releasing factor may be modulated by vasopressin. Nature 278:463–464, 1979.

194. Westendorf JM, Philips MA, Schonbrunn A. Vasoactive intestinal peptide stimulates hormone release from corticotrophic cells in culture. Endocrinology 112:550–557, 1983.

195. Gaillard RC, Grossman A, Gilks G, Ress LH, Besser GM. Angiotensin II stimulates the release of ACTH from dispersed rat anterior pituitary cells. Clin Endocrinol (Oxf) 15:573–578, 1981.

196. Chandler WF, Schteingart DE. Controversies in the management of Cushing's disease. Clin Neurosurg 33:553–562, 1986.

197. Chandler WF, Schteingart DE, Lloyd RV, McKeever PE, Ibarra-Perez G. Surgical treatment of Cushing's disease. J Neurosurg 66(2):204–212, 1987.

198. Crapo L. Cushing's syndrome: A review of diagnostic tests. Metabolism 28(99):955–977, 1979.

199. Nishida S, Matsuki M, Nagase Y, Horino M, Endoh M, Kakita K, Tenku A, Oyama H. Suppression of the plasma cortisol level by a single large dose of dexamethasone administered in the morning in Cushing's disease. Horm Metab Res 16:326–327, 1984.

200. Tyrrell JB, Findling JW, Aron DC, Fitzgherald PA, Forsham PH. An overnight high-dose dexamethasone suppression test for rapid differential diagnosis of Cushing's syndrome. Ann Intern Med 104(22):180–186, 1986.

201. Klibanski A, Zervas NT. Diagnosis and management of hormone-secreting pituitary adenomas. N Engl J Med 324(12):822–831, 1991.

202. Kaye TB, Crapo L. The Cushing syndrome: An update on diagnostic tests. Ann Intern Med 112(6):434–444, 1990.

203. Chrousos GP, Schulte HM, Oldfield EH, Gold PW, Cutler GBJ, Loriaux DL. The corticotropin-releasing factor stimulation test: An aid in the evaluation of patients with Cushing's syndrome. N Engl J Med 310:622–626, 1984.

204. Nieman LK, Chrousos GP, Oldfield EH, Avgerinos PC, Cutler GBJ, Loriaux DL. The ovine corticotropin-releasing hormone stimulation test and the dexamethasone suppression test in the differential diagnosis of Cushing's syndrome. Ann Intern Med 105:862–f866, 1986.

205. Peck WW, Dillon WP, Norman D, Newton TH, Wilson CB. High-resolution MR imaging of pituitary microadenomas at 1.5 T: Experience with Cushing's disease. AJR 152:145–151, 1989.

206. Zovickian J, Oldfield EH, Doppman JL, Cutler GBJ, Loriaux DL. Usefulness of inferior petrosal sinus venous endocrine markers in Cushing's disease. J Neurosurg 68(2):205–210, 1988.

207. Doppman JL, Krudy AG, Girton ME, Oldfield EH. Basilar venous plexus of the posterior fossa: A potential source of error in petrosal sinus sampling. Radiology 155(2):375–378, 1985.

208. McCance Dr, McIlrath E, McNeill A, Gordon DS, Hadden DR, Kennedy L, Sheridan B, Atkinson AB. Bilateral inferior petrosal sinus sampling as a routine procedure in ACTH-dependent Cushing's syndrome. Clin Endocrinol (Oxf) 302(2):157–166, 1989.

209. Mampalam TJ, Tyrrell JB, Wilson CB. Transsphenoidal microsurgery for Cushing disease: A report of 216 cases. Ann Intern Med 109(6):487–493, 1988.

210. Friedman RB, Oldfield EH, Nieman LK, Chrousos GP, Doppman JL, Cutler GBJ, Loriaux DL. Repeat transsphenoidal surgery for Cushing's disease. J Neurosurg 71(4):520–527, 1989.

211. Pieters GF, Hermus AR, Meijer E, Smals AG, Kloppenborg PW. Predictive factors for initial cure and relapse rate after pituitary surgery for Cushing's disease. J Clin Endocrinol Metab 69(6):1122–1126, 1989.

212. Lamberts SWJ, Birkenhager JC. The mechanism of the suppressive action of bromocriptine on ACTH secretion in patients with Cushing's and Nelson's syndrome. J Clin Endocrinol Metabol 51:307–315, 1980.

213. Hale AC, Coates PJ, Doniach I, Howlett TA, Grossman A, Rees LH, Besser GM. A bromocriptine-responsive corticotroph adenoma secreting alpha-MSH in a patient with Cushing's disease. Clin Endocrinol (Oxf) 28(2):215–223, 1988.

214. Tomita A, Suzuki S, Hara I, Oiso Y, Mizuno S, Yogo H, Kuwayama A, Kageyama N. Follow-up study on treatment in 27 patients with Cushing's disease: Adrenalectomy, transsphenoidal adenomectomy and medical treatment. Endocrinol Jpn 28(2):197–205, 1981.

215. Hirata Y, Nakashima H, Uchihashi M, Tomita M, Fujita T, Ikeda M. Effects of bromocriptine and cyproheptadine on basal and corticotropin-releasing factor (CRF)-induced ACTH release in a patient with Nelson's syndrome. Endocrinol Jpn 31(5):619–526, 1984.

216. Halperin I, Rodriguez MD, Cardenal C, Casamitjana R, Martinez Osaba MJ, Lienas V, Vilardell E. Treatment of pituitary macroadenomas secreting PRL, HGH or ACTH with long-acting bromocriptine. J Endocrinol Invest 10(3):277–282, 1987.

217. Krieger DT, Amorosa L, Linick F. Cyproheptadine-induced remission of Cushing's disease. N Engl J Med 293:893–896, 1975.

218. Litvin Y, Leiser M, Fleischer N, Erlichman J. Somatostatin inhibits corticotropin-releasing factor-

stimulated adrenocorticotropin release, adenylate cyclase, and activation of adenosine 3′, 5′-monophosphate-dependent protein kinase isoenzymes in AtT20 cells. Endocrinology 119(2):737–745, 1986.

219. Lamberts SW, Uitterlinden P, Klijn JM. The effect of the long-acting somatostatin analogue SMS 201–995 on ACTH secretion in Nelson's syndrome and Cushing's disease. Acta Endocrinol (Copenh) 120(6):760–7766, 1989.

220. Tyrrell JB, Lorenzi M, Gerich JE, Forsham PH. Inhibition by somatostatin of ACTH secretion in Nelson's syndrome. J Clin Endocrinol Metab 40(6):1125–1127, 1975.

221. Oki S, Nakai Y, Nakao K, Imura H. Plasma beta-endorphin responses to somatostatin, thyrotropin-releasing hormone, or vasopressin in Nelson's syndrome. J Clin Endocrinol Metab 50(1):194–197 1980.

222. Ruszniewski P, Girard F, Benamouzig R, Mignon M, Bonfils S. Long acting somatostatin treatment of paraneoplastic Cushing's syndrome in a case of Zollinger-Ellison syndrome. Gut 29(6):838–842, 1988.

223. Bertagna X, Favrod-Coune C, Escourolle H, Beuzeboc P, Christoforov B, Girard F, Luton JP. Suppression of ectopic adrenocorticotropin secretion by the long-acting somatostatin analog octreotide. J Clin Endocrinol Metab 68(5):988–991, 1989.

224. Schteingart DE, Tsao HS, Taylor CI, McKenzie A, Victoria R, Therrien BA. Sustained remission of Cushing's disease with mitotane and pituitary irradiation. Ann Intern Med 92(55):613–619, 1980.

225. Sonino N, Boscaro M, Merola G, Mantero F. Prolonged treatment of Cushing's disease by ketoconazole. J Clin Endocrinol Metab 61:718–722, 1985.

226. Halberg FE, Sheline GE. Radiotherapy of pituitary tumors. Endocrinol Metab Clin North Am 16(3):667–684, 1987.

227. Kjellberg RN, Kliman B, Swisher B, Butler W. Proton beam therapy of Cushing's disease and Nelson's syndrome. In: Black PM, Zervas NT, Ridgway EC, Martin JB (eds). Secretory Tumors of the Pituitary Gland. New York, Raven, 1984, pp 295–307.

228. Brabant G, Ocran K, Ranft U, von zur Muhlen A, Hesch RD. Physiological regulation of thyrotropin. Biochimie 71(2):293–301, 1989.

229. Kwekkeboom DJ, Hofland LJ, van Koetsveld PM, Singh R, van den Berge JH, Lamberts SW. Bromocriptine increasingly suppresses the in vitro gonadotropin and alpha-subunit release from pituitary adenomas during long term culture. J Clin Endocrinol Metab 71(3):718–724, 1990.

230. Magner JA. Thyroid-stimulating hormone: biosynthesis, cell biology, and bioactivity. Endocr Rev 11(2):354–385, 1990.

231. Cloutier MD, Hayles AB, Sprague RG. Pituitary tumor and Cushing's syndrome. Report of a case of an adolescent male with cutaneous melanosis after adrenalectomy. Am J Dis Child 112(6):596–599, 1966.

232. Morley JE. Neuroendocrine control of thyrotropin secretion. Endocr Rev 2(4):396–436, 1981.

233. Cooper DS, Klibanski A, Ridgway EC. Dopaminergic modulation of TSH and its subunits: In vivo and in vitro studies. Clin Endocrinol 18(3):265–275, 1983.

234. Dieguez C, Foord SM, Peters JR, Hall R, Scanlon MF. Interactions among epinephrine, thyrotropin (TSH)-releasing hormone, dopamine, and soma-

tostatin in the control of TSH secretion in vitro. Endocrinology 114(3):957–961, 1984.

235. Ferland L, Labrie F, Jobin M, Arimura A, Schally AV. Physiological role of somatostatin in the control of growth hormone and thyrotropin secretion. Biochem Biophys Res Commun 68(1):149–156, 1976.

236. Vale W, Rivier C, Brazeau P, Guillemin R. Effects of somatostatin on the secretion of thyrotropin and prolactin. Endocrinology 95(4):968–977, 1974.

237. Mess B, Ruzsas C, Jozsa R. The role of the central-nervous serotoninergic system in the regulation of the TRH-TSH-thyroid complex. Folia Morphol 25(2):206–207, 1977.

238. Gurr JA, Kourides IA. Regulation of thyrotropin biosynthesis. Discordant effect of thyroid hormone on alpha and beta subunit mRNA levels. J Biol Chem 258(17):10208–10211, 1983.

239. Chin WW, Shupnik MA, Ross DS, Habener JF, Ridgway EC. Regulation of the alpha and thyrotropin beta-subunit messenger ribonucleic acids by thyroid hormones. Endocrinology 116(23):873–878, 1985.

240. Franklyn JA, Wood DF, Balfour NJ, Ransden DB, Docherty K, Sheppard MC. Modulation by oestrogen of thyroid hormone effects on thyrotropin in gene expression. J Endocrinol 115:53, 1987.

241. Franklyn JA, Ahlquist N, Balfour N, King S, Sheppard MC. Testosterone and effects of thyroid status on pituitary and hepatic messenger (m)RNAs. Abstract T69. Washington, DC, 62nd Annual Meeting of the American Thyroid Association, 1987.

242. Ross DS. Testosterone increases TSHβ mRNA and modulates a-subunit mRNA differentially in the thyrotrope and the gonadotrope. Abstract 705. New Orleans, LA, 67th Annual Meeting of the Endocrine Society, 1988, p 177.

243. Hamilton CRJ, Adams LC, Maloof F. Hyperthyroidism due to thyrotropin-producing pituitary chromophobe adenoma. N Engl J Med 283(20): 1077–1080, 1970.

244. Hill SA, Falko JM, Wilson CB, Hunt WE. Thyrotrophin-producing pituitary adenomas. J Neurosurg 57(4):515–519, 1982.

245. Smallridge RC. Thyrotropin-secreting pituitary tumors. Endocrinol Metab Clin North Am 16(3):765–792, 1987.

246. Faglia G, Beck-Peccoz P, Piscitelli G, Medri G. Inappropriate secretion of thyrotropin by the pituitary. Horm Res 26:79–99, 1987.

247. Emerson CH. Central hypothyroidism and hyperthyroidism. Med Clin North Am 69(5):1019–1034, 1985.

248. Scheithauer BW, Kovacs KT, Laws ERJ, Randall RV. Pathology of invasive pituitary tumors with special reference to functional classification. J Neurosurg 65(6):733–744, 1986.

249. Girod C, Trouillas J, Claustrat B. The human thyrotropic adenoma: Pathologic diagnosis in five cases and critical review of the literature. Semin Diagn Pathol 3(1):58–68, 1986.

250. Wilson CB. A decade of pituitary microsurgery: The Herbert Olivecrona lecture. J Neurosurg 61:814, 1984.

251. McComb DJ, Ryan N, Horvath E, Kovacs K. Subclinical adenomas of the human pituitary. New light on old problems. Arch Pathol Lab Med 107(9):488–491, 1983.

252. Gesundheit N, Petrick PA, Nissim M, Dahlberg

PA, Doppman JL, Emerson CH, Braverman LE, Oldfield EH, Weintraub BD. Thyrotropin-secreting pituitary adenomas: Clinical and biochemical heterogeneity. Case reports and follow-up of nine patients. Ann Intern Med 111(10):827–835, 1989.

253. Blackman MR, Gershengorn MC, Weintraub BD. Excess production of free alpha subunits by mouse pituitary thyrotropic tumor cells in vitro. Endocrinology 102(2):499–508, 1978.

254. Ridgway EC, Kieffer JD, Ross DS, Downing M, Mover H, Chin WW. Mouse pituitary tumor line secreting only the alpha-subunit of the glycoprotein hormones: Development from a thyrotropic tumor. Endocrinology 113(5):1587–1591, 1983.

255. Shupnik MA, Greenspan SL, Mac Veigh MS, Ridgway EC. A non-responsive alpha-secreting thyrotropic tumor contains T3 receptors and a TSH beta gene. Mol Cell Endocrinol 44(3):279–298, 1986.

256. Ross DS, Kieffer JD, Shupnik MA, Ridgway EC. Pure alpha-subunit producing tumor derived from a thyrotropic tumor: Impaired regulation of alpha-subunit and its mRNA by thyroid hormone. Mol Cell Endocrinol 39(2):161–165, 1985.

257. Waldhausl W. Bratusch-Marrain P, Nowotny P, Buchler M, Forssmann WG, Lujf A, Schuster H. Secondary hyperthyroidism due to thyrotropin hypersecretion: Study of pituitary tumor morphology and thyrotropin chemistry and release. J Clin Endocrinol Metab 49(6):879–887, 1979.

258. Samuels MH, Wood WM, Gordon DF, Kleinschmidt-DeMasters BK, Lillehei K, Ridgway EC. Clinical and molecular studies of a thyrotropin-secreting pituitary adenoma. J Clin Endocrinol Metab 68(6):879–887, 1979.

259. Weintraub BD, Menezes-Ferreira MM, Petrick PA. Inappropriate secretion of TSH. Endocr Res 15(4):601–617, 1989.

260. Simard M, Mirell CJ, Pekary AE, Drexler J, Kovacs K, Hershman JM. Hormonal control of thyrotropin and growth hormone secretion in a human thyrotrope pituitary adenoma studied in vitro. Acta Endocrinol (Copenh) 119(2):283–290, 1988.

261. Beck-Peccoz P, Piscitelli G, Amr S, Ballabio M, Bassetti M, Giannattasio G, Spada A, Nissim M, Weintraub BD, Faglia G. Endocrine, biochemical, and morphological studies of a pituitary adenoma secreting growth hormone, thyrotropin (TSH), and alpha-subunit: Evidence for secretion of TSH with increased bioactivity. J Clin Endocrinol Metab 62(4):704–711, 1986.

262. Jaquet P, Hassoun J, Delori P, Gunz G, Grisoli F, Weintraub BD. A human pituitary adenoma secreting thyrotropin and prolactin: Immunohistochemical, biochemical, and cell culture studies. J Clin Endocrinol Metab 59(5):817–824, 1984.

263. Savastano S, Lombardi G, Merola B, Miletto P, Di Prisco B, Manco A, Beck-Peccoz P, Faglia G. Hyperthyroidism due to a thyroid-stimulating hormone (TSH)-secreting pituitary adenoma associated with functional hyperprolactinemia. A case report. Acta Endocrinol (Copenh) 116(4):452–458, 1987.

264. Koide Y, Kugai N, Kimura S, Kujita T, Kameya T, Azukizawa M, Ogata E, Tomono Y, Yamashita K. A case of pituitary adenoma with possible simultaneous secretion of thyrotropin and follicle-stimulating hormone. J Clin Endocrinol Metab 54(2):397–403, 1982.

265. McCutcheon IE, Weintraub BD, Oldfield EH. Surgical treatment of thyrotropin-secreting pituitary adenomas. J Neurosurg 73(5):674–683, 1990.

266. Reschini E, Giustina G, Cantalamessa Lperacchi M. Hyperthyroidism with elevated plasma TSH levels and pituitary tumor: Study with somatostatin. J Clin Endocrinol Metab 43(4):924–927, 1976.

267. Comi RJ, Gesundheit N, Murray L, Gorden P, Weintraub BD. Response of thyrotropin-secreting pituitary adenomas to a long-acting somatostatin analogue. N Engl J Med 317(1):12–17, 1987.

268. Beck-Peccoz P, Medri G, Piscitelli G, Mariotti S, Bertoli A, Barbarino A, Rondena M, Martino E, Pinchera A, Faglia G. Treatment of inappropriate secretion of thyrotropin with somatostatin analog SMS 201–995. Horm Res 29(2–3)121–123, 1988.

269. Guillausseau PJ, Chanson P, Timsit J, Warnet A, Lajeunie E, Duet M, Lubetski J. Visual improvement with SMS 201–995 in a patient with a thyrotropin-secreting pituitary adenoma. Letter. N Engl J Med 317(1):53–54, 1987.

270. Wemeau JL, Dewailly D, Leroy R, D'Herbomez M, Mazzuca M, Decoulx M, Jaquet P. Long term treatment with the somatostatin analog SMS 201–995 in a patient with a thyrotropin- and growth hormone-secreting pituitary adenoma. J Clin Endocrinol Metab 66(3):636–639, 1988.

271. Smallridge RC, Ahmann AJ, Fein HG. Long-term control of a TSH-secreting macroadenoma with a somatostatin analogue (SMS 201–995). Washington, DC, 62nd Annual Meeting of the American Thyroid Association, 1987, p 16.

272. McLellan AR, Connell JM, Alexander WD, Davies DL. Clinical response of thyrotropin-secreting macroadenoma to bromocriptine and radiotherapy. Acta Endocrinol (Copenh) 119(2):189–194, 1988.

273. Carlson HE, Linfoot JA, Braunstein GD, Kovacs K, Young RT. Hyperthyroidism and acromegaly due to a thyrotropin- and growth hormone-secreting pituitary tumor. Lack of hormonal response to bromocriptine. Am J Med 74(5):915–923, 1983.

274. Chanson P, Orgiazzi J, Derome PJ, Bression D, Jedynak CP, Trouillas J, Legentil P, Racadot J, Peillon F. Paradoxical response of thyrotropin to L-dopa and presence of dopaminergic receptors in a thyrotropin-secreting pituitary adenoma. J Clin Endocrinol Metab 59(3):542–546, 1984.

275. Guerrero LA, Carnovale R. Regression of pituitary tumor after thyroid replacement in primary hypothroidism. South Med J 76(4):529–531, 1983.

276. Santen RJ, Bardin CW. Episodic luteinizing hormone secretion in man. J Clin Invest 52:2617–2628, 1973.

277. Clarke IJ, Cummins JT. The temporal relationship between gonadotropin releasing hormone (GnRH) and luteinizing hormone (LH) secretion in ovariectomized ewes. Endocrinology 111:1737–1739, 1982.

278. Urban RJ, Johnson ML, Veldhuis JD. In vivo biological validation and biophysical modeling of the sensitivity and positive accuracy of endocrine peak detection. II. The follicle-stimulating hormone pulse signal. Endocrinology 128:2008–2014, 1991.

279. Belchetz PE, Plant TM, Nakai Y, Keogh EG, Knobil E. Hypophysial responses to continuous and intermittent delivery of hypothalamic gonadotropin-releasing hormone. Science 202:631–6333, 1978.

280. Marshall JC, Kelch RP. Low dose pulsatile gonadotropin-releasing hormone in anorexia nervosa—a model of human pubertal development. J Clin Endocrinol Metab 49:712–718, 1978.

281. Hoffman AR, Crowley WF. Induction of puberty in men by long term pulsatile administration of low dose gonadotropin-releasing hormone. N Engl J Med 307:1237–1241, 1982.

282. Crowley WF, McArthur JW. Simulation of the normal menstrual cycle in Kallman's syndrome by pulsatile administration of LHRH. J Clin Endocrinol Metab 51:173–175, 1980.

283. Leyendecker G, Wildt L, Hansmen M. Pregnancies following chronic intermittent pulsatile administration of GnRH. J Clin Endocrinol Metab 51:1214–1216, 1980.

284. Marshall JC, Kelch RP. Gonadotropin-releasing hormone: Role of pulsatile secretion in the regulation of reproduction. N Engl J Med 315:1459–1468, 1986.

285. Dalkin AC, Haisenleder DJ, Ortolano GA, Ellis TR, Marshall JC. The frequency of GnRH stimulation differentially regulates gonadotropin subunit mRNA expression. Endocrinology 125:917–924, 1989.

286. Estes KS, Simpkins JW, Kalra SP. Resumption with clonidine of pulsatile LH release following acute norepinephrine depletion in ovariectomized rats. Neuroendocrinology 35:56–64, 1982.

287. Gay VL, Plant TM. N-methyl D, L, aspartate elicits hypothalamic GnRH release in prepubertal male rhesus monkeys. Endocrinology 120:2289–2295, 1987.

288. Grossman A, Moult PJA, Gaillard RC, Delitala G, Toff WD, Rees LH, Besser GM. The opioid control of LH and FSH release—effects of a met-enkephalin analogue and naloxone. Clin Endocrinol 14:41–47, 1981.

289. Nippoldt TB, Reame NE, Kelch RP, Marshall JC. The roles of estradiol and progesterone in decreasing LH pulse frequency in the luteal phase of the menstrual cycle. J Clin Endocrinol Metab 69:67–76, 1989.

290. VanVugt DA, Lam NY, Ferin M. Reduced frequency of pulsatile luteinizing hormone secretion in the luteal phase of the rhesus monkey—involvement of endogenous opiates. Endocrinology 115:1095–1101, 1984.

291. Cook CB, Nippoldt TB, Kletter GB, Kelch RP, Marshall JC. Naloxone increases the frequency of pulsatile LH secretion in women with hyperprolactinemia. J Clin Endocrinol Metab 73:1099–1105, 1991.

292. Wang CF, Lasley BL, Lein A, Yen SSC. The functional changes of the pituitary gonadotrophs during the menstrual cycle. J Clin Endocrinol Metab 42:718–728, 1986.

293. Liu JH, Yen SSC. Induction of the mid-cycle gonadotropin surge by ovarian steroids in women. A critical evaluation. J Clin Endocrinol Metab 57:797–802, 1983.

294. Marshall JC, Case GD, Valk TW, Corley KP, Sauder SE, Kelch RP. Selective inhibition of follicle-stimulating hormone secretion by estradiol—a mechanism for modulation of gonadotropin responses to low dose pulses of gonadotropin-releasing hormone. J Clin Invest 71:248–257, 1983.

295. Ying SY. Inhibins, activins and follistatin: Gonadal proteins modulating the secretion of FSH. Endocr Rev 9:267–293, 1990.

296. Rivier C, Vale W. Immunoneutralization of endogenous inhibin modifies hormone secretion and ovulation rate in the rat. Endocrinology 125:152–157, 1989.

297. Snyder PJ. Gonadotroph cell adenomas of the pituitary. Endocr Rev 6(4):552–563, 1985.

298. Kwekkeboom DJ, de Jong FH, Lamberts SW. Gonadotropin release by clinically nonfunctioning and gonadotroph pituitary adenomas in vivo and in vitro: Relation to sex and effects of thyrotropin-releasing hormone, gonadotropin-releasing hormone, and bromocriptine. J Clin Endocrinol Metab 68(6):1128–1135, 1989.

299. Heseltine D, White MC, Kendall-Taylor P, De Kretser DM, Kelly W. Testicular enlargement and elevated serum inhibin concentrations occur in patients with pituitary macroadenomas secreting follicle stimulating hormone. Clin Endocrinol (Oxf) 31(4):411–423, 1989.

300. Peterson RE, Kourides IA, Horwith M, Vaughan ED, Saxena BB, Fraser RAR. Luteinizing hormone- and α-subunit-secreting pituitary tumor: Positive feedback of estrogen. J Clin Endocrinol Metab 52:692, 1981.

301. Snyder PJ, Sterling FH. Hypersecretion of LH and FSH by a pituitary adenoma. J Clin Endocrinol Metab 42(3):544–550, 1976.

302. Beckers A, Stevenaert A, Mashiter K, Hennen G. Follicle-stimulating hormone-secreting pituitary adenomas. J Clin Endocrinol Metab 61:525–528, 1985.

303. Daneshdoost L, Gennarelli TA, Bashey HM, Savino PJ, Sergott RC, Bosley TM, Snyder PJ. Recognition of gonadotroph adenomas in women. N Engl J Med 324(9):589–594, 1991.

304. Jameson JL, Klibanski A, Black P, Zervas NT, Lindell CM, Hsu DW, Ridgway EC, Habener JF. Glycoprotein hormone genes are expressed in clinically nonfunctioning pituitary adenomas. J Clin Invest 80:1472–1478, 1987.

305. Moses N, Goldberg V, Gutman R, Cacamo D. Combined FSH and LH secreting pituitary adenoma in a young fertile woman without primary gonadal failure. Acta Endocrinol (Copenh) 112(1):58–63, 1986.

306. Demura R, Kubo O, Demura H, Shizume K. FSH and LH secreting pituitary adenoma. J Clin Endocrinol Metab 45(4):653–657, 1977.

307. Snyder PJ, Johnson J, Muzyka R. Abnormal secretion of glycoprotein alpha-subunit and follicle-stimulating hormone (FSH) beta-subunit in men with pituitary adenomas and FSH hypersecretion. J Clin Endocrinol Metab 51(3):579–584, 1980.

308. Kourides IA, Weintaub BD, Rosen SW, Ridgway EC, Kliman B, Maloof F. Secretion of alpha subunit of glycoprotein hormones by pituitary adenomas. J Clin Endocrinol Metab 43(1):97–106, 1976.

309. Borges JL, Ridgway EC, Kovacs K, Rogol AD, Thorner MO. Follicle-stimulating hormone-secreting pituitary tumor with concomitant elevation of serum alpha-subunit levels. J Clin Endocrinol Metab 58(5):937–941, 1984.

310. Ridgway EC, Klibanski A, Ladenson PW, Clemmons D, Beitins IZ, McArthur JW, Martorana MA, Zervas NT. Pure alpha-secreting pituitary adenomas. N Engl J Med 304(21):1254–1259, 1981.

311. Koide Y, Kugai N, Kimura S, Fujita T, Kameya T, Azukizawa M, Ogata E, Tomono Y, Yamashita K. A case of pituitary adenoma with possible simultaneous secretion of thyrotropin and follicle-stim-

ulating hormone. J Clin Endocrinol Metab 54(2):397–403, 1982.

312. Reubi JC, Heitz PU, Landolt AM. Visualization of somatostatin receptors and correlation with immunoreactive growth hormone and prolactin in human pituitary adenomas: Evidence for different tumor subclasses. J Clin Endocrinol Metab 6591):65–73, 1987.

313. Vos P, Croughs RJ, Thijssen JH, van't Verlaat JW, van Ginkel LA. Response of luteinizing hormone secreting pituitary adenoma to a long-acting somatostatin analogue. Acta Endocrinol (Copenh) 118(4):587–590, 1988.

314. Sassolas G, Serusclat P, Claustrat B, Trouillas J, Merabet S, Cohen R, Souquet JC. Plasma alpha-subunit levels during the treatment of pituitary adenomas with the somatostatin analog (SMS 201–995). Horm Res 29(2–3):124–128, 1988.

315. Klibanski A, Shupnik MA, Bikkal HA, Black PM, Kliman B, Zervas NT. Dopaminergic regulation of alpha-subunit secretion and messenger ribonucleic acid levels in alpha-secreting pituitary tumors. J Clin Endocrinol Metab 66:96–102, 1988.

316. Vance ML, Ridgway EC, Thorner MO. Follicle-stimulating hormone- and alpha-subunit-secreting pituitary tumor treated with bromocriptine. J Clin Endocrinol Metab 61:580–584, 1985.

317. Lamberts SW, Verleun T, Oosterom R, Hofland L, van Ginkel LA, Loeber JG, van Vroonhoven CC, Stefanko SZ, de Jong FH. The effects of bromocriptine, thyrotropin-releasing hormone, and gonadotropin-releasing hormone on hormone secretion by gonadotropin-secreting pituitary adenomas in vivo and in vitro. J Clin Endocrinol Metab 64(3):524–530, 1987.

318. Roman SH, Goldstein M, Kourides IA, Comite F, Bardin CW, Krieger DT. The luteinizing hormone-releasing hormone (LHRH) agonist [D-Trp6-Pro9-NEt]LHRH increased rather than lowered LH and alpha-subunit levels in a patient with an LH-secreting pituitary tumor. J Clin Endocrinol Metab 58(2):313–319, 1984.

319. Sassolas G, Lejeune H, Trouillas J, Forest MG, Claustrat B, Lahlou N, Loras B. Gonadotropin-releasing hormone agonists are unsuccessful in reducing tumoral gonadotropin secretion in two patients with gonadotropin-secreting pituitary adenomas. J Clin Endocrinol Metab 67(1):180–185, 1988.

320. Zarate A, Fonseca ME, Mason M, Tapia R, Miranda R, Kovacs K, Schally AV. Gonadotropin-secreting pituitary adenoma with concimitant hypersecretion of testosterone and elevated sperm count. Treatment with LRH agonist. Acta Endocrinol (Copenh) 113(1):29–34, 1986.

321. Daneshdoost L, Pavlou SN, Molitch ME, Gennarelli TA, Savino PJ, Sergott RC, Bosley TM, River JE, Vale WW, Snyder PJ. Inhibition of follicle-stimulating hormone secretion from gonadotroph adenomas by repetitive administration of a gonadotropin-releasing hormone antagonist. J Clin Endocrinol Metab 71(1):92–97, 1990.

322. Klibanski A, Zervas NT. Diagnosis and management of hormone-secreting pituitary adenomas. N Engl J Med 324(12):822–831, 1991.

15

SURGICAL TREATMENT OF PITUITARY ADENOMAS

William F. Chandler

A discussion of the surgical treatment of pituitary adenomas must include a review of the clinical problems that compel patients to seek medical advice, as well as the various endocrine and imaging tests that are currently available to reach a specific diagnosis. With modern imaging technology it is possible not only to confirm that a pituitary mass is present, but also to help plan a specific surgical approach and provide the patient with a reasonable expectation of the result of surgery, both regarding endocrine status and tumor recurrence. Since lesions other than pituitary adenomas may occur in and about the sella, the differential diagnosis of parasellar lesions is considered.

CLINICAL AND ENDOCRINE EVALUATION

Clinical Signs and Symptoms

Patients with pituitary lesions may present with signs and symptoms related to a mass effect on the pituitary and its surrounding structures, to hypersecretion of hormones by the lesion itself or to a combination of both. Tumors or other mass lesions are generally greater than 1 cm in size before they produce symptoms related to compression. As a lesion enlarges, it may cause loss of function of the pituitary, usually manifested by a decrease in the secretion of hormones from the adenohypophysis. This may result in a loss of thyroid-stimulating hormone (TSH) and sub-

sequent hypothyroidism. A decrease in adrenocorticotropic hormone (ACTH) will result in Addison's disease, and a decrease in luteinizing hormone (LH) and follicle-stimulating hormone (FSH) will cause amenorrhea. A decline in growth hormone (GH) will only be noted clinically in children by a loss of normal growth progress. The one exception to this pattern is that generalized pituitary compression may cause a rise in prolactin (PRL), since the PRL inhibitory factor (dopamine) from the hypothalamus may be compromised by the compression. Generalized compression from within the sella rarely results in loss of antidiuretic hormone from the neurohypophysis and subsequent diabetes insipidus. Lesions that originate in the region of the pituitary stalk, however, often present with early signs of diabetes insipidus. Symptoms related to loss of pituitary function are usually insidious in onset, with the exception of a sudden hemorrhage within the sella, or so-called "pituitary apoplexy." Such hemorrhages are usually associated with the presence of a pituitary adenoma.

When mass lesions in the region of the pituitary enlarge they may also compress or invade nearby structures, causing a number of neurological symptoms. As tumors grow laterally from the sella, they encounter the various contents of the cavernous sinuses. These include the third, fourth, sixth and first two divisions of the fifth cranial nerves, as well as the internal carotid artery. Compression of cranial nerves III, IV or VI will cause diplopia, and compression of cranial

235

nerve V will cause ipsilateral facial numbness. Invasion or constriction of the carotid may result in carotid occlusion, which in rare cases may result in cerebral infarction. Growth of a tumor in the relatively unrestricted upward direction is much more common and will often result in compression of the optic chiasm with resultant loss of vision, typically a bitemporal visual field cut. Extensive upward intracranial growth may result in hypothalamic compression and/or compression of the third ventricle, causing hydrocephalus. Rarely, intracranial extension can result in cortical irritation and associated seizures. Downward growth of tumors into the sphenoid sinus is common and causes no clinical symptoms or signs.

The syndromes associated with hypersecretion of pituitary hormones by "functional" pituitary tumors will be discussed in more detail later. These include Cushing's disease (ACTH hypersecretion), acromegaly (GH hypersecretion), hyperprolactinemia (PRL hypersecretion) and Nelson's syndrome (ACTH hypersecretion after adrenalectomy). Rare cases of TSH-secreting adenomas have been documented, as well as cases of tumors secreting only the α subunit of the pituitary glycoproteins (those being TSH, LH, and FSH) (1). Traditionally, pituitary adenomas have been divided into "non-functioning" or "functioning" tumors, but it has become clear through immunohistochemical studies of the tumors that many "non-functioning" tumors are in fact endocrinologically active. Although these secreted hormones, such as α subunit, may not cause clinical symptoms or signs, they may serve as markers for the presence of the tumor pre- and post-treatment.

Endocrine Evaluation

The extent of the endocrine evaluation of a patient with a pituitary lesion depends on the urgency of the situation and whether a hypersecretion state is suspected. If the patient's vision is not declining rapidly and therefore time permits, a careful evaluation of endocrine status, including testing of pituitary reserve, is warranted. Although this is most critical after treatment, it is ideal to have complete pre-treatment evaluation for comparison. Pituitary endocrine evaluation should include the following baseline values:

PRL, GH, LH, FSH, testosterone (male), estrogen (female), cortisol, ACTH, electrolytes, glucose, and thyroid function tests, including TSH. Since baseline values may not reflect the ability of the pituitary to respond to stress, it is also important to test the reserve capacity of the pituitary. Currently the most efficient way to do this is with insulin-induced hypoglycemia combined with thyrotropin releasing hormone (TRH). Assuming the patient does not have a contraindication to transient hypoglycemia (i.e., ischemic heart disease, cerebrovascular disease, or seizure disorder), insulin is given in a dose of 0.10 to 0.15 U/kg such that the serum glucose falls below 40 mg%. In the patient with normal pituitary function, this causes a rise in cortisol to above 20μg/100 ml and a rise in GH to above 10 ng/ml. In patients with compromise of ACTH or GH production, such a response is not noted. The administration of TRH should normally cause a rise in both TSH and PRL. If indicated, gonadotropin releasing hormone (GnRH) may be administered to cause a rise in the gonadotropins, LH and FSH.

If urgent surgical decompression is indicated, the previously mentioned baseline values are obtained, and the patient is prepared for surgery with sufficient hydrocortisone to cover the possibility of inadequate cortisol reserve. Careful post-operative evaluation is then carried out to determine if long-term replacement therapy is needed. It should be stressed that if the patient receives post-operative radiation therapy, the status of the pituitary should be checked periodically over the following years, since pituitary function may slowly decline after radiation exposure.

If diabetes insipidus is suspected, urine specific gravity and serum sodium should be checked, and a careful evaluation of fluid intake and output done.

Cushing's Disease

Although the diagnosis of hypercortisolism (Cushing's syndrome) is often reached after physical examination by an astute physician, the physical manifestations are not always obvious, and often the precise diagnosis as to the cause of hypercortisolism is difficult to ascertain even with detailed endocrine and imaging tests. Cushing's syndrome often includes central obesity, hypertension, hirsutism, fatigue, easy bruisability, abdominal stria, "moon" facies, dorsal fat pad, and often depression or other mental changes. Less common abnormalities include headache, osteoporosis, diabetes mellitus, galactorrhea, edema, and amenorrhea. Often a patient will present without the classic "Cushingoid" appearance and only complain of severe fatigue or depression.

The etiology of hypercortisolism is an ACTH-secreting pituitary adenoma (Cushing's disease) in up to 80% of cases, with the remainder due either to an adrenocortical tumor or an ectopic neoplasm secreting ACTH and/or corticotropin releasing factor (CRF) (2). Pituitary-dependent hypercortisolism is much more common in women (80%), and an ectopic etiology more common in men (80%). Thus if an adult male presents with rapid onset of Cushing's syndrome, particularly with weight loss, an ectopic neoplasm must be strongly considered. It should also be kept in mind that increased cortisol levels may be due to primary depression, alcoholism, obesity or drugs such as estrogen and phenytoin (Dilantin).

Since up to 60% of patients with a pituitary etiology will have non-diagnostic imaging studies, the diagnosis often relies completely on endocrine testing (3). Multiple measurements of cortisol and ACTH to evaluate the diurnal pattern are important, but are often misleading. They are mainly of value when clearly elevated. Urinary free cortisol over 24 hours is an extremely important measurement and will not be elevated in obesity or with medication, but will be with depression or alcoholism. If the overnight dexamethasone screening test (1 mg at 10 P.M.) yields an 8 A.M. cortisol level of less than 5 μg/dl, then true hypercortisolism is rarely present. Generally patients with a pituitary etiology of hypercortisolism do not demonstrate suppression with the low-dose dexamethasone test (0.5 mg q 6 hours × eight doses) but do with the higher dose (2 mg q 6 hours × eight doses). There are exceptions, however, to both of these tests. Patients with adrenal or ectopic etiologies classically do not show suppression with either dose. When metyrapone is given, a rise in serum 11-deoxycortisol (or urinary 17-hydroxycortisol) is seen in normal or pituitary etiology patients. Unfortunately, a positive response does not absolutely rule out an adrenal or ectopic etiology. Perhaps the most specific diagnostic test is simultaneous measurement of ACTH levels in both inferior petrosal sinuses by transfemoral catheterization along with peripheral blood levels. This has produced very specific information about the existence of an ACTH-secreting pituitary tumor and even the laterality of the tumor (4). Along with this intensive endocrine workup, appropriate computed tomographic (CT) scanning of the adrenals and chest should be carried out to look for adrenal or lung tumors. An additional possible etiology—simple hyperplasia of the pituitary with ACTH hypersecretion—also exists.

Acromegaly

As with Cushing's syndrome, the diagnosis of acromegaly may be reached clinically when patients present with advanced stages of the disease. Enlargement of facial features and acral enlargement, however, may be subtle, and the presenting symptoms may be nonspecific (e.g., headaches, fatigue, arthralgias, decreased libido or amenorrhea). Patients often have hypertension, diabetes mellitus and early onset of atherosclerotic cardiovascular disease. It is critical that this disease be diagnosed and treated, since the mortality rate is 50% greater than expected at each decade over the age of 40 (5). With rare exceptions, the cause of acromegaly is a GH-secreting pituitary adenoma. As with other functioning adenomas, the tumors may be very small or large and invasive. Patients with larger tumors may, of course, present with visual loss. Rarely, elevated GH levels are secondary to GH-releasing hormone produced by ectopic tumor.

The endocrine diagnosis rests largely on serum GH levels, since 90% of patients will have levels over 10 ng/ml. Normally GH in a resting non-stressed patient is less than 5 ng/ml, but both normals and acromegalics may have levels between 5 and 10 mg/ml. Somatomedin C, or insulin-like growth factor (1GF I), which mediates the effect of GH on peripheral tissues, should also be measured in all situations. When the diagnosis is suspected but consistently elevated GH levels are not obtained, the glucose suppression test is the most useful diagnostic procedure. In normal patients, 1 to 2 hours after the oral administration of 100 gm of glucose, the GH level will fall well below 5 ng/ml. This suppression is not seen with GH-secreting adenomas, and often a paradoxical rise in GH is observed.

Hyperprolactinemia

Since 60% to 70% of PRL-secreting pituitary adenomas are microadenomas, the majority of patients will present with endocrine symptoms rather than local mass effects. In women, hyperprolactinemia usually causes amenorrhea and often galactorrhea, and thus young women more often seek medical evaluation early. In men, however, this early warning sign is not available, and they almost invariably present with macroadenomas, usually causing loss of libido, infertility or loss of vision. It should be kept in mind that the finding of amenorrhea or galactorrhea associated with an elevated PRL level does not always indicate the presence of a pituitary tumor. Table 15–1 lists the other possible causes of hyperprolactinemia. Most important among these are renal failure, hypothyroidism, or the presence of various drugs. Compression on the pituitary stalk by any type of mass lesion will result in the increased secretion of prolactin. Almost invariably, if the PRL level is over 150 ng/ml, a pituitary tumor is the etiology, but microadenomas often produce PRL levels of less than 100 ng/ml. The size of pituitary adenomas has been shown to correlate with the degree of PRL elevation, which may reach into the thousands of nanograms per milliliter. There are no reliable provocative tests to differentiate prolactinomas from other causes of hyperprolactinemia, so the diagnosis relies on ruling out other etiologies and attempting to image an adenoma.

Nelson's Syndrome

In 1958 Nelson _et al._ (6) identified a syndrome of progressive hyperpigmentation, visual field loss and amenorrhea associated with elevated ACTH levels related to a functional pituitary adenoma in a patient who had undergone bilateral adrenalectomy for hypercortisolism. This syndrome today generally represents a missed diagnosis of Cushing's disease that has been treated with adrenalectomy. Often these tumors are aggressive or frankly malignant.

IMAGING OF THE PITUITARY AND PARASELLAR REGION

Modern computerized imaging technology now provides us with remarkably detailed multiplanar images of the pituitary and parasellar structures. Magnetic resonance imaging (MRI) has evolved to be the first choice for diagnostic imaging and is often the only test needed to reach a therapeutic decision. MRI with intravenous infusion of a paramagnetic substance such as gadolinium will demonstrate intrasellar tumors down to 5 mm in size (Fig. 15–1) and will show the growth pattern of larger tumors (Fig. 15–2). MRI will reveal the extent of suprasellar and sphenoid sinus extension, as well as lateral extension into the cavernous sinuses. Cysts and hemorrhage can be differentiated, as can blood flowing within an aneurysm.

CT scanning also has a place in pituitary imaging and, if MRI scanning is unavailable, may well suffice as the only mode of imaging. CT scanning will show calcification better than MRI and thus is often helpful in imaging a craniopharyngioma. CT scanning, even with intravenous contrast, cannot differentiate an aneurysm, and thus MRI or angiography must be carried out if this is suspected.

Plain skull radiographs are not needed if the diagnosis has been reached by CT or MRI scanning, but they remain an important means of picking up incidental lesions. A pituitary macroadenoma (>10 mm) will cause enlargement of the sella turcica, and this can easily be noted on a plain lateral skull radio-

Table 15–1. Causes of Hyperprolactinemia

Pituitary disease
    Prolactinoma
    GH-secreting adenoma
    Pituitary stalk section
    Empty-sella syndrome

Hypothalamic disease
    Tumors
    Sarcoidosis
    Irradiation

Hypothyroidism

Chronic renal failure

Hepatic disease

Drugs
    Phenothiazines
    Tricyclic antidepressants
    Estrogen
    Opiates
    Reserpine
    Verapamil
    Others

Pregnancy

Stress

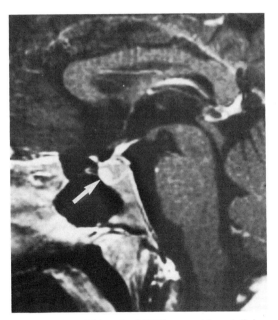

Figure 15–1. Mid-sagittal MRI scan with gadolinium demonstrating a 6-mm ACTH-secreting microadenoma in the anterior portion of the pituitary *(white arrow).* In this case the tumor enhances more than the pituitary.

graph. If this is noted on a radiograph performed for any reason, such as trauma, this should be followed up with a more detailed study such as MRI or CT scanning.

Angiography is only performed if an aneurysm is suspected or if a lesion is so large that occlusion or compression of the internal carotid artery is in question. Giant aneurysms can generally be ruled out with high-resolution MRI scanning.

DIFFERENTIAL DIAGNOSIS

Table 15–2 contains a list of the possible lesions that may occur within the sella or in the parasellar region. Pituitary adenomas head the list, since they are the most common lesion in this region and constitute 8% to 10% of all brain tumors. Occasionally they are cystic and thus are confused with other lesions. Craniopharyngiomas are the next most common tumor, and although usually more suprasellar in location may be exclusively intrasellar. They are more common in children but up to one third occur in adults. They are usually, but not always, cystic and are calcified in 70% of children and 40% in adults. Meningiomas are also generally more suprasellar and enhance very strongly on CT

and MRI. Rarely, they are exclusively intrasellar and are impossible to differentiate from an adenoma. Germinomas, or so-called "ectopic pinealomas," generally involve the pituitary stalk and usually present with diabetes insipidus. It is a general principle that if a patient presents with diabetes insipidus, one should think of a lesion other than a pituitary adenoma. Metastatic malignancies, commonly lung and breast, may be found in the pituitary, with 70% residing in the posterior pituitary. Optic nerve gliomas and hypothalamic gliomas may occasionally be confused with pituitary adenomas, as can be the rare granular cell tumor (choristoma). Dermoids and epidermoids may occur in an intrasellar location, and fifth nerve neuromas may compress the sella as well.

Rathke's cysts are benign congenital remnants that occur within the sella and can cause loss of pituitary function by compression. These can be confused on imaging studies with cystic adenomas or craniopharyngiomas and require biopsy and surgical decompression.

Inflammatory and granulomatous processes, including bacterial abscesses within the sella (7), should always be kept in mind. Sarcoidosis may invade the pituitary or its stalk as can the granulomas associated with

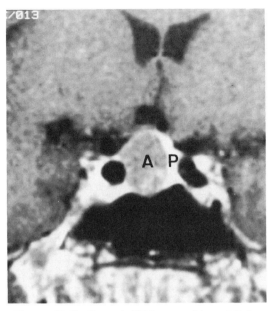

Figure 15–2. Coronal MRI scan with gadolinium showing a growth hormone–secreting macroadenoma (A). In this patient the adjacent compressed pituitary (P) enhanced with gadolinium more than the tumor.

Table 15–2. Differential Diagnosis of Intrasellar and Parasellar Lesions

Tumors
    Pituitary adenoma
    Craniopharyngioma
    Meningioma
    Germinoma
    Chordoma
    Granular cell tumor (choristoma)
    Neuroma (arising from cranial nerve V)
    Metastatic tumor
    Optic nerve glioma
    Dermoid tumor
    Infundibuloma
    Hypothalamic glioma

Cysts
    Rathke's cleft cyst
    Pituitary cyst

Inflammatory and granulomatous lesions
    Bacterial abscess
    Sarcoidosis
    Eosinophilic granuloma (histiocytosis X)
    Tuberculosis
    Mycoses
    Granulomatous hypophysitis

Aneurysm

Hamartoma

Empty-sella syndrome

Pituitary apoplexy

histiocytosis X. Hamartomas may involve the pituitary stalk and hypothalamus and are impossible to differentiate from invasive gliomas on imaging studies.

Aneurysms, usually from the internal carotid arteries but occasionally from the basilar artery, may appear within the sella and must be ruled out preoperatively with MRI or angiography.

The empty-sella syndrome is generally only an anatomic variation and rarely causes symptoms. This conditions exists when the diaphragma sella is incompetent, and the sella is filled with cerebrospinal fluid (CSF). The constant pulsation of the CSF will gradually enlarge the sella. Patients with headaches or head trauma may undergo a skull radiograph or CT scan and be found to have an enlarged sella. With high-resolution CT or MRI scanning, usually the elongated stalk may be seen to reach the sellar floor, thus ruling out a cystic lesion.

Pituitary apoplexy only rarely causes symptoms but may cause a profound and emergent situation. Infarction and hemorrhage, usually in a pituitary adenoma, causes sudden intrasellar expansion with severe headache and rapid loss of pituitary function, resulting in hypotension. There may also be sudden loss of vision and the development of cranial nerve palsies. Treatment in severe cases involves the administration of steroids and surgical decompression of the sella.

SURGICAL TREATMENT AND RESULTS

The initial treatment of most pituitary adenomas is surgical, although exceptions will be mentioned later and are discussed in detail in Chapter 14. Along with surgical removal or decompression of pituitary adenomas, additional treatment in the form of radiation therapy or medical therapy may be indicated. Even with modern imaging techniques, the unequivocal diagnosis of an adenoma is not reached until tissue is obtained. It is not unusual during a transsphenoidal procedure to be surprised at what is identified at the time the dura is opened. I have found abscesses, dermoids, meningiomas, metastases, Rathke's cleft cysts and even craniopharyngiomas when I was fully expecting to find a pituitary adenoma. As can be seen in Table 15–2, the list of possible parasellar lesions is long, and it is not within the scope of this chapter to delineate the surgical treatment for each lesion.

Over 95% of pituitary adenomas can be approached via the transsphenoidal route. This is usually accomplished via a sublabial incision and a transseptal approach to the sphenoid. Once the sphenoid sinus has been entered, the operating microscope is brought in, the anterior wall of the sella is carefully drilled away and the dura surrounding the pituitary is identified. The dura is opened, and if a macroadenoma is present, tumor is usually seen directly beneath the dura. If a microadenoma is present, the surgeon must carefully dissect around and often within the pituitary to identify the small tumor.

Contraindications to this approach, and therefore indications for a frontal craniotomy, include (1) massive suprasellar extension, (2) extensive lateral intracranial extension and (3) a rare dumbbell-shaped tumor with a tight constriction at the level of the diaphragma sella. If a craniotomy is necessary, this generally involves a right subfrontal approach to the optic nerve and chiasm, and the tumor is removed in a piecemeal fashion using the operating microscope and microinstruments. Access to the sella is gained between the optic nerves, in front of the chiasm or between the ipsilateral optic nerve and carotid artery. After substantial tumor removal, the pituitary stalk and even the basilar artery can be visualized.

With either surgical approach, the patients are carefully prepared with pre-operative and intra-operative hydrocortisone. This is true regardless of whether it has been proved that the patient has Addison's disease. It is also important to ascertain that the patient is euthyroid. If the patient is hypothyroid, replacement therapy should be provided well in advance of surgery to reduce anesthetic risk.

Non-functioning Adenomas

For the purposes of this chapter, the term "non-functioning adenomas" will refer to tumors that do not have clinically relevant hormone secretion. It is understood that many clinically silent adenomas will have immunocytochemical evidence of hormone production or even measurable blood levels of hormone overproduction.

Since patients with non-functioning adenomas usually present with the effects of a mass lesion, these tumors are rarely microadenomas. Although their sizes range from being exclusively intrasellar to having extensive intracranial involvement, these tumors are almost all approached by the transsphenoidal route. The goals of surgery for non-functioning macroadenomas include (1) establishment of a diagnosis, (2) decompression of surrounding structures and (3) attempt at gross total removal of tumor tissue. The first goal is usually accomplished easily, and although most tumors turn out to be adenomas, surprise findings are not unusual. The second goal of decompression is also usually accomplished readily, since most tumors are soft and easily decompressed. Less than 5% of the time an adenoma will be fibrous, making decompression difficult. Evidence for this decompression is demonstrated by the consistent finding that 75% to 80% of patients with visual field loss show recovery after transsphenoidal decompression (8). The third goal of total tumor resection is much more difficult to accomplish with macroade-

nomas. It has been demonstrated that most (88% to 94%) macroadenomas invade at least the dura, and many grossly invade surrounding structures (9). This invasion makes complete surgical resection impossible, and therefore these patients need to be followed indefinitely with high-quality imaging to look for signs of tumor progression or recurrence.

It was common practice in the past to provide postoperative radiation to all macroadenomas, but with today's high-resolution imaging, most neurosurgeons are content to watch for tumor progression and reserve focal radiation for situations of definite progression. There currently is no medical treatment for non-functional adenomas.

Cushing's Disease

Once it has been established that the etiology of a patient's hypercortisolism is a pituitary lesion, the treatment of choice is transsphenoidal exploration of the pituitary. Since only 40% to 50% of such patients will have positive imaging studies, many of these patients require a careful systematic exploration of the sellar contents by an experienced pituitary surgeon (3). Microadenomas secreting ACTH may be very small and are often located deep within the gland itself. If a tumor is not evident on opening the dura and examining all surfaces of the pituitary, then incisions must be made into the gland and an internal exploration carried out. These tumors are usually in one lateral aspect of the pituitary, and the choice of which side to explore first may be guided by the results of the pre-operative petrosal sinus sampling for ACTH levels, as described earlier. If no tumor is identified, then a decision must be made as to whether to resect all or a portion of the gland. If the endocrine evidence is convincing for a pituitary origin and the patient has no desire to have children, then total hypophysectomy is warranted. If the petrosal sinus sampling clearly indicates laterality of the ACTH secretion, then an appropriate hemi-resection of the gland is carried out. We have one example in which a 2-mm ACTH-secreting microadenoma was identified with immunocytochemical techniques within the resected pituitary of a patient in whom tumor could not be identified during surgery (3). The patient was in complete remission after removal of the gland containing this proven microadenoma. Macroadenomas are treated with maximum tumor resection, but in these situations it is more difficult to accomplish endocrine remission. Obviously patients with adrenal or ectopic lesions are treated by resection of tumors in these locations.

The author's experience (3) as well as the experience of others (10–13) has demonstrated that about 75% of patients explored will have a microadenoma as the source of ACTH secretion. The postoperative remission rate in these patients is 88% to 96% (3, 10–13), and the long-term recurrence rate appears to be no more than 5% (14). Therefore, selective microsurgical tumor resection in patients with microadenomas is clearly the current treatment of choice.

Approximately 10% to 20% of patients explored will have macroadenomas, and the post-operative remission rate in these patients has been reported to range from 33% to 61% (3, 10–13). Many of these patients will receive postoperative radiation therapy, which will provide remission in some of the surgical failures. Those who fail to remit with both surgery and radiation will require either a surgical adrenalectomy or medical suppression of adrenal function. In a small percentage of patients who have undergone adrenalectomy, the pituitary tumor will continue to grow and secrete ACTH, thus producing Nelson's syndrome.

In the remaining 10% to 15% of patients explored, no tumor will be found, and a hypophysectomy will not be advisable because of a desire for pregnancy. Some of these patients will later be found to have ectopic tumors or turn out to have small unidentifiable pituitary adenomas (3).

Acromegaly

Like Cushing's disease, acromegaly is a condition that ultimately threatens the life of the patient. For this reason it must be treated aggressively, even at the expense of normal pituitary function. Over the past two decades a variety of medical, surgical and radiation therapies have evolved that have proven effective in lowering GH levels. No one treatment is uniformly effective, and often a combination of treatment is necessary. The goal of treatment is to lower the circulating GH and insulin-like growth factor levels to within a normal range and to reduce the size of a mass lesion that is causing symptoms by compression.

Unfortunately, only 20% to 34% of GH-secreting tumors are microadenomas (5, 15–17), thus making microsurgical tumor resection less effective than in Cushing's disease. When a microadenoma is selectively removed transsphenoidally, endocrine remission may be expected in 80% to 88% of cases (5, 15–17). When a macroadenoma is resected, immediate post-operative remission is reported in 30% to 68% of cases (5, 15, 16). The rate of remission is adversely affected by higher pre-operative GH levels and larger invasive tumors (18). Pre-operative treatment of macroadenomas with somatostatin analogue may improve post-operative remission rates (19).

Radiation therapy has proven moderately effective either as a primary mode of treatment or to augment partial surgical resection. Proton beam heavy particle therapy has been used by Kliman et al. in 510 patients, 428 of whom have been followed for between 1 and 20 years (20). Analysis of these patients reveals that there is a progressive fall in GH levels beginning immediately after treatment and continuing for up to 20 years. At 2 years, 47.5% of patients have a GH level less than 10 ng/ml, and at 4, 10 and 20 years, the rate is 65%, 87.5% and 97.5%, respectively. If a GH level of less than 5 ng/ml is considered a "cure," then 75% of patients are cured at 10 years and 92.5% at 20 years. Conventional radiation therapy has been demonstrated to provide very comparable results (10-year post-treatment levels: <10 ng/ml in 81% and <5 ng/ml in 69%) (21).

Bromocriptine, a dopamine agonist, has been demonstrated by Besser and Wass to lower GH levels in 71% of 126 patients (15). Unfortunately, GH levels of less than 10 ng/ml were achieved in only 14% of patients. However, they did note "clinical response" in up to 95% of patients. This does not currently appear to be an effective primary treatment, but may help control GH and insulin-like growth factor levels as an adjuvant therapy.

A somatostatin analogue has been used on an experimental basis and has been demonstrated to significantly reduce GH and insulin-like growth factor levels in most patients. This treatment, however, provides only minimal tumor shrinkage, and GH levels rise again immediately after stopping the drug.

This drug may prove to be useful as a pre-operative treatment or in surgical failures (19).

The recurrence of GH-secreting tumors appears to be only 4% after successful surgery (14) and less than 1% after radiation (20).

Given the variety of treatment modalities outlined above, a rational therapeutic approach is to surgically resect tumors when possible and to provide radiation therapy to those in which a remission cannot be achieved. Somatostatin analogue is used as an adjuvant therapy in selected patients.

Prolactinomas

PRL-secreting adenomas are the most common functioning pituitary tumors but remain the most controversial with regard to treatment. The controversy exists because, unlike ACTH- or GH-secreting adenomas, there is a reasonably effective medical treatment available in the form of dopamine agonists. The treatment options include medical therapy, usually with bromocriptine, transsphenoidal surgical resection, radiation therapy or, in some cases, no treatment. Because different considerations are involved with different size tumors, the treatments will be discussed according to size.

Macroadenomas

The goal in treating a patient with a large PRL-secreting adenoma is to decompress the optic pathways, if involved, and to reduce the PRL levels to normal. Surgery is effective in improving vision in 80% of cases (22), but vision has also been reported to improve in patients treated with bromocriptine (23). The ability of surgery to reduce PRL levels to normal has generally been disappointing. The uniform finding of various investigators has been that the ability to normalize PRL is greatly reduced if the PRL level is greater than 200 ng/ml or the tumor size is over 10 mm. Hardy (24) normalized only 21% of patients with PRL levels over 200 ng/ml, and Randall et al. (22) normalized only 30% of patients with macroadenomas.

Treatment of macroadenomas with bromocriptine will reduce PRL levels significantly in almost all patients and to normal ranges in over 46% (23). In 90%, the size of the tumor is decreased to some degree, and in many, the decrease is dramatic. It is also true, with rare exceptions, that the tumor will return to the original size once bromocriptine is stopped. It is recognized that up to 25% of patients with macroadenomas will have an increase in tumor size during pregnancy, whereas this is true in less than 1% of patients with microadenomas (23).

Sheline et al. (25) have shown, in a mixture of PRL and nonfunctioning tumors, that at 10 years the recurrence rate is 21% after radiation plus surgery, 29% with radiation alone and 91% with only surgery. These facts demonstrate the effectiveness of radiation therapy and the lack of effectiveness of surgery alone.

Based on these facts, the treating physician's obligation is to discuss the treatment options with the patient in detail and to decide on a course of action. My choice is to recommend transsphenoidal debulking of the tumor in an attempt to achieve remission in up to 30% of patients. Usually bromocriptine is used for 3 to 4 weeks pre-operatively to reduce the size of the tumor. If a large, aggressive, invasive tumor is encountered, then post-operative radiation therapy is recommended. If remission is not achieved but the tumor is grossly removed, then bromocriptine is used alone post-operatively. Surgery is particularly recommended if pregnancy is desired, since expansion of the tumor during pregnancy (off bromocriptine) is likely to occur, possibly jeopardizing vision. It should be emphasized that careful follow-up with CT or MRI scanning is required for the lifetime of the patient, since rapid tumor growth may occur. The recurrence rate of macroadenomas is from 25% to 75% at 5 years (14, 25, 26), so adjunctive therapy is clearly indicated if the post-operative PRL level begins to elevate.

Microadenomas

The surgical treatment of PRL-secreting microadenomas results in post-operative remission in a much higher percentage of patients. Hardy reports remission in 77% (24), Richards and associates in 77% (27) and Randall et al. in 72% (22). Randall et al. found that 88% were in remission with PRL levels <100 ng/ml, and only 50% had PRL levels > 100 ng/ml (22). The incidence of new post-operative hypogonadism was only 1%. Landolt et al. found an 81% remission rate without bromocriptine pretreatment, but only a

33% rate with pretreatment (28). They demonstrated convincingly that bromocriptine causes fibrosis within the tumor and attributed the lower remission rate to this fibrosis (29). At the present time, medical treatment is a safe and effective primary treatment but may lessen the chance of long-term surgical "cure" by causing fibrosis. As in macroadenomas, long-term continued therapy is indicated, since PRL levels rapidly rise with cessation of dopamine agonists. Pregnancy poses less risk to patients with microadenomas, since tumor expansion and visual loss are very rare.

The recurrence rate in patients initially in remission after microsurgical tumor removal has been somewhat disappointing, compared with that for other functioning tumors. Recurrences have uniformly been found to be higher in patients with post-operative PRL levels in the upper end of the normal range. Charpentier *et al.* (30) reported a recurrence rate of 17%, Rodman *et al.* (31) a rate of 17%, Laws (14) a rate of 24% and Serri *et al.* (26) up to 50% in 4 years. Radiation therapy does not play a role in the treatment of microadenomas, unless they recur in an aggressive manner.

My current approach to PRL-secreting microadenomas that can be visualized on imaging studies is to carefully explain the medical and surgical options to the patient. Surgery is offered as a primary option, since it allows the possibility of long-term remission without continued medical therapy. In the final analysis, patients must make an educated choice between primary medical or surgical treatment.

Little objective data exist regarding surgical exploration of patients with presumed microadenomas. Unlike patients with Cushing's disease or acromegaly, most patients with hyperprolactinemia and normal imaging studies have not been studied. Once other causes of hyperprolactinemia have been ruled out, dopamine agonists are generally tried to lower PRL levels. These patients need to be carefully followed with imaging studies and measurement of PRL levels. The long-term occurrence of obvious adenomas is unknown, but appears to be as low as 5% (32).

REFERENCES

1. Klibanski A, Ridgeway EC, Zervas NT. Pure alpha-subunit-secreting pituitary tumors. J Neurosurg 59:585–589, 1983.

2. Chandler WF, Schteingart DE. Controversies in the management of Cushing's disease. In: Little JR (ed). Clinical Neurosurgery. Vol 33. Baltimore, Williams and Wilkins, 1986, pp 553–562.

3. Chandler WF, Schteingart DE, Lloyd RV, McKeever PE. Surgical treatment of Cushing's disease. J Neurosurg 66:204–212, 1987.

4. Oldfield EH, Chrousos GP, Schulte HM, Schaaf M, McKeever PE, Krudy AG, Cutler GB, Loriaux DL, Doppman JL. Preoperative lateralization of ACTH-secreting pituitary microadenomas by bilateral and simultaneous inferior petrosal venous sinus sampling. N Engl J Med 312:100–103, 1985.

5. Weiss MH. Acromegaly: Selection parameters and operative results. In: Carmel PW (ed). Clinical Neurosurgery. Vol 27. Baltimore, Williams and Wilkins, 1980, pp 31–37.

6. Nelson DH, Meakin JW, Dealy JB, Matson DD, Emerson K, Thorn GW. ACTH-producing tumor of the pituitary gland. N Engl J Med 259:161–164, 1958.

7. Bjerre P, Riishede J, Lindolm J. Pituitary abscess. Acta Neurochir (Wien) 68:187–193, 1983.

8. Ebersold MJ, Quast LM, Laws ER, Scheithauer B, Randall RV. Long-term results in transsphenoidal removal of nonfunctioning pituitary adenomas. J Neurosurg 64:713–719, 1986.

9. Selman WR, Laws ER, Scheithauer BW, Carpenter SM. The occurrence of dural invasion in pituitary adenomas. J Neurosurg 64:402–407, 1986.

10. Boggan JE, Tyrrell JB, Wilson CB. Transsphenoidal microsurgical management of Cushing's disease. J Neurosurg 59:195–200, 1983.

11. Hardy J. Cushing's disease: 50 years later. Can J Neurol Sci 9:375–380, 1982.

12. Kuwayama A, Kageyama N. Current management of Cushing's disease. Part II. Comtemp Neurosurg 7:1–6, 1985.

13. Salassa RM, Laws ER, Carpenter PC, Northcutt RC. Cushing's disease—50 years later. Am Clin Climatol Assoc (Trans) 94:122–129, 1982.

14. Laws ER. Frontiers in pituitary surgery. Presented at the Congress of Neurological Surgeons Meeting, New Orleans, LA, September, 1986.

15. Besser GM, Wass JAH. The medical management of acromegaly. In: Black PM, Zervas NT, Ridgway EC, Martin JB (eds). Secretory Tumors of the Pituitary Gland. New York, Raven Press, 1984, pp 155–168.

16. Laws ER, Piepgras DG, Randall RV, Abboud CF. Neurosurgical management of acromegaly. Results in 82 patients treated between 1972 and 1977. J Neurosurg 50:454–461, 1979.

17. Tindall GT, Tindall SC. Transsphenoidal surgery for acromegaly: Long-term results in 50 patients. In: Black PM, Zervas NT, Ridgway EC, Martin JB (eds). Secretory Tumors of the Pituitary Gland. New York, Raven Press, 1984, pp 175–178.

18. Laws ER. The neurosurgical management of acromegaly. In: Black PM, Zervas NT, Ridgway EC, Martin JB (eds). Secretory Tumors of the Pituitary Gland. New York, Raven Press, 1984, pp 169–173.

19. Barkan AL, Lloyd RV, Chandler WF, Hatfield MK, Gebarski SS, Kelch RP, Beitens IZ. Preoperative treatment of acromegaly with long-acting sondostatin: Shrinkage of invasive pituitary macroadenomas and improved surgical remission rate. J Clin Endocrinol Metab 67:1040–1048, 1988.

20. Kliman B, Kjellberg RN, Swisher B, Butler W. Proton beam therapy acromegaly: A 20-year expe-

rience. In: Black PM, Zervas NT, Ridgway EC, Martin JB (eds). Secretory Tumors of the Pituitary Gland. New York, Raven Press, 1984, pp 191–211.

21. Bloom B, Kramer S. Conventional radiation therapy in the management of acromegaly. In: Black PM, Zervas NT, Ridgway EC, Martin JB (eds). Secretory Tumors of the Pituitary Gland. New York, Raven Press, 1984, pp 179–190.

22. Randall RV, Laws ER, Abboud CF, Ebersold MJ, Kao PC, Scheithauer BW. Transsphenoidal microsurgical treatment of prolactin-producing pituitary adenomas. Mayo Clin Proc 58:108–121, 1983.

23. Thorner MO, Evans WS, Vance ML. Medical management of prolactinomas: I. In: Black PM, Zervas NT, Ridgway EC, Martin JB (eds). Secretory Tumors of the Pituitary Gland. New York, Raven Press, 1984, pp 53–64.

24. Hardy J. Transsphenoidal microsurgery of prolactinomas. In: Black PM, Zervas NT, Ridgway EC, Martin JB (eds). Secretory Tumors of the Pituitary Gland. New York, Raven Press, 1984, pp 73–81.

25. Sheline GE, Grossman A, Jones AE, Besser GM. Radiation therapy for prolactinomas. In: Black PM, Zervas NT, Ridgway EC, Martin JB (eds). Secretory Tumors of the Pituitary Gland. New York, Raven Press, 1984, pp 93–108.

26. Serri O, Rasio E, Beauregard H, Hardy J, Somma M. Recurrence of hyperprolactinemia after selective transsphenoidal adenomectomy in women with prolactinoma. N Engl J Med 309:280–283, 1983.

27. Richards AM, Bullock MRR, Teasdale GM, Thomson JA, Khan MI. Fertility and pregnancy after operation for a prolactinoma. Br J Obstet Gynecol 93:495–502, 1986.

28. Landolt AM, Keller PJ, Froesch ER, Mueller J. Bromocriptine: Does it jeopardize the result of later surgery for prolactinomas? Lancet 1:657–658, 1982.

29. Landolt AM, Osterwalder V. Perivascular fibrosis in prolactinomas: Is it increased by bromocriptine? J Clin Endocrinol Metab 58:1179–1183, 1984.

30. Charpentier G, dePlunkett T, Jedynak P, Peillon F, LeGentil P, Racadot J, Visot A, Derome P. Surgical treatment of prolactinomas. Short- and long-term results, prognostic factors. Horm Res 22:222–227, 1985.

31. Rodman EF, Molitch ME, Post KD, Biller BJ, Reichlin S. Long-term follow-up of transsphenoidal selective adenomectomy for prolactinoma. JAMA 252:921–924, 1984.

32. Boyd AE, Hamilton D, Murray BG, Goldberg D. Medical management of prolactinomas: II. In: Black PM, Zervas NT, Ridgway EC, Martin JB (eds). Secretory Tumors of the Pituitary Gland. New York, Raven Press, 1984, pp 65–72.

16

FUTURE PROSPECTS IN THE DIAGNOSIS AND TREATMENT OF PITUITARY ADENOMAS

RICARDO V. LLOYD

Since the 1970s there have been many advances in the diagnosis and treatment of pituitary disorders. The development of many sophisticated methods to diagnose pituitary disorders pre-operatively, the medical and surgical treatment of adenomas and other lesions and the sophisticated techniques used in the analysis and final histopathologic diagnosis of pituitary abnormalities have contributed to the understanding of the pathophysiology of pituitary disorders. Cell culture, immunohistochemistry, electron microscopy and molecular biological analyses of pituitary adenomas have provided new insights into the biology of these neoplasms. What can be anticipated for the next decade and beyond? Based on many recent developments, the 1990s should be as exciting and challenging as the previous 20 years.

New diagnostic imaging procedures should continue to improve the detection of pituitary microadenomas and other pituitary disorders. Although computed tomography (CT) and magnetic resonance imaging (MRI) are excellent for detection of macroadenomas or pituitary adenomas greater than 10 mm in diameter (1–3), there are some limitations in the detection of microadenomas. The use of gadolinium as a contrast agent should continue to improve the detection of microadenomas (4, 5). MRI has been used to diagnose

rare cases of congenital hypopituitarisms in which ectopic posterior pituitary was seen as a bright spot and correlated with the size of the anterior pituitary remnant (6). These studies show promise for the future application of these techniques in the diagnosis of pituitary disorders. The management of incidental pituitary adenomas detected by improved diagnostic imaging techniques is constantly undergoing revision (7).

The management of prolactin-secreting pituitary adenomas with bromocriptine and other ergot alkaloids has had a dramatic effect on the medical management of pituitary adenomas (8, 9). Long-acting non-ergot dopamine agonists such as CV 205–502 show great promise in the treatment of patients with large prolactinomas (10). The use of long-acting somatostatin analogues such as octreotide for the treatment of growth hormone (GH) adenomas has been associated with reduction of GH secretion in 90% of patients with acromegaly (11). The use of this drug and of longer acting analogues that will be developed in the future should improve the medical treatment of patients with acromegaly and gigantism.

Surgical treatment of pituitary adenomas and other disorders and new approaches such as surgical decompression for pituitary tumor apoplexy by urgent transsphenoidal surgery should continue to provide advances in this field (12, 13).

Molecular biological techniques have had a great impact on the diagnosis of endocrine disorders. Recombinant DNA technology with Southern analysis to determine inheritance patterns and to detect gene deletions such as the GH gene in some subtypes of GH deficiency should provide methods of more rigorously characterizing some endocrine disorders (14). Although linkage analysis is currently used to characterize the multiple endocrine neoplasms (MEN) type I and IIa, which have been mapped to chromosomes 11 and 10, respectively, the genes for these familial diseases should be cloned in the near future. This will facilitate development of specific screening tests to identify patients with these disorders. Because many patients with MEN I develop pituitary adenomas, cloning of the gene should help in the diagnosis and treatment of these patients.

The histopathologic diagnosis of pituitary disorders will be greatly enhanced with the continued development of sophisticated diagnostic modalities (15–18). For example, the rare disorder of mammosomatotroph hyperplasia causing gigantism was diagnosed in a child by a combination of hormone assays, cell culture studies, receptor analysis and immunohistochemical studies at the light and electron microscope levels (16). The use of the polymerase chain reaction (PCR), in which DNA is greatly amplified to increase the sensitivity for detecting target DNAs of interest, will continue to be a powerful method of analyzing mutations and regulatory defects in pituitary adenomas. Studies in the characterization of various GH adenomas with mutant G_S proteins have provided a sensitive way to analyze subtypes of adenomas with respect to tumor size and secretory activity and have implicated specific oncogenes in the regulation of GH tumor secretion (17, 18). Recent applications of the PCR technique revealed *ras* mutations in a recurrent, highly invasive prolactinoma, but not in 18 other adenomas, suggesting that *ras* mutations may provide a marker for highly invasive tumors (19).

With continued advances in the pre-operative diagnosis, medical and surgical treatment of adenomas and in the histopathologic analysis of these neoplasms, we can anticipate an ever-expanding body of knowledge about the biology and management of adenomas and other pituitary disorders.

REFERENCES

1. Miller DL, Doppman JL. Diagnostic imaging procedure. In: Kovacs K, Asa SL (eds). Functional Endocrine Pathology. Cambridge, MA, Blackwell Scientific, 1991, pp 56–70.
2. Davis PC, Hoffman JC Jr, Spencer T, Tindall GT, Braun IF. MR imaging of pituitary adenoma: CT, clinical, and surgical correlation. AJR *148*:797–802, 1987.
3. Kucharczyk W, Davis DO, Kelley WM, Sze G, Norman D, Newton TH. Pituitary adenomas: High-resolution MR imaging at 1.5 T. Radiology *161*:761–765, 1986.
4. Dwyer AJ, Frank JA, Doppman JL, Oldfield EH, Hickey AM, Cutler GB, Loriaux DL, Schiable TF. Pituitary adenomas in patients with Cushing's disease: Initial experience with Gd-DTPA-enhanced MR imaging. Radiology *163*:421–426, 1987.
5. Doppman JL, Frank JA, Dwyer AJ, Oldfield EH, Miller DL, Nieman LK, Chrousos GP, Cutler GB Jr, Loriaux DL. Gadolinium DTPA enhanced MR imaging of ACTH-secreting microadenomas of the pituitary gland. J Comput Assist Tomogr *12*:728–735, 1988.
6. Brown RS, Bhatia V, Hayes E. An apparent cluster of congenital hypopituitarism in central Massachusetts: Magnetic resonance imaging and hormonal studies. J Clin Endocrinol Metab *72*:12–18, 1991.
7. Molitch ME, Russell EJ. The pituitary "incidentaloma." Ann Intern Med *112*:925–931, 1990.
8. McGregor AM, Scanlon MF, Hall R, Hall K. Effects of bromocriptine on pituitary tumour size. Br Med J *2*:700–703, 1979.
9. Molitch ME, Elton RL, Blackwell RE, Caldwell B, Chang RJ, Jaffe R, Joplin G, Robbins RJ, Tyson J, Thorner MO. Bromocriptine as primary therapy for prolactin-secreting macroadenomas: Results of a prospective multicenter study. J Clin Endocrinol Metab *60*:698–705, 1985.
10. Khalfallah Y, Claustrat B, Grochowicki M, Flocard F, Horlait S, Serusclat P, Sassolas G. Effects of a new prolactin inhibitor, CV 205–502, in the treatment of human macroprolactinomas. J Clin Endocrinol Metab *71*:354–359, 1990.
11. Melmed S. Acromegaly. N Engl J Med *322*:966–977, 1990.
12. Welbourn RB. The evolution of transsphenoidal pituitary microsurgery. Surgery *100*:1185–1190, 1986.
13. Arafah BM, Harrington JF, Madhoun ZT, Selman WR. Improvement of pituitary function after surgical decompression for pituitary tumor apoplexy. J Clin Endocrinol Metab *71*:323–328, 1990.
14. Jameson JL, Arnold A. Clinical review 5: Recombinant DNA strategies for determining the molecular basis of endocrine disorders. J Clin Endocrinol Metab *70*:301–307, 1990.
15. Giannattasio G, Bassetti M. Human pituitary adenomas. Recent advances in morphological studies. J Endocrinol Invest *13*:435–454, 1990.

16. Moran A, Asa SL, Kovacs K, Horvath E, Singer W, Sagman U, Reubi J-C, Wilson CB, Larson R, Pescovitz OH. Gigantism due to pituitary mammosomatotroph hyperplasia. N Engl J Med *323*:322–327, 1990.

17. Landis CA, Harsh G, Lyons J, Davis RL, McCormick F, Bourne HR. Clinical characteristics of acromegalic patients whose pituitary tumors contain mutant G_s protein. J Clin Endocrinol Metab *71*:1416–1420, 1990.

18. Landis CA, Masters SB, Spada A, Pace AM, Bourne HR, Vallar L. GTPase inhibiting mutations activate the α chain of G_s and stimulate adenylyl cyclase in human pituitary tumours. Nature *340*:692–696, 1989.

19. Karga HJ, Alexander JM, Hedley-Whyte ET, Klibanski A, Jameson JL. Ras mutations in human pituitary tumors. J Clin Endocrinol Metab *74*:914–919, 1992.

Index

MAJOR PROBLEMS IN PATHOLOGY

- **Problems in Breast Pathology** *(Azzopardi)* Order #W1463-9
- **Surgical Pathology of the Salivary Glands** *(Ellis, Auclair & Gnepp)* Order #W3224-6
- **Pathology of Neoplasia in Children and Adolescents** *(Finegold)* Order #W1337-3
- **Thin Needle Aspiration Biopsy** *(Frable)* Order #W3835-X
- **Pathology of the Uterine Cervix, Vagina and Vulva** *(Fu & Reagan)* Order #W7493-3
- **Pathology of Incipient Neoplasia, 2nd Edition** *(Henson & Albores-Saavedra)* Order #W6457-1
- **Surgical Pathology of the Lymph Nodes and Related Organs** *(Jaffe)* Order #W1027-7
- **Surgical Pathology of Non-Neoplastic Lung Disease, 2nd Edition** *(Katzenstein & Askin)* Order #W1852-9

- **Surgical Pathology of the Thyroid** *(LiVolsi)* Order #W5782-6
- **Tumors of the Lung** *(Mackay, Lukeman & Ordóñez)* Order #W5807-5
- **Pathology of AIDS and HIV Infection** *(Nash & Said)* Order #W1540-6
- **The Renal Biopsy, 2nd Edition** *(Striker, Olson & Striker)* Order #W3040-5
- **Immunomicroscopy: A Diagnostic Tool for the Surgical Pathologist** *(Taylor)* Order #W8770-9
- **Cardiovascular Pathology** *(Virmani, Atkinson & Fenoglio)* Order #W3232-7
- **Mucosal Biopsy of the Gastrointestinal Tract, 4th Edition** *(Whitehead)* Order #W3287-4
- **Surgical Pathology of Bone Marrow: Core Biopsy Diagnosis** *(Wittels)* Order #W1434-5
- **Disorders of the Spleen** *(Wolf & Neiman)* Order #W2503-7

Enroll today!
See reverse side for details.

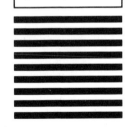